Inconceivable Iran

Fertility, Reproduction and Sexuality

Understanding the complex and multifaceted issue of human reproduction has been, and remains, of great interest both to academics and practitioners. This series includes studies by specialists in the field of social, cultural, medical, and biological anthropology, medical demography, psychology, and development studies. Current debates and issues of global relevance on the changing dynamics of fertility, human reproduction, and sexuality are addressed.

Recent volumes:

Volume 50
Inconceivable Iran: To Reproduce or Not to Reproduce?
Soraya Tremayne

Volume 49
Good Enough Mothers: Practicing Nurture and Motherhood in Chiapas, Mexico
J.M. López

Volume 48
How Is a Man Supposed to Be a Man? Male Childlessness – a Life Course Disrupted
Robin A. Hadley

Volume 47
Waithood: Gender, Education, and Global Delays in Marriage and Childbearing
Edited by Marcia C. Inhorn and Nancy J. Smith-Hefner

Volume 46
Abortion in Post-revolutionary Tunisia: Politics, Medicine and Morality
Irene Maffi

Volume 45
Navigating Miscarriage: Social, Medical and Conceptual Perspectives
Edited by Susie Kilshaw and Katie Borg

Volume 44
Privileges of Birth: Constellations of Care, Myth and Race in South Africa
Jennifer J.M. Rogerson

Volume 43
Access to Assisted Reproductive Technologies: The Case of France and Belgium
Edited by Jennifer Merchant

Volume 42
Making Bodies Kosher: The Politics of Reproduction among Haredi Jews in England
Ben Kasstan

Volume 41
Elite Malay Polygamy: Wives, Wealth and Woes in Malaysia
Miriam Koktvedgaard Zeitzen

For a full volume listing, please see the series page on our website:
http://www.berghahnbooks.com/series/fertility-reproduction-and-sexuality

INCONCEIVABLE IRAN
To Reproduce or Not to Reproduce?

Soraya Tremayne

berghahn
NEW YORK • OXFORD
www.berghahnbooks.com

First published in 2023 by

Berghahn Books

www.berghahnbooks.com

Library of Congress Cataloging-in-Publication Data

Names: Tremayne, Soraya, author.
Title: Inconceivable Iran : to reproduce or not to reproduce? / Soraya Tremayne.
Description: New York : Berghahn Books, 2023. | Series: Fertility, reproduction and sexuality : social and cultural perspectives ; volume 50 | Includes bibliographical references and index.
Identifiers: LCCN 2022019214 (print) | LCCN 2022019215 (ebook) | ISBN 9781800736719 (hardback) | ISBN 9781800736726 (ebook)
Subjects: LCSH: Fertility, Human--Iran. | Human reproduction--Iran. | Human reproductive technology--Iran. | Families--Iran.
Classification: LCC HB1046.4.A3 T74 2022 (print) | LCC HB1046.4.A3 (ebook) | DDC 304.6/32--dc23/eng/20220801
LC record available at https://lccn.loc.gov/2022019214
LC ebook record available at https://lccn.loc.gov/2022019215

British Library Cataloguing in Publication Data

A catalogue record for this book is available from the British Library

ISBN 978-1-80073-671-9 hardback
ISBN 978-1-80073-672-6 ebook

https://doi.org/10.3167/9781800736719

For Bruce

Contents

Illustrations

Figures

Tables

PREFACE

Culture is what remains after one has forgotten everything else.
—Édouard Herriot, French statesman 1872–1957

This book is written for those generally believing that the Iranian culture is disappearing under the impact of social transformation. It argues that changes in social behavior and attitude do not equal the weakening or disappearance of the core cultural values that underpin society. Instead, the book maintains that the strength of these values lies in their adaptability and in the way they interact selectively with innovation. It provides evidence by studying those social institutions that surround reproduction, such as marriage, family, kinship, patriarchy, fertility, and population fluctuation. This book is not about whether modernity and tradition clash but rather how they work together to fit the agendas of their recipients. Soheila Shahshahani's study, "Wedding Ceremony in Turmoil," published in the journal *Anthropology of the Middle East* in 2007, encapsulates the ways in which the institution of marriage in Iran has adapted to modernity. According to Shahshahani's research, the core of the marriage ritual has been preserved although sequences have been changed to fit the working agendas of the bride and groom.

By implication, therefore, I take a different approach to the study of change by exploring what has not changed. Most of the chapters in this volume have been published in other books and journals since 2006, and their selection is meant to show the depth and extent of the process of change over time. Having carried out research for more than four decades, I have the advantage of being, simultaneously, both an insider and outsider to Iran. After being born and spending my early adult life in Iran, I grew up to naturally "know" my own culture. At the same time, as an anthropologist having spent most of my adult life outside Iran, I am able to adopt an objective outsider's approach by making explicit the factors that are intrinsic to everyday life and thus invisible to those living among them. I am also fortunate to have had the opportunity to spend several years living among and studying different cultures across the globe. Long exposures to such varied, if not contrasting, cultures, such as those of Nigeria, Romania, Malaysia, Hong Kong, and the United Kingdom, led me to question profoundly some of my own prejudices and value judgments. This has meant re-visiting assumptions about my own culture, viewing them with fresh eyes. I believe that the anthropological research technique of participant observation is a powerful adjunct to quantitative surveys, which have become the norm for so many studies on Iran and which often, as articulated by an old Iranian saying, "take people to the spring but bring them back thirsty." My findings neither endorse nor reject the practices described, such as child marriage, but merely reveal the underlying motivations behind their persistence.

I am aware that this book may provoke varied responses from those who are patient enough to read it, ranging from: those who disagree strongly, providing counter arguments and correctives such as, "You don't live here and don't understand"; to those who shrug their shoulders, implying that this book states the obvious; to those who think that I am missing the full picture. Some may also point out that I have neglected to explore the role of Iran's theocratic regime in perpetuating these practices. While this assertion may be partially true, this is not the book's objective. However, as always, I remain open to critique and prepared to learn from alternative perspectives.

Acknowledgments

As always, in writing a book one owes a debt of gratitude to many people, from colleagues and friends to family. While it is not possible to name everybody involved in such undertaking, my special thanks go to the few without whose help this book would not have seen the light of day. I would like to thank Marion Berghahn, who initially encouraged me to put this collection on the anthropology of reproduction in Iran together. My warm thanks also go to Tom Bonnington, the Associate Editor of Berghahn Books in Oxford, for his patience and invaluable help throughout. I am grateful to the publishers, who agreed to the publication of some of the chapters that had been published by them previously, details of which are included at the end of the relevant chapters. These are Indiana University Press, New York University Press, Elsevier, Oxford University Press, and Springers. My thanks go to Dr. Mohammad Mehdi Akhondi, who co-authored Chapter 11 with me. My thanks also go to my valued colleague, Philip Kreager, for his warm support and enthusiasm. However, my greatest heartfelt thanks go to my colleague and dear friend, Marcia Inhorn, without whose encouragement and help this book project would not have been conceived. She has remained a staunch supporter throughout, and I cannot thank her enough. Also, a big special thanks go to her for the suggestion of the title. My warmest thanks go to Bonnie Rose Schulman for her meticulous editorial work and patience throughout. I am indebted to my friend and colleague, Soheila Shahshahani, an anthropologist of Iran, without whose invaluable support some of my fieldwork in Iran would not have taken place. I cherish the times spent discussing my findings and benefiting from her generously sharing her insights with me. I remain indebted to the people, who, by allowing me to live among them for long periods of time and by willingly giving up their valuable time and open heartedly sharing their life experiences, form the backbone of these studies. I will also always remember their expressions of astonishment or amusement at some of the "strange" questions I asked them. Finally, I cannot end the list without mentioning the contribution of my family, who, through their interest and also by asking "strange" and unexpected questions, have made me re-visit some of my own assumptions, an exercise during which we also had hours of fun.

Introduction

The past two decades have produced an abundance of writing on societal change in Iranian culture. These studies usually emerge under the banner of social sciences, with some claiming to be in-depth ethnographies. They are the result of surveys, questionnaires, or interviews with a limited number of respondents, or they come in the form of focus groups, alongside some fieldwork. Most of this scholarship asserts that trends in socio-economic development, modernization, and globalization have served to transform the country's fundamental cultural institutions and core values. This volume aims to take a more comprehensive approach by asserting, through the lens of reproduction, how Iranian cultural norms and practices have prevailed, in essence if not in form, despite these global and local shifts. It maintains that many of these studies are missing the larger picture; they lack comprehensive and longitudinal perspective. For example, research that explores changes in marriage patterns in Iran often neglects to examine the institution of marriage itself and further fails to situate marriage in its broader cultural Iranian context. One such study interprets marriage arrangements between couples who met on the internet in Iran as an example of modernity undermining tradition. However, this study overlooks the full trajectory of these relationships, which often disintegrate during ensuing traditional marriage contract negotiations. According to most of these studies, societal change implicitly serves to disrupt or erode cultural norms and values. While these works have merit, they tend to miss the more nuanced, longer-term, and profound dynamics involved in interactions between modernity and tradition. As Thomas Hylland Eriksen (2010) in *Small Places, Large Issues* argues, "'modernity' and 'tradition' are not mutually exclusive and can exist side by side" (274), and "although there are bound to be tensions and contradictions within complex societies

. . . it is the resilience of cultures that ensures their perpetuation and/or their revival rather than any coercion, whether political or religious, imposed by any outside factors" (321). My own findings, spanning more than three decades of research, concur with this view and confirm that the essence of cultural norms and practices in Iran endures, despite changes in form. As history has shown time and again, cultures do not disintegrate under pressures of modernity, war, revolution, authoritarianism, or any other form of aggression and coercion. Rather, outside threats often serve to reinforce local traditions; many anthropological studies show that when cultures are exposed to outside innovations, they select and mold them to suit their needs. As Maya Unnithan-Kumar (2010: 163) explains regarding the infiltration of global technologies into traditional societies, "technologies in themselves do not bring about social transformation but it is in how they are made socially meaningful that their power lies."

Focusing the lens of this approach on Iran, the chapters in this volume were selected based on their shared theme of reproduction. Revealing the complex dynamics of encounters between modernity and tradition, they illustrate how no single factor, be it development, modernity, globalization, conservatism, or state policy, determines or shapes established cultural institutions. Rather, it is the versatile and multifaceted ways in which people respond to—and engage with—innovations that determine the extent to which change can penetrate and alter a culture.

Why Reproduction?

The selection of reproduction as the common theme in this collection stems from several factors. First, since the Islamic Revolution in 1979, reproduction has been the state's primary target of reform. The authorities consider reproductive values and practices to have been destabilized by modernity and seek a return to what they see as their traditional roots. As a result, the norms and practices that surround reproduction have been subject to more upheaval than any other institution in society and have remained the most contentious item on the agendas of the theocratic state and its opponents at both ideological and generational levels. The state's prioritization of reproduction over all other institutions is understandable, since it is reproduction, as the embodiment of family, kinship, marriage, and fertility, that underpins society and ensures its stability. Second, despite the state's extensive efforts to return and confine reproductive practices to their traditional forms, these practices seem to have undergone more drastic changes than any other institution in society. Research on the nature and extent of these changes in reproductive practices sheds light on the nature and extent of social and cultural change in the country in general. Third, a more in-depth analysis of shifts in the structure of kinship and family, which today seems to be disintegrating at an alarming rate in Iranian society—consider, for example, the country's high divorce rate ("Marriage Threefold of Divorce" 2020)—leads to a better understanding of the dynamics of the interaction between modernity and tradition. Fourth, although Iran is not a monolithic culture and is home to considerable cultural diversity, Iranians share strong and deep-rooted values on issues of reproduction, family, and kinship—values that seem to apply to all layers of society, from rich to poor and from rural to urban. Likewise, against the sizeable number of successive younger generations deviating from parental authority and traditional norms, there exists an equal number who remain compliant. Often, when faced with conflicting values and aspirations, both generations try to compromise on a modus vivendi to maintain the harmony of the community. For example, more and more girls from conservative families are losing their virginity before marriage. This act of transgression provokes violent reactions, even murder, as depicted in Chapters 1 and 3 in this volume.[1] However, many of these young girls are saved by being able to resort to hymenoplasty—in some cases more than once—to remain "acceptable" future wives.[2] The paramount importance of virginity and its persistence is also clearly illustrated in recent research among Iranians in the diaspora (Zavieh 2017). The compromises made to protect these girls also range from their mothers helping them seek hymenoplasty, to some highly religious female doctors, whom I have met during my research, who were prepared to compromise their own religious beliefs and perform hymenoplasty on unmarried girls. The rate of hymenoplasty had increased so much by 2006 that one of the leading sources of emulation, Ayatollah Mohammad Sadeg Rouhani,[3] in answering the question of whether hymenoplasty was allowed, promptly issued a *fatwa* (religious edict) allowing it. Finally, reproduction, as the nucleus of my own longitudinal research, has provided me with abundant data to counter the claims of those studies that conclude that Iranian culture has radically changed.

Background

The Islamic Revolution of 1979 served as a critical juncture for seemingly profound change in Iran. The past four decades have witnessed a complicated relationship between the theocratic state and its ideological opponents, particularly among the younger generations, who are the main agents of change. The state remains consistent in its resolve to save the country from the invasion of "corrupt Western cultural imports" and to return it to its "traditional" roots. In the process, it has repeatedly employed coercive and brutal measures to enforce its ideology, built on its interpretation of Islamic law. Over the past forty years, Iranians have experienced the emergence of conservative, pragmatic, reformist, and moderate presidents, and, most recently in 2021, of an ultraconservative cleric. Any efforts by the two reformist and moderate presidents to bring about meaningful change were thwarted by the current political structure of the Guardianship of the Jurisprudence. However, Iranian society, especially the generations born after the revolution, has not remained passive in the face of these fluctuations. Rather, these young people, a considerable number from among the conservative groups themselves, have gradually moved away from their parents' ideological and/or political stances and are striving to create their own vision of an ideal society. While opponents to the regime from all political, social, and educational backgrounds remain vocal and active even at the cost of their own lives, another equally if not more effective weapon of resistance lies in the responses of ordinary people who manage to go about their everyday lives, either ignoring or finding ways to bypass the dictates of the authorities. In his seminal book *Life as Politics: How Ordinary People Change the Middle East,* Asef Bayat (2009, 2013) explains how this type of resistance can erode the effectiveness of the state's politics.

Moreover, while the Iranian state has the power to control political opponents by brutal means, its grip is loosening on the younger generation, which is increasingly defying the rules of behavior, morality, ethics, gender relations, and sexuality, imposed by the Guardians of the Revolution. The authorities, in their search to keep pace with these changes and regain control, are anxious to adjust their strategies to "guide" the young in the "right" direction. In her insightful book *Iran Re-Framed: Anxieties of Power in the Islamic Republic,* Narges Bajoghli (2019), through her decade-long research among the "media producers" of the state, describes in meticulous detail the new strategies adopted by the authorities "to court Iranian youth."

As explained in Chapters 4 and 8, the social and economic policies implemented by the state in the first two decades after the revolution, which included a massive and successful educational program and policies aimed to slow population growth in the 1980s, further deepened the rift between the two camps. In the process, the dynamics of the relationship between the state and its challengers shifted, and it is now often the educated and socially and politically aware youth who, through their provocative and defiant acts, take the lead and spur the state into action. By the beginning of the millennium, twenty years after the revolution, the introduction and nearly immediate ubiquity of internet technologies gave most of the younger generation easy and unfettered access to the outside world. Today, apolitical youth want to enjoy simple daily freedoms: to have fun, to mix with the opposite sex, and to live a life in public free of government surveillance, harassment, and oppression.

There is little doubt that Iranian society has undergone major change over the past few decades, despite the dictatorial policies of the authorities. However, the ethnographic research in this volume explores the extent to which these social changes have altered the core cultural values that are the building blocks of Iranian society. These chapters question whether social change is identical to cultural transformation. As Furlong and Cartmel (2007) in *Young People and Social Change: New Perspectives* also show, the assumption that social change equals cultural transformation is not unique to conservative societies but applies also to developed and pluralistic communities. In a discussion of the changes brought about by modernity in the context of capitalism, social class, and gender, they write, "We accept that experiences of young people have changed quite radically over the last three decades, yet suggest that in the age of 'high modernity' life chances and processes of social production remain highly structured" (Furlong and Cartmel 2007: 3). Moreover, they assert, "While structures appear to have fragmented, changed their form and become increasingly obscure, we suggest that life chances and experiences can still largely be predicted using knowledge of individuals' locations within social structures: despite arguments to the contrary" (Furlong and Cartmel 2007: 2).

The Book

The chapters in this book are a selection of essays that have been published in different academic volumes and journals over the past fifteen years, between 2006 and 2021. Reflecting more than three decades of research on reproduction in Iran, these chapters explore the dynamics of the institutions that serve as the social expression of reproduction, including family, marriage, kinship, patriarchy, fertility, and the relationship between the state and the nation. They are presented in an order that aims to explore the impact of change over time on the values of reproduction in Iran.

The book is divided into four parts, each of which approaches a different aspect of the topic of reproduction in Iran. The chapters are closely interconnected, and there is an inevitable amount of repetition of topics between them, especially on infertility and assisted reproductive technologies (ARTs). However, in dealing with the same themes, each chapter offers a fresh view on the topic.

Part I of this volume focuses on the meaning of modernity and its impact on three of the foundational constituents of Iranian culture, namely "face" (*aberu*), early marriage, and patriarchy. Chapter 1 analyzes the role "face" plays in individuals' interactions with the outside world, which culminate in one maintaining, gaining, or losing face and on which one's reputation and position in the public sphere depend. Deeper among the factors affecting face also lie the notions of honor and shame and their inextricable links with the public position of a person and his/her wider network of kin. While the research for Chapter 1 was gathered in 2004, Iranian attitudes toward face remain unchanged. As current reports show, face continues to form an important part of a family's and individual's public persona. The examples of face put forth in this volume represent a widespread phenomenon. As the findings of one study show, "Iran already had high levels of violence against women, with reported 8,000 so-called honor killings between 2010 and 2014" and that "about 20 percent of all murders and 50 percent of family murders in East Azerbaijan Province are related to sexual and honor issues" (Pirnia, Pirnia, and Pirnia 2020). According to recent reports, sixty women fell victim to honor killings in the southern province of Khouzestan in the past two years.[4] Furthermore, honor killings are not carried out exclusively in cases of women bringing shame upon their families but can also apply to men deviating from what is considered the social and sexual norm, including cases of male homosexuality.[5] For example, in May 2021, a well-known Iranian filmmaker was murdered by his parents, allegedly for remaining unmarried at the age of forty-seven ("Iranian Film Director Murdered by Family" 2021). Although human rights activists condemn these acts of violence and conservative authorities often express support for sentencing the perpetrators, these cases are rarely pursued seriously (Fassihi 2020). Most authorities come from conservative backgrounds; they tacitly endorse this behavior, believing that it is for the family alone to address. While overstepping cultural and sexual norms continues to provoke violent responses among conservative families, the occurrence of such violent reactions is less common among secular and less conservative groups in society, who tend to adopt more subtle strategies to bury the shame of family "transgression." Other chapters in the book provide examples of face playing a decisive role, such as in cases of runaway children or infertility and its persisting stigma.

Chapter 2 addresses the phenomenon of early or child marriage in Iran and examines the assumptions of policymakers who believed that educating women would empower them and cause them to delay marriage, thus solving the problem of child marriages.[6] The initial research for this chapter was carried out in 2004 in Yazd, based on its ranking as the most conservative town in the country due to its low rate of divorce. On returning to the same city four years later, a new set of statistics was released, ranking it as having the fourth highest rate of divorce in the country. I asked the director of the newly opened State Welfare Organization Center, which offers counseling to vulnerable men and women, what brought about such a drastic change. He explained that the Center was receiving 30,000 telephone calls per month, mainly from women, most of whom were desperate to initiate divorce but were afraid of their fathers and brothers who threatened to kill them if they did so. Obviously, these women hoped that the Center would release them from the "prison" of marriage. Recent studies carried out in 2020 in Yazd confirm that the main causes of divorce remain violence against women, the interference of family members into the newly married couples' relationships, and infertility (predominantly in cases of female infertility), which drives men to seek other wives (Bidaki et al. 2020). Likewise, the ten-year-old girls I knew in 2004 have since attended universities and are economically independent; they are now supposedly "empowered" and therefore no longer forced to marry early. Now in their late twenties, many of these young women remain unmarried and are still living with their parents. Although such a delay in the age of marriage is partly by choice, the prospects of finding a marriage partner are also more limited due to a variety of reasons, which are further discussed in Chapters 2, 6, and 8. As leading an independent life away from the family remains out of the question for young unmarried women, predominantly those living in small towns, remaining unmarried means that these young women's lifestyles have not kept pace with the socio-economic changes over the past two decades. Interestingly, back in 2004, numbers of consanguineous marriages were decreasing, and marriages with outsiders had become more frequent. Two decades later, with the divorce rates soaring, many families blame this instability on the decrease in consanguineous marriage, which had traditionally strengthened relationships within the kin group through the bond of mutual duty and obligation. However, as various studies show, despite this decrease, the practice of consanguineous marriage remains prevalent. For example, one survey carried out in 2017 reports that, of the 1,535 couples interviewed in both urban and rural areas, 74.3 percent had consanguineous relationships and 62.3 percent were between first cousins (Nouri et al. 2017).

While social trends point to an increase in the number of young women in Iran who choose to delay marriage or remain single, most eventually marry and form families. The endurance of traditional reproductive practices is not unique to Iran. For example, on the topic of delayed marriage, Marcia C. Inhorn and Nancy J. Smith-Hefner (2021: 394) conclude that "in the majority of cultural contexts . . . (a) marriage is still a given, (b) childbearing is still expected within the bounds of marriage, and (c) both are closely linked to the achievements of social adulthood." This is also confirmed by longitudinal studies of women cohabiting with their partners, a practice referred to as "white marriage." Discussions in Chapter 5 of this volume show how, in the long term, marriage is the only realistic option for most of these women. Alternative prospects remain bleak if the cohabitation comes to an end, as many do. However, men in this form of "marriage" are not doomed in the same way as women are if the relationship ends.[7]

In the meantime, recent reports on early marriage show that not only does the practice continue, but it may even be on the rise:

> According to figures from the Iran Statistics Center, in the three-month period from March 20, 2020, more than 7,000 girls aged ten to fourteen years were married, with one girl aged less than ten also registered as married. The same body found that the mothers of 346

> children born in that period were not yet fifteen years old, with mothers aged fifteen to nineteen giving birth to some 16,000 babies. Additionally, it counted 131 divorces involving a wife aged less than fourteen years, and 2,650 divorcées aged fifteen to nineteen years.[8]

Chapter 3 is a study of the impact of globalization on fatherhood in Iran. It examines the role of fatherhood in a predominantly patrilineal and patriarchal society among men caught at the crossroads of modernity and the preservation of their identities and privileges. While the findings confirm the persistence of patriarchal practices in one form or another, they also show how traditions are exploiting modernity in creative ways. Among more liberal, secular, and educated fathers, control ranges from showing affection to family members and ensuring that the family remains financially and otherwise dependent on them, to trying to gain full knowledge of the behavior of family members, through the help of surveillance technologies that allow them to spy on their wives' and children's online activities. At the same time, among a large section of conservative groups in society, whether educated or otherwise, control is often exercised more forcefully and even violently.

While some scholars point to weakening patriarchal values and decreasing gender inequalities, discussed in Chapter 2, the case studies in this chapter confirm that, for men, fatherhood remains the culmination of their personhood and identity, from manhood to masculinity and sexuality. Regardless of diminishing patriarchal values and powers, to date, a considerably large number of families remain dependent on fathers or their close male relatives for support. Such dependence not only stems from the persisting cultural perceptions of the role and place of women in society, but is perpetuated by the country's legal system, which denies women equal access to resources, financially and legally, reducing any power they might have over their families. For example, the number of female heads of household, which has risen sharply in Iran, has in no way given women the power to control their families. These women face challenges that men in their positions do not; among these are farmers who are routinely denied ownership of land that had belonged to their husbands, and access to key amenities, such as loans or machinery. The assumption by some scholars that these women are now in control of their families is contradicted by reports from various official sources indicating that such a change is "a shift from a relatively normal special trend into a social problem" (Statistical Research and Training Center 2014). Finally, Chapter 3 discusses how patriarchal practices, often involving violence, are not only controlled and carried out by men, but incorporate the full endorsement and cooperation of women, too. This more holistic look at gender relations remains under-researched by students of Iranian culture.

The chapters in Part II explore the various population policies of different Iranian states through a historical lens, showing their frequent policy reversals concerning the nation's reproductive life. These chapters examine Iran's population policies under two monarchies and under the current Islamic Republic. Chapter 4, first published in 2004, analyzes Iran's highly successful anti-natalist policies of the late 1980s. It argues that these anti-natalist programs were successful for two reasons: first, the program was well-coordinated; second, it was mindful of the fact that asking families to have fewer children ran counter to the cultural and religious imperatives of reproduction, and thus it adopted convincing strategies that remained harmonious with these practices. Chapter 5 explores the outcomes of these anti-natalist policies two decades later, when the 2011 census showed that population growth had fallen to below replacement level. This study examines the state's reversal from its previous policies to its subsequent pronatalist ones, as the state aims to increase its population from around 84 million to 150 million by 2050. To encourage growth, policies initially offered several incentives and disincentives, which failed to gain the cooperation of the generation of reproductive age; despite these efforts, the population continued to decline. While this chapter analyzes the factors responsible for the state's failure to encourage larger families, it also shows through case studies that, regardless of the resistance of young couples to respond to the state's plea for more children, most end up having at least one child, not to satisfy the state, but under persistent pressure from their kin group and society in general. Chapter 6 is a study of the state's most recent pronatalist policies, introduced as a result of the failures of the previous ones. The latest policies, which were legalized in November 2021, soon after the election of an ultra-conservative president in August 2021, are extremely coercive if not draconian. The new measures ban all forms of contraception in the hope of forcing married couples to reproduce. The state has gone so far as to sanction the use of a dating app called Hamdam (meaning "companion") to find potential matches for its users (Teh 2021). This chapter also examines the process by which the treatment of infertility, which had been ignored by previous state policies, has been incorporated into the current population policies, as part of the state's body politic. These findings also counter the state's simplistic claim that socio-economic factors are to blame for the population decline. It asserts that resistance to having more children stems from a multitude of factors, which are also discussed in Chapters 5, 6, and 8.[9] These factors include the younger generation's resentment for being treated as reproductive pawns and for being expected to reverse their reproductive values and practices, which reflect those the state itself had instilled two decades earlier.

The chapters in Part III discuss the high prevalence of infertility in Iran and the persistence of the stigma of barrenness, both of which explain the country's enthusiastic reception of assisted reproductive technologies (ARTs). The studies in this section examine the effect of ARTs on family and kinship and their impact on the extent to which the values and practices attached to reproduction have been altered in the process. Chapter 7 demonstrates the successful, but unhappy, outcome of resorting to ARTs in cases whereby modernity meets with tradition; it cites, for example, cases of infertile men who received sperm from third-party donors and subsequently subjected their wives to years of violence. A number of issues arise from the case studies in this chapter, which highlight: the persistence of gender inequality; the tenacity of values among men on manhood and masculinity; the persistence of women forced to bear the brunt of infertility; and the dilemma of maintaining "purity" of "lineage" that arises when an infertile couple is faced with resorting to a stranger's gametes or remaining childless. Chapter 8 addresses the relationship between religion and gender in Islam and explores the impact of the Islamic Republic's policies on education and the legitimization of ARTs on women. Women find themselves in a Catch-22: while education and the ability to make reproductive choices seem to have liberated and empowered women in many respects, cultural barriers act as obstacles, and women are often brought to a halt by a wall of cultural norms and values with limited room to maneuver. Interestingly, this chapter also shows that, although women have not remained passive in the face of cultural, legal, and political restrictions and have surmounted many of these obstructions, ultimately they too, when faced with these decisions, seek refuge in marriage and family as a strategy to protect some of their hard-won freedoms. Chapter 9, through the study of infertility treatment clinics, shows the persistence of two of the most basic aspects of reproduction, namely the major stigma attached to the inability to reproduce and the paramount importance of continuity of lineage through biological relatedness. The study of infertile couples illustrates how core values surrounding reproduction and kinship persist in essence despite changes in form. In seeking fertility treatment and considering their options, infertile couples, who need gamete donation, invariably choose their blood relatives as donors to ensure the continuity of their blood line and the perpetuation of the traditional forms of family and kinship. Ironically, as this study reveals, such practices result in the emergence of new forms of kinship and relatedness, which contradict the strict Islamic instructions regarding the prohibition of social and sexual interaction between close blood relatives (*mahramiat*). Conceiving with gametes from blood relatives also has implications for the structure of the traditional family.

The chapters in Part IV discuss the introduction of ARTs to Iran and the role played by Shia Islamic jurists in legitimizing their use for infertility treatment. The studies provide insights into the way these technologies have been interpreted, endorsed by religious leaders, and used by their recipients to perpetuate their cultural values attached to reproduction. Chapter 10 examines the introduction of reproductive technologies to Iran and their legitimization by Shia Islamic jurists. It analyzes the process by which Islamic jurists interpret the significance of reproduction in Islam and thus issue a wide—often contradictory—array of *fatwas*, which shaped the practice of ARTs for all parties involved. Unlike the Sunni leadership, which has banned all third-party gamete donation for infertility treatment, Iran's Shia jurists have found solutions within Islamic texts to legitimize all forms of ARTs (Inhorn and Tremayne 2012). This chapter further points to the flexibility created by contradictory verdicts, as well as the ensuing uncertainty and confusion that leave these practices in a state of flux. Chapter 11 explains the history of the introduction of IVF technology to Iran and elaborates on the process by which some Shia jurists found ways to permit third-party gamete donation. One solution involves re-casting the definition of lineage from biological relatedness to an agreement between the gamete donor and recipient whereby the donor forgoes his right to ownership of the child, a condition that had been the original premise in legitimizing third-party donation. While this redefinition seems to suit and satisfy all parties by appearing to uphold the imperative of the purity of lineage without breaching any religious or cultural taboos, in reality it deviates sharply from this imperative. Finally, Chapter 12 discusses how the preferences of third-party gamete recipients have shifted over time, from relying on blood relatives to actively and secretly seeking anonymous third-party donors, in order to claim their own ability to conceive and thus appear to abide by the imperatives of protecting their blood lines. This chapter further examines the inherent conundrum of third-party donation in general and anonymous donation in particular for the politico-religious authorities. On one hand, the drive for population growth means that infertility treatment is high on the state's agenda and that resorting to donors will help increase the number of children born using ARTs. On the other hand, this practice conflicts with every existing Islamic rule, even those that define the parameters of third-party donation.

Taken together, these chapters indicate that modernity and globalization have not succeeded in upending Iran's fundamental institutions. Instead, the incorporation of innovations into the country's social fabric has only revealed the consistency of these core reproductive values. Through the lens of reproduction, this volume explores the interplay between these innovations and the fundamental institutions surrounding reproduction, such as marriage, lineage, patriarchy, and "face" in Iranian culture. As these ethnographic essays show, in embracing new technologies with open arms, Iranians remain guided by their core cultural values and accommodate or even manipulate those aspects of modernity that best fit into their own molds.

Notes

1. See also Afary (2009).
2. In Iran, a woman who has never been married or, by definition, who has never engaged in sexual intercourse, is referred to as a "girl." Moreover, some of these women are in fact girls as young as fourteen years old.
3. https://en.wikipedia.org/wiki/Mohammad_Sadeq_Rouhani
4. https://www.radiofarda.com/a/honor-murder-khuzestan-iran-statistics/31636333.html
5. For example, see Yurcaba (2021).
6. For more information on recent studies on child marriage in Iran, see Montazeri et al. (2016).
7. For more on the practice of white marriage in Iran, see Vatandoust and Sheipari (2020).
8. https://www.radiofarda.com/a/gender-discrimination-in-iran-girls-textbooks/31635422.html; see also "Child Marriage in Iran" (2021) and "Sharp Increase in Child Marriages" (2021).
9. See also "Iran's Demographic Crisis" (2020).

References

Afary, Janet. 2009. *Sexual Politics in Modern Iran*. Cambridge and New York: Cambridge University Press.

Bajoghli, Narges. 2019. *Iran Re-Framed: Anxieties of Power in the Islamic Republic*. Stanford: Stanford University Press.

Bayat, Asef. 2009. *Life as Politics: How Ordinary People Change the Middle East*. Stanford: Stanford University Press.

———. 2013. *Life as Politics: How Ordinary People Change the Middle East*, 2nd edn. Stanford: Stanford University Press.

Bidaki Reza, Hadi Ghazalbash, Sogol Alsaidi, Zahra Ghazalbash, Azadeh Barkhoordarian Ahmadabadi, and Golraste Kholasezade. 2020. "Frequency Distribution of Divorce Causes in Yazd City." Social Behaviour Research and Health, Shahid Sadoughi, University of Medical Sciences, School of Public Health, Yazd. Retrieved 5 October 2021 from http://sbrh.ssu.ac.ir/article-1-129-en.pdf.

"Child Marriage in Iran: Is 13 Too Young? Some Are Even Younger." 2021. *Worldcrunch*, 29 March. Retrieved 27 January 2022 from https://worldcrunch.com/culture-society/child-marriage-in-iran-is-13-too-young-some-are-even-younger.

Eriksen, Thomas Hylland. 2010. *Small Places, Large Issues*. Pluto Press.

Fassihi, Farnaz. 2020. "A Daughter Is Beheaded, and Iran Asks if Women Have a Right to Safety." *New York Times*, 7 June. Retrieved 5 October 2021 from https://www.nytimes.com/2020/06/07/world/middleeast/honor-killing-iran-women.html.

Furlong, Andy, and Fred Cartmel. 2007. *Young People and Social Change: New Perspectives*, 2nd edn. Open University Press.

Inhorn, Marcia C., and Nancy J. Smith-Hefner, eds. 2021. *Waithood: Gender, Education, and Global Delays in Marriage and Childbearing*. Oxford and New York: Berghahn Books.

Inhorn, Marcia C., and Soraya Tremayne, eds. 2012. *Islam and Assisted Reproductive Technologies: Sunni and Shia Perspectives*. Oxford and New York: Berghahn Books.

"Iranian Film Director Murdered by Family in So-Called 'Honor Killing.'" 2021. *Arab News*, 19 May. Retrieved 27 January 2022 from https://www.arabnews.com/node/1861396/middle-east.

"Iran's Demographic Crisis: 'How Can I Have Children When I Can Barely Make Ends Meet?'" 2020. *Financial Times*, 22 August. Retrieved 27 January 2022 from https://www.ft.com/content/c1bd20d6-f019-40ba-9ee7-b23e6150bf6c.

"Marriage Threefold of Divorce in Iran." 2020. *Tehran Times*, 21 December. Retrieved 27 January 2022 from https://www.tehrantimes.com/news/456031/Marriage-threefold-of-divorce-in-Iran.

Montazeri, Simin, Maryam Gharacheh, Nooredin Mohammadi, Javad Alaghband Rad, and Hassan Eftekhar Ardabili. 2016. "Determinants of

Early Marriage from Married Girls' Perspectives in Iranian Setting: A Qualitative Study." *Journal of Environmental and Public Health*. Retrieved 9 October 2021 from https://downloads.hindawi.com/journals/jeph/2016/8615929.pdf.

Nouri, Narges, Nayereh Nouri, Samane Tirgar, Elham Soleimani, Vida Yazdani, Farzaneh Zahedi, and Bagher Larijani. 2017. "Consanguineous Marriages in the Genetic Counseling Centers of Isfahan and the Ethical Issues of Clinical Consultations." *Journal of Medical Ethics and History of Medicine* 10(12).

Pirnia, Bijan, Fariborz Pirnia, and Kambiz Pirnia. 2020. "Honour Killings and Violence against Women in Iran during the COVID-19 Pandemic." *The Lancet* 7(10).

"Sharp Increase in Child Marriages." 2021. *Middle East Eye*, 2 December. Retrieved 27 January 2022 from https://www.middleeasteye.net/news/iran-conservatives-sins-rehab-clinic-open-press-review.

Statistical Research and Training Center. 2014. "Health and Socioeconomic Status of Female-Headed Households: Support Policies and Programs." Retrieved 27 January 2022 from https://iran.unfpa.org/sites/default/files/pub-pdf/Female-Headed%20Households.pdf.

Teh, Cheryl. 2021. "Iran Wants to Boost Marriage Rates with a State-Approved Dating App that Mandates All Its Users Take a Psychology Test." *Insider*, 14 July. Retrieved 5 October 2021 from https://www.insider.com/iran-releases-state-sanctioned-dating-app-users-take-psychology-tests-2021-7#:~:text=The%20Iranian%20government%20has%20released,four%20years%20after%20they%20marry.

Unnithan-Kumar, Maya. 2010. "Female Selective Abortion—Beyond 'Culture': Family Making and Gender Inequality in a Globalising India." *Journal of Culture, Health and Sexuality* 12(2): 153–166.

Vatandoust, Gholam Reza, and Maryam Sheipari. 2020. "Beyond the *Shari'a*: 'White Marriage' in the Islamic Republic of Iran." In *Iranian Romance in the Digital Age: From Arranged Marriage to White Marriage*, ed. Janet Afary and Jesilyn Faust, 55–79. I. B. Tauris.

Yurcaba, Jo. 2021. "Gay Iranian Man Dead in Alleged 'Honor Killing,' Rights Group Says." NBC News, 11 May. Retrieved 5 October 2021 from https://www.nbcnews.com/feature/nbc-out/gay-iranian-man-dead-alleged-honor-killing-rights-group-says-n1266995.

Zavieh, Zahra Ghassemi. 2017. "Reproducing the Virginity Imperative: Women's Collusion and Men's Complicity among Young Iranians Living in Montreal." MA thesis. Montreal, CA: Concordia University.

Part I

Modernity, Discord, Compliance

Chapter 1

CHANGE AND "FACE" IN MODERN IRAN

The Middle East is perhaps the most difficult region of the world for Westerners to comprehend. We are more familiar with its stereotypes, often inaccurate, than with its specificity. The area seems rife with contradictions.

—Donna Lee Bowen and Evelyn A. Early,
Everyday Life in the Muslim Middle East

Most of everyday life is a mix of the old and the new. The cultural system that holds it all together for Muslim Middle Easterners is a rich tapestry woven with strands of Islamic and local customs in a historic framework. Everyday culture blends classic and local religious traditions to solve problems—finding a job, raising children, mending a quarrelling community, combating inflation. It is in this arena that people work out cultural conflicts between tradition and modernity or religiosity and secularism wrought by the rapid changes in the Middle East.

—Donna Lee Bowen and Evelyn A. Early,
Everyday Life in the Muslim Middle East

Introduction

Few would dispute that everyday life in Iran today is shaped by a blend of the old and the new, and at an increasingly rapid pace. Contrary to general outside impressions and perceptions, present-day Iran, although dominated by an authoritarian and Islamist ruling establishment, is not a closed or monolithic society with uniform thinking and behavior. In Iranian society today, there are more differences in lifestyles, values, views, and behavior among various groups than there are similarities. Divergent views have emerged in a distinctly visible way at all levels in the society, and I shall elaborate on these further. However, in spite of the seemingly relative ease with which Iranians adopt the "new" and adapt to change, the underlying factors behind their choices remain deeply rooted in common cultural values, many of which have remained intact and are shared by almost all Iranians, regardless of their social, ethnic, or religious background.

In the following chapter, I shall try to show that in the encounter between the old and the new, "face" (in Persian *aberu*, literally meaning the "water of one's face") acts as a key agent, a checkpoint and a brake to set the boundaries for what is culturally permissible within the "new" context. "Face" plays a determining role in the selection of what to adopt and how to adapt to change. The "new" has to be made to fit into the existing cultural mold and accord with acceptable norms to preserve cultural practices and thereby cultural identity. "Face" cannot be defined per se and in isolation from the more profound cultural tenets that uphold a society. As the public manifestation and culmination of those values, it is similar to what Gilsenan (1993: 157–158) summarizes as the feature of "lying": "[a] fundamental element, not only of a specific situation and individual actions, but also of the cultural universe as a whole." Although "face" represents broad concepts of honor, shame, and power relations among others, I do not intend to explore these here. Instead, I shall focus on exploring the role "face" plays in the context of modern Iran and its everyday life.

Where Does the Openness Come From?

A brief history on where the changes that lead to an encounter between the old and the new come from in today's Iran will be helpful. After the Islamic Revolution in 1979, many traditional values, which had gradually been suppressed in the name of development and modernity, were revived and found a new voice. This revival, which advocated a return to traditional social and cultural values, gave rise to new debates, not only between the religious and secular groups, but also among the religious groups themselves. The latter sought to reinterpret their ideologies within a new framework, which accommodated, justified, or rejected inter alia social, cultural, and economic change, gender relations, and the relationship between religion and politics. Such a division has led to an unprecedented openness in society. For example, while the conservative religious groups have continued to take every opportunity to discuss and encourage a return to conservative and traditional ways of thinking and living, the more liberal religious thinkers have tried to find a more "enlightened" version of Islamic ideology, one that can accommodate religious values and modernity. "Even those with clerical education are increasingly inclined to question what the leading political clerics say and do" (Keddie 2003: 316). In order to adjust religious law (*sharia*) to the requirements of modern life, *ijtihad* (interpretation of *sharia*) has been used as a mechanism to allow the issuing of *fatwas* (religious decrees) to make such adjustments possible wherever they are deemed necessary.[1] Considering the pervasive nature of Islam and its involvement in giving instructions for daily life, *fatwas* are not limited to major issues such as politics or religious laws. As I shall explain below, they also concern everyday life and cover a wide range of issues, from the permissibility of consuming treated sewage water (*fatwa* no. 09944 by Ayatollah Khamenei) to the ruling on keeping arms crossed during prayer with Sunni brothers (*fatwa* no. 4191 by Ayatollah Khamenei on "Praying and eating with Ahl al Tasannun," meaning Sunnis).[2] Change, leading to further openness, has also resulted from reforms and the introduction of new policies in various spheres of Islamic life. Some of these reforms are internal, while others derive from global decisions agreed upon at international gatherings. To implement social policies successfully, policymakers have had to communicate with the people, familiarize them with new ideas and seek their participation. The accompanying education and creation of public awareness have inevitably led to an irreversible openness in society and to a shift in the balance of relationships at all levels, including gender and generation. A clear example of these reforms are the population policies aimed at reducing population growth, which had to address women as the main agents of implementation and give them rights in contradiction with the original ideologies of the Islamic Republic. The implementation of these policies proved an irreversible process and opened important horizons in the field of gender relations, since they gave women the license to make decisions in one of the most important aspects of their lives, i.e., that of reproduction. Addressing women on the importance of controlling their fertility and reducing the number of children they have, as well as allowing them access to free contraceptive means, proved a drastic measure in altering relationships within the family and between the genders. To date, many men from conservative and traditional groups do not approve of such measures, but they are no longer in a position to reject them openly, especially since the program was endorsed by the clerics at the highest level (Hoodfar 1995). However, even today many men do not allow their wives access to contraceptives, and women have to resort to them secretly.

There are many other areas in which the implementation of modern policies has clashed with traditions and caused serious disruptions. One such example pertains to the Convention on the Rights of the Child (CRC) of 1998, which defines "anybody under the age of eighteen as a child." Though a signatory to this convention, Iran reserved the right not to implement those clauses that were against Islamic law. In Islam, the definition of a child is contextual and varies depending on what is expected of a child at different stages of his/her growth. A child can be an adult in one context and a child in another. For example, according to Islam, girls reach puberty at the age of nine and boys at fifteen. In this respect, they are seen as having reached physical maturity and are considered adults; however, they are not considered mentally mature and still need a guardian until they reach mental maturity, usually around eighteen. The definition of age can also vary in other contexts, such as the age for voting (fifteen years old), for legal employment (fifteen years old), and for obtaining a driving license or a passport (eighteen years old). The contradictions between the CRC's understanding of childhood and that of Islam are many (Ebadi 1997, 2002; Tremayne 2004). Though its implementation has proved problematic, the convention has nevertheless given rise to new debates on the definitions of different age categories and the mutual rights and obligations related to them.

There are also other spheres—human rights, environmental issues, certain scientific areas—that introduce new ideas and have an impact, whether officially accepted or not. The result is an ongoing questioning of values within the society. Global trends, such as urbanization, improvement in education and health, and technological and scientific innovations, have resulted in major changes that present new challenges to old values. Finally, the openness of Iranian society is also stimulated by external sources, including access to the Internet, satellite television, travel, and tourism.

"Face"

In a society such as Iran, which is constantly on the move and where changes are taking place at a fast pace, people do not remain passive. In taking decisions as to whether and how to adopt change, "face" plays an important part in checking and shaping cultural responses. Face is one of the manifestations of Iranian culture that has not been weakened by the challenges of modernity and the introduction of the "new" in society. Whereas the concept of face is generally well-known, and every culture has its own definition of what constitutes face, its meanings can be more critical and extensive in some cultures than others. While the loss of face in the West may mean embarrassment, it frequently means much more than this in Middle Eastern cultures. There, loss of face often causes deep humiliation, which in turn can lead to loss of credibility and entail other social and economic consequences. In extreme cases, it can provoke strong reactions, violence, and even a blood feud. Essentially, face is closely linked to failure, or what is perceived as failure in meeting public expectations. Face is related to the position of a person in society and, by implication, to the position of his/her family. The more senior a person, the more face he/she has to preserve or lose. Awareness of one's social position and of the appropriate related behavior is an imperative in all social interactions. Therefore, every decision taken must consider the social consequences as far as the status and respectability of the family are concerned. Apart from being lost, face can also be maintained, gained, given, restored, or saved. While face becomes particularly apparent at major life events such as marriage, birth, divorce, death, and similar happenings, and where every effort is being made to preserve it, face also remains a preoccupation in the smaller matters of everyday life, such as shopping (for example, failing to buy a sufficient quantity of market produce, not being able to distinguish good quality from bad, not driving a hard bargain—all result in contempt by the seller and a loss of face by the buyer), gift-giving (these can be big gifts, but they should never be too small), or tipping the taxi driver (giving the wrong tip is to be avoided). In other words, individuals have to constantly consider their position in their interactions with others, and since social interaction is fluid by nature, they have to reconsider their strategy in every new situation. This subconscious process is at work during all interactions with others, especially in public.

In what follows, I shall give some examples to illustrate the extent to which face remains a major consideration in actions relating to the adoption of the "new" where it affects everyday life, as well as in some areas where advanced technological or global policies have an impact on everyday life. To do so, I have chosen two different sets of examples. The first set is selected to demonstrate the application of modern medical technology, its legitimization within the framework of Shia Islam, and the way face determines the form and extent of its use. In this connection, the case of transsexuals is also looked at, in spite of the relatively small number of people it involves. This choice was made to emphasize that while technological and religious barriers to undergo sex change have been removed, norms and face prevent its widespread practice. Attention is also given to street and runaway children as a vulnerable group and the reactions that face provokes in such a situation. The conclusions reached with regard to the first set of examples relate to the disruptions caused by social reforms and their effect on the family. The second set of examples, perhaps less dramatic, is based on a recent field study I undertook in the spring and summer of 2004 in a small conservative city in central Iran.

Infertility Treatment

The relationship between reproduction and face is so intertwined and complex that its discussion deserves a chapter of its own. To touch on it briefly, it could be said that the ability to reproduce forms a major aspect of face in Iranian society. For many people, having a girl as the first child is a loss of face; having too many children, and therefore being deemed ignorant and backward in the modern context, is a loss of face; having a disabled child is a loss of face (examples still exist of rural parents who, out of shame, chain and hide disabled children in cowsheds[3]). But not being able to have any children at all is a major loss of face. Infertility in Iranian culture, which still places very high value on having one's own children, remains a stigma. Infertile couples have always resorted to every means available to cure their infertility. Traditionally, they have resorted to healers, magic, and doctors. However, for the past ten years, many private clinics and public hospitals have started offering infertility treatment through the use of new reproductive technologies (NRT). These have proved so successful, and the demand for them has been so high, that in 1993 Ayatollah Khamenei issued a *fatwa* allowing the use of NRT. This was followed by the legalization of the practice in 2003. Many infertility treatment centers are offering the most advanced methods, and Iran is rated as very progressive in this field by specialists who visit the country. During a recent visit to Iran, Dr. Safaa Al-Hassani, the head of the ART Medical Center of USHCL University in Germany, commented that "the current facilities for treatment of infertility in Iran are comparable to those of the ART Medical Center in Germany, which are much higher than the global standards." He also added that "the infertility rate in Iran is high . . . between 10 to 15 percent of couples are infertile. There is hardly any other disorder across the nation with such a high rate of incidence."[4]

Based on Shia law, the 2003 legislation on infertility treatment is clear in its scope, specifying that egg and sperm donations can take place only between a wife and a husband.[5] In the case of the wife's infertility, a temporary marriage—or, to use the term coined by Jane Khatib-Chahidi (1981), a "fictive marriage"[6]—is arranged between the husband and an egg donor (usually for one day) to legitimize the donation. If it is the husband who is infertile, the couple receives an embryo from another married couple, since a married woman cannot marry a second man. It is beyond the scope of this chapter to go into the details of the adaptation of Shia law concerning infertility. Also, our focus here is rather on how people adapt the technology and the law in everyday life to suit their particular needs and to save face (Tremayne 2005). However, while the law allows infertility treatment within acceptable Shia practices and the most advanced methods of treatment are available to infertile couples, in reality the reasons that underpin the infertile couples' reproductive decisions and choices stem more from cultural values. These values are not informed by medical knowledge and reproductive technologies but by a deeply rooted cultural understanding of what constitutes kinship, family relationships, incest, and sexuality that predominates over scientific and medical considerations. For Iranian infertile couples, face becomes one of the determining factors in the understanding of the use of in vitro fertilization and gamete donation and in the decisions they make regarding these issues. In general, admitting infertility is highly embarrassing and is avoided, if at all possible. Many infertile couples who can afford to do so go abroad to circumvent the inevitable repercussions of such admission: an endless accounting of their situation and a close check being kept on every one of their moves. They often choose to bypass some of the limitations imposed by Shia law, such as the restriction on receiving sperm or eggs from strangers. A true story is recounted in infertility treatment clinics about one such couple, who did not reveal their real reason for traveling. When they returned with the wife pregnant, nobody suspected that they had received treatment until the baby was born—and it was black! It is not difficult to imagine the consequences in such an instance and the loss of face involved. Usually, infertile couples reveal their infertility only if they seek help from one of their relatives. An infertile man not wishing to admit the fact and also not wishing to receive another couple's embryo might secretly make arrangements for his brother to donate his sperm without his wife's knowledge.[7] A woman may also secretly ask another woman—a sister, perhaps, or even a stranger with whom she has become friends in the waiting room of the clinic—to donate eggs and pass them off as her own rather than letting her husband enter a "fictive marriage" even for only one day. Since brothers-in-law and sisters-in-law are *na-mahram*[8] to each other, using their sperm or egg without the necessary ceremony legalizing this action would be unlawful (Khatib-Chahidi 1981: 125), but efforts to prevent the outside world from finding out about the treatment are driven primarily by regard for face.

Another method of assisted conception is surrogacy. Currently, there are no specific laws either for or against surrogacy, and three cases have recently come to the fore. With its practice continuing, public debate has been stimulated, and eventually a *fatwa*, followed by a law, is likely to be issued to legitimize surrogacy. However, while the technology exists and its practice is not banned, in reality very few women would volunteer to become surrogate mothers, since this is in conflict with cultural principles. As one woman put it, "I am willing to do it [be a surrogate mother], but I am afraid of inquisitive people who may not believe that I am just a 'rented mother.'" "Rented mothers," so far, have been mostly relatives or reliable acquaintances, since it is easier for them to convince others within the family network that they are not carrying an illegitimate child. Although becoming a surrogate mother is a profitable undertaking, the loss of face involved has so far prevented a lot of women from engaging freely in it.[9]

Transsexuality

Another interesting example of how face acts as a brake, preventing advanced medical technologies from reaching those who need them, is that of transsexuality.[10] Transsexuality is an issue that even in the West is not yet fully understood and accepted by the public. As in the case of NRT, surgeons in Iran carry out operations on transsexuals, even attracting customers from neighboring countries. The practice started twenty years ago after representatives of the medical community met with Ayatollah Khomeini and explained what it means to be a transsexual. Ayatollah Khomeini issued a *fatwa* allowing the surgery to be carried out, and his successor, Ayatollah Khamenei, has also endorsed this practice.

Today in Iran, these operations take place openly.[11] A person wishing to undergo a transsexual operation is led through a well-established and elaborate procedure. The necessary medical and legal steps are taken. A coroner and a judge examine the patient and give him/her a certificate from the court to allow him/her to dress as a man or woman for eighteen months before the surgery in order to ascertain that he/she wishes to change sex. A social worker is assigned to counsel the parents, since their permission for such an operation is required. Funds have been allocated by some of the charities for a limited number of individuals who cannot afford such costly operations. However, while transsexuality is officially recognized as an illness, socially it remains stigmatized. Parents of transsexuals, especially those from the more conservative layers of society, react fiercely to the problem and often throw their children out of the house. Men[12] have a particularly difficult time, since Iranian society does not distinguish between homosexuality and transsexuality, and transsexuals have often been arrested for homosexuality and sentenced. In one case, a transsexual man, having endured frequent arrests and sentencing, and having been rejected by his family, had to flee the country and seek asylum. He did so with his family's help, since his life was considered in danger; however, the family was even more anxious to eliminate the shame by helping him escape.[13] Women in need of surgery come forward less often, even though they do not have to suffer humiliation similar to that of men since they can disguise their condition more easily. Many of them prefer to go through life as they are rather than seek treatment and suffer the social consequences.

Transsexual surgery is not widely known by the public, and those who are aware of the possibility cannot always afford it. Even if surgery takes place, the future remains grim for most male transsexuals. They are either rejected by their families, end in prostitution, or join a dance group or similar activities, all of which condemn them in the eyes of society. An alternative option for men who have become women[14] is to become a temporary wife to a man who marries for purely sexual purposes. The feeling of shame for having a transsexual child is so great that even the educated non-conservative groups consider it a massive loss of face. A mother's account of the agonies her transsexual son had to endure, and the harassment meted out by the police and society in general before he was diagnosed, reflects the prevalent attitudes toward transsexuals.[15] After their son was diagnosed, she and her husband were tormented for months as to how to break the news to their relatives. Transsexuality remains a stigma regardless of social and educational background in Iranian society.

Runaway Children

Some recently introduced social policies and reforms have unwittingly exposed aspects of family life that have traditionally been considered as strictly private matters, thereby violating the sanctity of family relationships. Policies concerning the protection of family and women's rights and the rights of the child have created conflict and confusion, not only between the new reforms and traditions, but also between modern policies and Islamic law itself.

The tension emerging from the incompatibility between social reforms and traditional practices has resulted in severe disruptions in family life, especially as far as children are concerned. Measures undertaken by new policies to improve the situation of children with regard to violence and abuse are in contradiction with customary practices and religious interpretations, which give the parents the right to control their children as they see fit. However, in the application of the law concerning children's rights and the protection provided by the legal system, it is essential to understand the Islamic view of the family and the rights it accords to parents over their children.

Until a few years ago, cases of child abuse within the family rarely came to public attention. New laws about the rights of the child[16] together with improvements in education and health (especially for girls), physical mobility between urban and rural areas, access to media, as well as a growing awareness of alternatives to bad treatment at home, continue to create major clashes within families between men and women and parents and children. Young women and children are the main casualties of these conflicts, and one way of coping is to run away from home. In telling their stories, some runaway and street children have revealed the most intimate details about their family lives (e.g., violence, beatings, rape by close relatives and parents) and exposed them publicly.[17] The authorities' first reaction to runaway children is to send them back home. This stems partly from a genuine desire to reunite the children with their families and partly from the inadequacy of provisions for protecting such children.

Parents meet the return of their runaway children with extremely fierce reactions. Their loss of face is so great that in most cases either they refuse to take the children back, or they subject them to even harsher treatment, purely to punish them for the shame they have inflicted on the family. Such occurrences are reported in the Iranian papers almost on a daily basis: in one case, a child was sent back home eight times before the authorities took her in. In almost all such instances, it is face that takes precedence over the welfare of the child, as far as the parents are concerned. One striking example is that of a young woman who had been sold as a child by her parents. When her adoptive parents were killed in a car crash, she was returned to her birth parents, who then forced her to marry a much older man. He had five children and constantly subjected her to violence. She divorced him but was rejected by her parents for doing so. Having secured herself a job in a town, she was remarried, this time to a man who turned out to be a violent drug addict. After divorcing him, too, she continued working and had no contact with her parents. One day she received a visit from her mother, who told her that they had forgiven her and invited her to pay them a visit. When she arrived at her parents' home, they poured petrol over her, set her on fire and beat her with a stick for bringing shame upon the family by divorcing twice. She was rescued by neighbors and taken to hospital where she died after telling her story.[18] In another instance, the father of a runaway girl, who had been informed by the police of her whereabouts, visited his daughter's shelter carrying a butcher's knife to slaughter her and to "wash the stain of shame from the family."[19] If the authorities had not acted quickly, he would have killed her. Some parents, upon learning that their daughter is in a shelter, agree to take the child back only "if she is not spoiled," that is, if she has not lost her virginity.

The Everyday Context of "Face"

Whether the occasion is sad or happy, face can be lost, maintained, given, restored, or diminished in a multitude of ways and remains a determining factor in all social events. For example, getting divorced is still viewed as a failure, and thousands of people, more women than men, tolerate abuse, violence, mental stress, and other miseries out of reluctance to ask for divorce and the fear of losing face. On a much smaller scale, when death occurs in a family, the names of the relatives announcing the death in the daily paper appear in order of closeness to the deceased. The ranking of relatives is decided upon by the person closest to the deceased, who is often distraught and can easily get the order wrong. This then leads to a major loss of face for both the person making the decision and the person whose name has been left out or is in the wrong place. Families are totally unforgiving in such instances and have been known not to talk to each other for years afterward. Marriage, divorce, birth, and gift-giving also involve face and remain the topic of conversation and complaint (*gueleh*) for a long time, as many faces can be affected in the process.

"Face" in a Conservative Town

The following examples illustrate what constitutes "face" in the daily life of a conservative society that is also exposed to all the changes mentioned earlier. They arose from recent fieldwork I carried out in Yazd (in central Iran) in 2004.[20] Yazd has been officially classified as the most conservative city in Iran on the basis of having the lowest divorce rate in the country. However, I think that, in essence, most of what I observed there can be extended to the majority of families in most parts of Iran, albeit to varying degrees in form and extent.

One of the families I studied consisted of a husband and wife and their two daughters, aged fifteen and ten. With a conservative man as its head, the family seems to epitomize the picture of patriarchy to perfection. The female members are under the total control of the husband. They wear the veil for every occasion that entails contact with *na-mahrams* and are not allowed out without a *mahram* companion. The family lives on a modest income, and meals, served at totally irregular hours, are simple and without frills. The husband is a clerk at a brick-distributing company, and the wife runs a hairdressing salon from home. The wife and husband are cross-cousins, the husband being the son of the wife's mother's brother (*dokhtar ameh va pesar dayi*). In spite of a frugal lifestyle, the family has air conditioning, sophisticated music and video equipment, and access to satellite television. Although we did not watch a great deal of television when I visited them, it was clear that having these amenities was more important than using them. Eating small meals, or not at all, matters less since nobody needs to know, but not having a mobile phone, satellite television, or video machine is a sign of poverty and a matter for loss of face.

The wife's marriage to her cousin was arranged purely to save her mother's face. According to the wife, she was coerced into marrying her husband because "[her] mother told [her] that her brother had asked for [her] hand for his son." Her mother added: "Although this is your decision, I think that you should agree. This is the first time my brother has asked me for a favor, and I cannot refuse his request, since he will lose face and I can never look him in the eye again." Her paternal uncle, who oversaw the family affairs after her father's death, also supported her mother's views. But it was not until after constant indirect pressure and the marriage arrangements were going ahead that both her mother and uncle insisted that she did not have to marry if she didn't want to. By then, though, it was too late to call off the marriage. Although her husband is her cousin, the wife considers him and his entire family as "people of low culture" (*mardom-e ba farhang-e pâin*). Having married him has "diminished the status" that she enjoyed in her mother's home. "Low culture" for her is associated with wearing the veil and with the way women are treated in his family. She is contemptuous of her sisters-in-law and is convinced that they are out to humiliate her. Every morning starts by reassessing her actions based on those of her in-laws. She interprets every one of their actions as an intentional effort to make her lose face, be it by asking her to do their hair or offering to make clothes for her children (to make her feel inadequate). She then adjusts her plan and her next move based on her assumption of their intentions. One of the many examples of this was when she went on a pilgrimage to the holy city of Mashhad, the shrine of Imam Reza. On her return, as is customary, her relatives came with an armful of presents. Some of their presents were far too small and were meant to show her that her pilgrimage was not that important. However, the one that caused real offence was from one sister-in-law who had brought her some water glasses made in Iran. "She (the sister-in-law) could have easily bought some Japanese glasses," explained the wife. "I sent the glasses back and have told them not to visit my house again. I have also told everybody about it." By giving the wrong present, both parties have lost face, and the sister-in-law is now excluded from the woman's circle.

Before my departure, I invited a family to eat out and decided to give the children a chance to choose where they wanted to dine. They chose a new pizza restaurant, instead of one of the upmarket restaurants that are old places converted into glossy establishments serving traditional meals. The look of disbelief on the adults' faces made it clear that I had made a grave mistake and had lost their respect by even considering consulting the children. As a senior and educated woman, I was the focus of attention and considered a role model. By asking the children's opinion, not only had I not used my own superior judgment, but also I had not paid due attention and respect to the parents. Once a mistake of this nature is made, there is little hope of recovering from it quickly, if at all. Throughout my stay, I was walking a tightrope, which did not allow room for misjudgments. One is supposed to "know" the unspoken rules. I hope to recover my face on my next trip!

One way of maintaining face in today's Iran is to appear knowledgeable and well informed on current issues. Iranians are used to following role models and are reluctant to express personal views in public, which may contradict what is advocated by those who "know better." My research in Yazd involved spending many days in one of the maternity hospitals to study early marriage. In my casual discussions with the staff, I enquired whether any members of their families had been married under the age of fifteen. The answer was invariably phrased along the following lines: "It is true that this was practiced in the past by people of low culture, but where I come from people don't marry their children at an early age anymore. Some still do, but they are people in the next village." They even gave me the names of those villages. Almost everybody I interviewed made similar statements, from the doctors to their secretaries to the hospital porters.

As time went by, and I made more progress in my research, it became apparent that in almost all the villages early marriage was still practiced, and in some its incidence was considerable. The reason for denial of the practice by people in the hospital was that over the past few decades an extensive campaign has been launched to discourage early marriage, which entails early and multiple pregnancies.[21] The practice is viewed as "backward,"[22] and disapproval of it raises the status of the individual concerned. Nevertheless, while many of my respondents secretly approve of early marriage and practice it, they would not admit it for fear of being viewed negatively by an outsider. I gradually found a face-saving formula by conveying the message that early marriages had taken place in my family, too, that not everything was negative about them, and that I did not look down on people who practiced early marriage. Once reassured, they came forward in large groups and volunteered information about themselves and their families on both girls' and boys' early marriages. They even introduced me to many of their relatives who had had early marriages, so that I now have a wealth of data, thanks to having saved so many faces.

Familiarity with new ideas can also improve one's face. Even some of the clerics whom I interviewed were anxious to demonstrate their familiarity with modern ideas and debates. During a meeting with a lecturer in divinity at the university, trying to find a common language and start on a friendly note, I began by telling him that as an anthropologist I do not consider all traditions as outdated and would like to see some of them preserved. Without hesitation, the cleric answered: "Most traditions are outdated and must be replaced by new ideas." He clearly was anxious to show that he was a modern cleric. However, at the same time he stated that, following Islamic ideology, he fully approved of early marriage for girls and queried the definition of "early" marriage, as did several other clerics whom I interviewed. "When a girl is ready to be married, it is not too early for her to get married," they told me, with the cleric being the judge of what "ready" is.

One area of constant debate is marriage: early marriage, late marriage, coerced marriage, temporary marriage, divorce, infertility due to late marriage, and so on. One woman acquainted me with the details of a recent family scandal. A few months previously, somebody had brought the news that one of her sisters had been the temporary wife (*sigheh*) of a married man, who is also her boss, for over two years. She had managed to deceive the family by continuing to live with her mother. Although temporary marriage is a legal and legitimate form of marriage and is permitted under Shia Islam, it is looked down upon by self-respecting families, who do not consider it acceptable that a decent unmarried girl would enter into such an arrangement. It was obvious that the entire extended family had lost face in a serious way, especially since half of the town seemed to know about the affair before they did. Temporary marriage is not viewed as a serious undertaking by men and does not provide the necessary protection for women or their children.[23] Certainly, for most families, their daughter's first marriage is not, and should not be, a temporary one, even though some such unions remain permanent and the couple lives together as wife and husband for many years. The family of the woman in question at first reacted by trying to negotiate and bring the girl to her senses by asking her to divorce the husband, which she refused to do. The next stage was to ask her to insist on becoming the man's permanent wife, which she also refused to do on the grounds that as the man was already married, she would always be treated as a second-class citizen, and her status would be diminished even further. She said that she was perfectly happy as she was and loved the man and he loved her. But love and happiness are not concepts easily understood when it is a question of the family's face. The girl's brothers were informed. They came in full force and at first talked to her, then shouted at her and resorted to violence, but nothing persuaded her to separate from her husband. Left with no other choice, the brothers tied their sister up and imprisoned her in a cellar for several days until she consented to become the permanent wife to her husband. The man agreed to divorce his first wife and marry her. The family's face was bruised but saved.

The opposite to the above was the case of the husband's younger sister, who is twenty-nine years old and single, living at home and looking after her parents. She, too, felt that she had lost face in society for not having been able to find a husband. While all her five older sisters had married under the age of fifteen, she was still at home with no prospect of marriage. She mentioned that her parents had not forced her to marry young because society had changed and now looked down on those who practiced early marriage. They had agreed for her to complete secondary school, but she was not allowed to go to university. As a result, she had lost all her chances of marrying young. By moving to town she had lost the prospect of meeting a marriage partner in their village, and by not being allowed to continue her education, she had also missed her chances of meeting a prospective husband at the university, which, of late, has become a common place for finding a marriage partner.

Living in such a closed society, women have very few opportunities for physical exercise. For women in this particular layer of society, even walking means having a man accompany them, which is not always practical. My suggestion of swimming met with fierce reaction from the men. A criminal gang had apparently started a profitable business by sending women with small cameras to women's swimming pools, where they would take pictures of swimmers in their swimsuits. They then either blackmailed these women or sold their pictures in the city.[24] Such an incidence constitutes an ultimate loss of face and becomes an issue of honor.

A final example, which comes first-hand and took place recently in England, testifies to the extent to which face still dictates the actions of individuals of all generations when interacting with other Iranians, even outside Iran. Two young Iranian brothers were sent from Iran to visit a friend of mine in England. He took them to buy some fish and chips, and while he was in the queue, the older brother beat up his younger brother, causing a great deal of disturbance. When asked why he caused such trouble, the boy answered, "My brother made my entire family in Iran lose face by asking for a large portion of chips. He behaves as if my mother has not fed us well."

Conclusion

As suggested at the beginning of this chapter, at one level Iran is a relatively open society, one that embraces change willingly. Rather than rejecting "new" elements outright, all groups in society, including the conservative or even reactionary ones, make use of them for their own purposes and justify change through religious interpretation. However, at a deeper level, Iran remains a closed society, whose strong cultural ties act as unifying factors by monitoring and controlling the degree of interaction between the old and the new. They allow only a well-defined space for maneuver to each individual, depending on his/her position in society, thereby determining to what extent he/she can deviate from the norms (i.e., adopt the "new"). Face, as one such regulating agent, acts as a brake to prevent the disappearance of fundamental values.

However, the more senior, wealthy, and powerful the individuals are, the tighter the space for social maneuver, as far as maintaining their face is concerned. They are bound by obligations and expectations imposed upon them by society. This obviously does not imply powerlessness, but it shapes the way power is used to preserve face. In doing so, face controls the actions and decisions taken by individuals in all public aspects of their lives, regardless of class, age, ethnic origin, or gender.

Acknowledgments

This chapter was published originally as "Change and 'Face' in Modern Iran," *Anthropology of the Middle East* 1(1): 25–41, Berghahn Journals (2006). I should like to thank Anna Enayat, Camillia El-Solh, and Jane Khatib-Chahidi for their valuable comments on this chapter.

Notes

1. Literature on *ijtihad* written by Shia scholars is rich. For a brief reference, see Richard (2003).
2. For details of Ayatollah Khamenei's *fatwas*, see his websites. The information cited is from http://islam-pure.de/imam/fatwas/fatwas04.htm.
3. Personal interviews with welfare officers, Iran, June 2004.
4. These are figures quoted by Dr. Safaa Al-Hassani, without any source

being given for them, in a speech he made to a workshop held in Avicenna Specialized Medical Center in February 2003. Reported by *Sharq Daily Newspaper*, 4 February 2003.

5. Although the *fatwa* to allow infertility treatment was given by Ayatollah Khamenei, it does not meet with the approval of all the other senior clerics. For a different view on both NRT and transsexuality, see Mir-Hosseini (1999: 34–47).
6. For more information on "fictive marriage," whereby temporary marriage is arranged but no sexual contact takes place, see Khatib-Chahidi (1981: 112–135).
7. There are also other reasons, such as kinship and inheritance, that determine the preference for receiving a donation from one's brother or sister, in spite of this being against the law. Having the baby of one's in-law without prior legitimate arrangements is viewed as committing incest (*zena*).
8. *Na-mahram* is a person of the opposite sex who is a potential marriage partner. *Mahram* is the opposite of *na-mahram*. The *mahrams* include father/mother, brother/sister, son/daughter, and husband/wife (Khatib-Chahidi 1981).
9. Reported by *Sharq Daily Newspaper*, 31 January 2004.
10. This chapter was published in 2006, when the term "transsexuality" was often used interchangeably with "transgender." Today, we draw more of a distinction between these terms. Pioneering scholar Afsaneh Najmabadi (2005, 2014) covers the topics of gender and transsexuality in Iran in her groundbreaking books.
11. Personal interviews with Professor Bahram Mir-Djalali, January 2004.
12. Because this chapter appeared as an article almost twenty years ago, some of the terminology surrounding transsexual and transgender people is outdated. What are described here as "men" are now understood to be "transgender women." Similarly, "women," as described here, are "transgender men."
13. I have personal knowledge of the case.
14. Described here as "men who have become women," we now understand these individuals to be transgender women who have received gender affirming therapy or surgery.
15. The Gully, 2001. Available at www.thegully.com/essay/gaymundo/010508transgender.html.
16. With the Child Abuse Bill, passed by the Iranian parliament in June 2002, the authorities expressed hope that child abuse will be considered a crime against society. Iran-e-emrooz Khordadd 1381 (May 2002). See also www.iranianchildren.org.majlis_702.html.
17. A report by the head of the welfare organization in Iran on runaway children states that in the first six months of the Iranian calendar 1382 (2003), fifteen thousand runaway children have been collected from

the streets of Tehran and two other provinces (reported by *London Kayhan*, 3 October 2003).

18. *London Kayhan*, 13 November 2003.
19. Reported by *Sharq Daily Newspaper*, June 2004.
20. For the choice of the place and arranging the contacts, I am deeply grateful to Soheila Shahshahani.
21. Before the 1979 Revolution, the minimum age of marriage was sixteen for girls; after the Revolution, the Islamic law lowered it to nine for girls and fifteen for boys. Although it is legal to marry at those ages according to Islamic law, in practice, due to an extensive family-planning program, the age of marriage has gone up and the rate of early marriages has gone down. Although during the first few years after the Revolution the campaign for discouraging early marriage and early pregnancy stopped, in 1986 the new family-planning program in Iran started an extensive and ongoing campaign regarding the reproductive health of young people. Hence the reluctance to admit the practice of early marriage.
22. Erica Friedl (1989: 14) recounts a midwife's visit to a remote village, where the midwife lectured the women on the blessings of the pill and said that "having more children than one could well care for was backward. Even the Shah has only four." "Here in the village we are like cows. Every year another calf, always in milk," she added.
23. For more details on temporary marriage, see Haeri (1989).
24. The website Hadeseh also reported similar incidents in other cities. See www.hadeseh.com/b/archives/004000.php [in Persian], 21 October 2004.

References

Bowen, Donna Lee, and Evelyn A. Early, eds. 1993. *Everyday Life in the Muslim Middle East*. Bloomington: Indiana University Press.

Ebadi, Shirin. 1997. "The Legal Punishment of Murdering One's Child." http://www.inq7.net/opi/2003/dec/16/opi_mltan-1.htm.

———. 2002. "Serious Steps Taken to Enforce Children's Rights Convention," IRNA (Iranian News Agency), 26 May.

Friedl, Erika. 1989. *Lives in an Iranian Village: Women of Deh Koh*. Washington, DC, and London: Smithsonian Institution Press.

Gilsenan, Michael. 1993. "Lying, Honor, and Contradiction." In *Everyday Life in the Muslim Middle East*, ed. Donna Lee Bowen and Evelyn A. Early, 157–169. Bloomington: Indiana University Press.

Haeri, Shahla. 1989. *Law of Desire: Temporary Marriage in Iran*. London: I.B. Tauris.

Hoodfar, Homa. 1995. "Population Policy and Gender Equity in Post-Revolutionary Iran." In *Family, Gender and Population in the Middle East:*

Policies in Context, ed. Carla Makhlouf Obermeyer, 105–135. Cairo: American University of Cairo Press.

Keddie, Nikki R. 2003. *Modern Iran: Roots and Results of Revolution*. New Haven and London: Yale University Press.

Khatib-Chahidi, Jane. 1981. "Sexual Prohibitions, Shared Space and Fictive Marriages in Shi'ite Iran." In *Women and Space: Ground Rules and Social Maps*, ed. Shirley Ardener, 112–135. London: Croom Helm.

Mir-Hosseini, Ziba. 1999. *Islam and Gender: The Religious Debate in Contemporary Iran*, revised ed. London: I.B. Tauris.

Najmabadi, Afsaneh. 2005. *Women with Mustaches and Men without Beards: Gender and Sexual Anxieties of Iranian Modernity*. Berkeley and Los Angeles: University of California Press.

———. 2014. *Professing Selves: Transsexuality and Same-Sex Desire in Contemporary Iran*. Durham, NC: Duke University Press.

Richard, Yann. 2003. "Contemporary Shi'i Thought." In *Modern Iran: Roots and Results of Revolution*, ed. Nikki R. Keddie, 188–212. New Haven and London: Yale University Press.

Tremayne, Soraya. 2004. "'And Never Shall the Twain Meet': Reproductive Health Policies in the Islamic Republic of Iran." In *Reproductive Change, Agency and the State: Cultural Transformations in Childbearing*, ed. Maya Unnithan-Kumar, 181–202. Oxford and New York: Berghahn Books.

———. 2005. "The Moral, Ethical, and Legal Implications of Egg, Sperm and Embryo Donation in Iran." Reproductive Disruptions: Childlessness, Adoption and other Reproductive Complexities Conference, Ann Arbor, Michigan, 19–22 May. University of Michigan.

Chapter 2

Modernity and Early Marriage in Iran

A View from Within

The past few decades have witnessed important changes in the patterns of marriage in the Middle East and North Africa. These changes are well documented by specialists from various disciplines and from diverse perspectives (see Hopkins 2003; Singerman and Hoodfar 1996; Tucker 1993; Moghadam 1993; Afshar 1993; Abbasi-Shavazi, McDonald, and Hosseini-Chavoshi 2003). They stem from a multitude of reasons molded by modernity and globalization, which include inter alia rapid urbanization and physical mobility; better access to education, especially for girls; the transformation of the relationships between the generations and genders; the shift from extended to nuclear family and the loss of larger family networks; the emergence of new opportunities and aspirations in the choice of marriage partners; changes in the marriage and divorce laws, giving women new rights; a considerable increase in the rate of divorce; and finally the inclusion and participation of women in the labor market. The extent of the change, however, varies not only from country to country but in different areas within each country.

In spite of the great diversity in marriage patterns in the region, marriage itself remains fundamental to the social identity of all women, regardless of their achievements in other spheres of life, and pressure on women to marry persists. A recent study by De-Jong et al. (2005) reviewing the sexual and reproductive health situation of young people in the Arab countries and Iran emphasizes that marriage remains central to any discussion in the region of the sexual and reproductive health of young people "because of the universal valuation of marriage and the taboos and religious sanctions against pre-marital and extra-marital sexual relations" (52). While acknowledging the differences in the patterns of marriage, DeJong et al. (2005: 52) identify certain recent general trends as being "rising age at marriage for both sexes; early marriage still a problem in pockets of all societies; high incidence of consanguineous marriages; persistence but decline in polygamy in some countries; higher numbers of single women; and resurgence of forms of non-conventional marriage."

Whereas the rise in the age of marriage has attracted sufficient attention by researchers and is relatively well understood, some of the other general trends, including early marriage and legally unprotected forms of marriage, remain under-researched (DeJong et al. 2005: 54). As an example of unconventional forms of marriage, DeJong et al. (2005) refer to temporary marriage (*mut'a*), a form of marriage practiced by the Shia Muslim and actively encouraged by the Iranian political leaders since the Islamic Revolution in Iran, and point to the recent spread of this practice among the Sunni, albeit in a different form.

The rise in the age of marriage is viewed as a positive sign particularly for women, which Fargues (2003), as cited in DeJong et al. (2005), summarizes as follows: "it [rise in age] is protective against early childbirth and associated with greater educational and employment opportunities" (53). The role of education is also singled out by others as the most important factor in preventing early marriage (Hamamsy 1994). In general, education has been viewed as an indicator of social modernization and all-empowering institution liberating women from gender inequality and discrimination. Implicit in the urge for education for girls is also their economic and social empowerment, and the lack of participation of women in the labor market is blamed on their lack of education (see Fargues 2003). DeJong et al.'s (2005: 51) review mentions that, in the Middle East and North Africa, "gender disparities in social opportunities are wide, and indeed the region ranks next to last behind Sub-Saharan Africa on the UN Development Programme gender empowerment measure," more than half of Arab women are illiterate, and the region has the world's lowest rate of female participation in the labor force at 26 percent. However, the rate of female employment varies from country to country. In Iran, in spite of a remarkably high literacy rate for women between the ages of ten and twenty-four, which has risen from 48 percent to 92 percent in the past two decades (DeJong et al. 2005: 51), the rate of female employment remains low at around 12 percent (Abbasi-Shavazi, McDonald, and Hosseini-Chavoshi 2003: 19).[1]

In spite of the considerable rise in the age of marriage and a decline in early marriage, the practice persists in the region as a whole and may even be on the rise in some areas (DeJong et al. 2005; UNICEF 2001; Forum on Marriage and the Rights of Women and Girls 2000). During the past decade, the practice of early marriage has witnessed an increasing interest and an unequivocal condemnation by human rights activists, advocates of gender equality, policymakers and planners, and health practitioners. Policies to eradicate the practice are often made on the basis that early marriages are coercive, that they stem from poverty and lack of education, especially for girls, and that by empowering girls and young women they will stop. An understanding of the impact of social transformations on early marriage is essential to the understanding of the modern context of early marriage. Simply linking a rise in literacy level to a decline in early marriage misses the fact that early marriage is no longer just a matter of education. Instead, the practice has adapted itself to modernity and its imperatives. Girls can and do go to school and get married early, and they are not necessarily empowered after leaving school.

The International Conference on Population and Development (ICPD) in 1994 was convened at a time of growing consensus about the complexities of the relationship between education, work, fertility, and family planning and the fact that improving just one aspect of life (e.g., education alone) does not necessarily empower women (Tremayne 2001: 7). Nevertheless, the feminist agendas remain emphatic on the role of education in empowering women. Several factors affect education as a means of liberation for women. First, consideration should be given to the concept of "empowerment" itself, which is ridden with complexities and needs careful examination and redefinition (Kabeer 2005: 14). Also, early marriage in many parts of the world has adopted a modern face while retaining its conservative structure, and the new face can be misleading with apparent empowerment. Finally, the inevitable clash resulting from the encounter between the new form and old practice has provoked new and unexpected reactions, which in many instances has left girls even more vulnerable than before. Can we therefore say that new rules are being set up in the process, and if so, whether these are indicative of the apparently fundamental changes we are witnessing with regard to family and gender relations?

The Modern View of Early Marriage

"Early" or "child" marriage, whereby either or both the bride and groom (usually the bride) is under the age of eighteen,[2] remains contentious. While these marriages have been practiced for centuries in many parts of the world, it is only during the past decade that they have become the target of an active campaign by various human rights advocates and national and international agencies across the world to stop their practice.

Various agencies on human rights and the rights of the child, such as UNICEF (2001), the Forum on Marriage and the Rights of Women and Girls (2000), and the International Center for Research on Women (2003), refer to the harmful effects of early marriage due to its physical and psychosocial effects on adolescent health and reproduction, especially for girls (sexual exploitation of young girls, the impact on their reproductive health, and early and multiple pregnancies), the denial of human rights such as education and access to economic independence, and finally, the risks of violence and abandonment. From a biomedical perspective, risks of early pregnancy are well documented and include premature labor complications during delivery, low birth weight of babies, and poor survival chances for newborns. Mothers under the age of fifteen are five times as likely to die during labor as women in their twenties. While the high death rate is not solely linked to the low age of mothers—and poor socioeconomic conditions that prevent them from having access to antenatal and obstetrics care are listed also as contributory factors—physical immaturity has been identified as "the key risk for the under 15s" (UNICEF 2001: 11).

Several reasons for the practice of early marriage have been offered, and literature on the subject suggests that most early marriages continue to be coerced and are often a strategy for economic survival (Forum on Marriage and the Rights of Women and Girls 2000: 10), poverty is the key motivation behind the practice (UNICEF 2001: 6), and there may be an increase in early marriage among populations under stress (UNICEF 2001: 6). Although early marriage involves both boys and girls, the focus of the human rights activists remains on girls and their well-being since the consequences of early marriage can be more serious for girls, who are more likely to be subject to coercion and health risks (UNICEF 2001: 11). However, early marriage does not happen in isolation from other social bonds and obligations. Viewed in its broader social and cultural context it takes on a different meaning, and local communities often demonstrate a different understanding and do not necessarily consider it a violation of their personal rights. "Rights," as approached by global conventions in the context of marriage, effectively means the ability of individuals to make decisions on their fertility, reproductive health, and sexual freedom in isolation from their other bonds and obligations in society. The reality is that the way men and women perceive, manage, and negotiate the various forces exerted on their lives (which are paramount in any measures to improve their health and rights) is embedded within the wider construction and negotiation of social identity. The relationship between power, marriage, kinship, and gender is shown to be intertwined and to affect the interaction between individuals, the community, and the state. Power taken in both its aspects of repressing as well as constructing identities (to use Foucauldian analysis) needs to be built into the equation when seeking solutions to early marriage (see also Locke and Zhang 2004; Petchesky and Judd 1998).

Few studies have addressed the reasons for the survival of early marriage in spite of progress achieved in the areas of education and a rise in female employment, or the possible consequences of giving up the practice and its impact on the family, the children themselves, and their wider social network. Little is known of the choices open to those who do not marry very young and whether the new solutions are providing fairer conditions in terms of human rights. The extent to which girls benefit from delaying their marriages and following the education path, which in many cases is provided in a vacuum for the sake of education per se, remains unknown. As Kabeer (2005: 23–24), in an assessment of the Millennium Development Goals, mentions, "Women's access to education may improve their chances of a good marriage or their capacity to sign their names on a document, but unless it also provides them with the analytical capacity and courage to question unjust practices, its potential for change will be limited." Finally, the nature of the accommodation and adjustment to modernity by the institutions that practice and control early marriage remains misunderstood.

The connection made between education, delay in the age of marriage, and the economic empowerment of women is not as straightforward as it may appear and does not necessarily lead to the ideal solution of liberating girls from their marriage and kinship bonds. Even when the persisting patriarchal values accommodate modernity by trading the early marriage for a few more years of education, "a token gesture of paternalist benevolence," as Kabeer (2005: 23) puts it, the prevailing social and cultural demands for girls, including their own desire to get married and not to miss their chance at marriage, act as an incentive and create unforeseen circumstances well beyond the expectations of the advocates of human rights.

This study provides a view from within a community in which early marriage continues to be practiced: on whether early marriages are necessarily coerced and/or driven by poverty, as well as the impact of education upon early marriage. Although the data presented are part of a larger study undertaken in Yazd in central Iran in 2004, many of the findings can be extended to most other conservative communities in Iran, since they also draw on previous data collected in Ardebil (Azarbaijan) and Tehran between 2000 and 2004 and on other relevant research carried out by Iranian scholars. The study includes perspectives from various parties involved in the practice of early marriage, i.e., three generations of women from extended families and their kin group, local clerics, and health professionals. That this chapter focuses on women does not imply that early marriage for boys does not exist. A visit to the barracks in any town or the seminaries in religious cities in Iran reveals the wide extent of early marriage among boys. The conscripts' families marry them off for a variety of reasons, including an attempt to gain exemption from the army by claiming family responsibilities (although they often serve in the army anyway). Young religious students of the seminaries get married early under pressure from the religious community.

The Case of Iran

No study of early marriage in present-day Iran can be understood without an understanding of Shia practices. Iran, with a theocratic regime, closely follows *sharia* (Islamic law) and presents a special case as far as early marriage or child marriage is concerned. The age of marriage is a much-disputed subject in the Islamic Republic and is closely linked to the definition of childhood. What constitutes childhood according to *sharia* differs from that of the Convention on the Rights of the Child (CRC) of 1988, which describes "anybody under the age of eighteen as a child" and to which Iran is a signatory. When the delegation from the Islamic Republic of Iran signed the CRC, it reserved the right not to implement those sections that were against the Islamic practices of the country. It maintained that *sharia* provides clear instructions for the responsibilities and conduct of people, which in some instances do not accord with international agreements. One such exception was the practice of early marriage. It is therefore not surprising that no official action has been taken to prevent the practice following the signing of the CRC.

The definition of a child, according to the law, is not restricted to a certain age and differs from context to context. A child can be a child in one context and an adult in another. For example, a girl is eligible to marry at eight years and nine months and a boy at fourteen years and seven months, when they are supposed to have reached puberty and can reproduce. However, they are not considered mentally mature and require a guardian until they reach mental maturity, the judgment of which is more elaborate (Ebadi 2002, 2003b). Although Article 1041 of the Civil Law specifies that the legal age of marriage is fifteen for girls and eighteen for boys, after the Islamic Revolution the minimum age of marriage was dropped to that approved by *sharia* (see above). In August 2003, after much pressure from the female members of the Iranian parliament (*majilis*), the age of marriage was raised to thirteen for girls, but a clause was added stating that earlier marriage would be allowed if the girl's guardian and a judge or medical doctor considered that the girl was ready for marriage. Effectively, this means that the application of the law is not compulsory.

From what precedes, it is clear that the contradictions between *sharia*, the human rights approach (both on human rights and health grounds), and the modernizing policies of the government (see Tremayne 2004) as they impinge on day-to-day realities provide fertile ground for a study of whether and to what extent policies, laws, and conventions affect the practice of early marriage and whether they are responsible for any changes that have taken place in this sphere.

Extent of Early Marriage in Iran

The exact extent of the practice of early marriage is not known in Iran and is likely to be considerably higher than the official statistics suggest (for statistics on early marriage, see IDHS 2000 and Kian-Thiébaut 2005). One reason for lack of reliable information in this area is partly due to the discrepancies in the data collection methods (Mehryar 1998a). A second and important factor affecting the accuracy of the information on marriage in general and early marriage in particular is the practice of temporary marriage (*mut'a* or *sigheh*), which is unique to the Shia sect and has been practiced in Shia Iran for centuries (Haeri 1989). A considerable number of early marriages continue to take place,[3] some of which are changed to permanent marriage when the children become adults. Others remain temporary and either dissolve at the end of the contract or with the couple living together without changing their status to a permanent one. A temporary marriage need not be registered (although it can if the parties involved wish it to be), and witnesses are not required. Interesting statistics were released in 2004 by the General Registration Office of Iran mentioning that the figures for registered temporary marriages showed an increase of 20 percent as compared to the previous year.[4]

Temporary marriage or *mut'a*, meaning a marriage of pleasure, is a contract between a man and an unmarried woman in which the couple agrees to be married for a specified length of time and a fixed sum of money is given to the temporary wife. The time agreed could be anywhere from one hour to ninety-nine years. At the end of the contract the temporary spouses may part company without any divorce ceremony, but many continue to live together for life. In Haeri's (1989: 2) words, "Ideologically, Shia doctrine distinguishes temporary marriage, *mut'a*, from permanent marriage, *nikāḥ*, in that the objective of *mut'a* is sexual enjoyment, *istimita*, while that of *nikāḥ* is procreation, *tulid-i-nasl*."

The children born as a result of temporary marriage are recognized as legitimate and theoretically have status equal to their siblings born of permanent marriage. "Here lies the legal uniqueness of *mut'a*, that which distinguishes it from prostitution, despite their striking resemblance" (Haeri 1989: 2). Haeri distinguishes the permanent marriage as a contract of sale and temporary marriage as contract of lease. In this sense, because the objective of a temporary marriage is sexual enjoyment, *sigheh* women are often considered temporary sexual partners, thus suggesting a close structural association to prostitution. The temporary marriage does not provide the protection or social prestige women seek, as it often takes place in secrecy, and the very word *sigheh* has a pejorative connotation in society. Temporary wives are not treated as equals to permanent wives, and *sigheh* marriages for women are highly stigmatized. However, in addition to temporary marriage being used for the purpose of sexual pleasure, it is also used to legitimize early marriage with full approval of the parents, and in this case it does not carry the same stigma as the marriage for purely sexual pleasure. In the few decades leading to the Islamic Revolution, the minimum age of marriage was raised to fifteen for girls (Article 1041 of the civil code), and the registration of marriage became compulsory. At that time, early marriage was still practiced to a considerable extent by conservative layers of the society, both urban and rural. Parents prohibited under the civil code from registering the marriages of their underage daughters resorted to temporary marriage, which the couple changed into a permanent one upon reaching the legal age.

To return to the extent of the practice of early marriage, research by academic and governmental agencies reveals that the number of early marriages in some provinces is high and the practice admitted publicly. For example, in some rural areas of Sistan and Baluchestan, children as young as seven are known to have been given in marriage, but the figure for towns in the same provinces is between eleven and twelve years for girls (confidential report by sociologists for UN agencies). The prevalence of attitudes toward early marriage is also confirmed by other studies. In Baluchestan, where the age of marriage is still one of the lowest in the country, one university student interviewed about his views on the age of marriage stated that "the most suitable age of marriage for girls is eight or nine years old. As soon as a girl can count her fingers, she is ready for marriage." My earlier interviews with marriage consultants in the province of Ardebil also confirmed the existence of similar attitudes in many villages in that area. Firsthand observation from provinces such as Khousestan, Kordestan, and Khorasan confirms time and again the same attitudes and behavior. Examples abound of the forms the practice takes, from two octogenarian men exchanging their fourteen-year-old daughters in Kordestan (confidential report by sociologists for the UN agencies) to a report of an early marriage between a thirteen-year-old boy and his sixteen-year-old cousin in Khousestan whereby both parties expressed total happiness at being married and mentioned that early marriage is customary in the province and takes place regularly.[5]

Studies show that the changes in the rise in the age of marriage (the mean age of marriage for women in Iran was 22.4 according to the 1996 census) and the continuation of early marriage are related to a multitude of factors that do not stem from laws imposed by the ruling religious authorities, government, or by global agreements reached at international conventions. These external factors only affect these practices in an indirect way and by innuendo. Changes in the age of marriage tend to follow their own internal dynamics. For example, the practice of early marriage in the rural and tribal areas was widespread before the Revolution in 1979 in spite of the law setting the minimum age of marriage at fifteen, but the indications were that it was declining due to a variety of social reasons (Mehryar 1998b; Mehryar and Tajdini 1998). Likewise, the rate of early marriage continued to drop after the Revolution in spite of the encouragement of the clerics, who follow the Islamic instructions in relation to the age of marriage (Mehryar 1998b; Tremayne 2004).

The cultural context in which early marriage occurs seems to be similar almost everywhere in Iran. The prevalence of patriarchal systems, the persistence of traditional values with regard to family and marriage among conservative communities, and the endorsement by the ruling clerics are some of the historical reasons behind the practice. Although "modernity" has entered many spheres of life, attitudes toward early marriage have not kept pace with this change. Economic hardship and an increase in poverty, cited as key factors in the continuation and increase in the rate of early marriage, may have reinforced the attitudes toward early marriage, especially in some areas where family ties have been affected by change.

Reliable statistics are hard to come by, but limited research shows that, contrary to the general belief that early marriages are prevalent in rural and tribal areas, early marriage takes place at a higher rate in some urban areas (IDHS 2000: 38), especially those that have remained more conservative and traditional and/or have retained a strong sense of ethnic or religious identity. A recent report estimates that as much as 53 percent of the total numbers occurs in urban areas.[6] Kian-Thiébaut's (2005: 52) study of various ethnic and linguistic groups estimates the average rate of early marriage at 16 percent, with Baluchestan at 32 percent as the highest, and Guilan at under 0.5 as the lowest (see also IDHS 2000).

Early Marriage in the Town of Yazd

As mentioned earlier, data used in this chapter derive from a larger project and were collected during fieldwork on the sociocultural transformations that have taken place within the family with regard to reproductive health values. The research was carried out in Yazd, situated in central Iran with 326,776 inhabitants. Yazd seemed a particularly suitable choice for the study of early marriage. In many respects, it epitomizes the interface between tradition and modernity and their ensuing paradoxes. In a comparative study of four provinces in Iran, Abbasi-Shavazi, McDonald, and Hosseini-Chavoshi (2003) conclude that Yazd has retained most of its traditional and religious characteristics in spite of approaching one of the highest levels of socioeconomic development in the country (16) and that it has a high level of female literacy at 81 percent[7] and a low level of employment (19; see also Abbasi-Shavazi and Askari-Nodoushan 2005). Yazd also has the lowest rate of divorce in Iran, which classifies it as the most conservative town in the country (350 divorces for 8,868 marriages—one in twenty-five). The comparative figures for Tehran for the same year were 17,956 divorces for 104,496 marriages—1 in 6) (Statistical Center of Iran 2000).[8] Abbasi-Shavazi's findings reveal that women in Yazd place more emphasis on education as a means of enhancing marriage for girls rather than for the purpose of employment, and that the expression of more conservative attitudes by women in Yazd is consistent across all indicators chosen. Yazd maintains relatively conservative attitudes with regard to early marriage despite the fact that its education levels are actually higher than in any of the other four provinces (Abbasi-Shavazi, McDonald, and Hosseini-Chavoshi 2003: 18); one of the interpretations in Abbasi-Shavazi's research is that "Yazd has family-religious values that may have counterbalanced the effects of its higher education levels." Although patriarchal values do not get a mention in the above study, the present study shows that they remain the strongest driving force behind the persistence of conservative values, which are not necessarily Islamic but are reinforced by Islamic values.

The present research in Yazd focused on highly conservative families in which modernity exists alongside patriarchal and religious values. Of course many men and women from Yazd no longer follow the traditional way of life, and some have gone on to have successful and distinguished careers, but the community studied here reflects the more conservative layers of the society. In this sense, it may be more similar to several other conservative communities in Iran such as Khousestan, parts of Azarbaijan, Kordestan, Sistan, and Baluchestan than to the more liberal ones in Yazd itself. Men in the study included clerks in private companies, long-distance lorry drivers, builders, junior civil servants, goldsmiths, office managers, and some unemployed. Their wives either worked from home as dressmakers or hairdressers or were engaged in cottage industries (e.g., preparing dried herbs for other households, small-scale carpet weaving, etc.) or did not have any income-generating occupation.

Methodology

Two main sources were used to identify women who had married early. A study of the archives of Mojibian Hospital, the oldest private maternity hospital in town, was undertaken. The main aim of the study, however, was not to obtain statistics and percentages but to identify women who had given birth under the age of fifteen and therefore married early.

The second source for the in-depth study and day-to-day observation was the host family. The wife and husband, who were cross-cousins, came from large families of eleven and nine brothers and sisters respectively, and introduction to their extended network of relatives allowed access to a considerable number of case studies.

To extract data from the hospital archives, the limit of early marriage was set at fifteen years of age, and by studying the archives between 1971 and 2004 at five-year intervals, 537 cases of women who had given birth under the age of fifteen over the past thirty-three years were identified. Fifty cases were selected for interviews, and those women were invited to come to an initial interview. This led to invitations to their homes, which in turn led to meeting their mothers, daughters, or granddaughters, and some of the husbands or sons also agreed to be interviewed. Such large gatherings allowed observation of the changes in the attitudes toward early marriage among different generations of women. It also made it possible to investigate early marriage of men in the same families.

Some basic and preliminary facts from the hospital archives showed that the minimum age of mothers who had given birth was twelve years. Fourteen of the cases had a second baby before reaching fifteen. Thirty-two had Caesarean sections. In one extreme case, a twelve-year-old had given birth to quadruplets, all of whom died after a few hours. The analysis of the data for the 537 cases showed that 404 of the cases were normal deliveries, and 101 cases ended in termination of the pregnancy. These figures seem to be consistent with those for other countries (UNICEF 2001: 36). In addition, several of the hospital staff volunteered similar information from their own families, and it became evident that two decades ago such pregnancies were more the norm than the exception.

Much of the data used for this chapter is the result of several weeks of meeting and discussing issues related to early marriage with women who belonged to the same kin group, mainly first and second cousins, some of whom formed three generations of grandmothers, mothers, and daughters, and most of whom married under the age of fifteen. Other participants were relatives of the first group and of different age groups. Of the forty women who took part in discussions, all but two had married their cousins.[9]

Coercion and Violence

One of the objectives of the research was to understand the context of early marriage as far as coercion was concerned. Had all these women of different generations been "beaten" into submission to being married off, and had their rights been violated?

The accounts by the first and second generations of women were almost identical in that making one's own decisions about marriage was not even thought of. "We were just told that we were going to be married to our cousin or the next-door neighbor's son, and that was it. We did not even think of resisting it any more than resisting our parents' other wishes and commands in other matters." In many cases the marriage had been decided at birth, when the umbilical cord had been cut in the name of the future husband. No violence had taken place, since none of the girls had resisted. They said that "at that age, the idea of saying no was inconceivable, even in retrospect. If we did not get married, we would have brought great shame upon our family." Breaking a promise or refusing a long-standing agreement between two families would have led to bloodshed and feud. A female medical doctor from Baluchestan, in a separate study, said that she herself had consented to an arranged marriage for the fear of family feud and that her superior education had been overshadowed by her kinship obligations.[10] Obligations to the family and kin group seem to have remained untouched and continue to be the greatest determining factor in any decision made in relation to marriage. The word coercion in such an instance seems somewhat inappropriate because it is not perceived as such but rather as fulfilling a heavy obligation to the family. In addition, the only prospect for a girl from a conservative family a few decades ago was to get married.

The main difference between the first- and second-generation women, interestingly, was that the majority of the second generation had married at an even younger age than their mothers, from between twelve and fourteen years. These marriages coincided with an increase in urbanization in the 1970s; moving away from the close-knit communities into the less well-known surroundings in towns required securing girls' protection, which may have played a role in earlier marriage. These changes also coincided with the Islamic Revolution of 1979, the abolition of the minimum age of marriage, and the relaxation of the marriage law, dropping the minimum age of marriage to nine for girls and the ruling clerics' encouragement to marry early (Tremayne 2004). The civil disturbances surrounding the Revolution itself may have been a contributing factor in bringing forward the age of marriage. Lack of reliable data makes it impossible to know whether there was an increase in numbers of early marriages at this point, but the drop in the age of marriage among the group studied seems consistent with the suggestion that early marriages often increase at a time of crisis and in societies under pressure (UNICEF 2001).

The second generation was more reflective about coercion. For this group, their mild resistance had been diffused in a variety of ways by the family. Their accounts were frequently that of persuasion and lack of other choices rather than coercion. Persuasion itself was applied indirectly and gently guided the girl to come to a decision herself. Akram (not her real name), one of the women in the group, said that her mother had asked her to marry her mother's nephew. When she resisted the idea because she thought that "his family were people of low culture" (in spite of being her cross-cousins), the mother said, "It is up to you, but this is the first time that my brother has asked me for a favor. I don't know how to refuse him." The negotiations continued with her paternal uncles, who, in the absence of her dead father, were consulted. They all supported the mother and mentioned that Akram should be considerate of her mother's position vis-à-vis her brother, as her mother would lose face by turning down her brother's request. However, everybody's last words were "it is up to you." She also said, "I was promised by my husband's family that he will allow me to continue my studies if I married him, but once he married me, he insisted that I should stay at home, and I agreed because in those days studying was not such an important issue." Although Akram married the cousin sixteen years ago, she is still angry and resentful because she feels that "[she] made the decision in the end, and nobody forced [her] into the marriage."

The slightly higher level of education among the second generation of women seemed to be a determining factor in shaping their outlook on coerced marriage. Those who were completely illiterate or had little education agreed with their mothers that marriage was their only choice since they had no other way of living and that remaining unmarried would have been socially unacceptable and an economic imposition on the family. Unmarried girls above thirteen years of age were stigmatized as "something being seriously wrong with her" and as being "spoiled goods."[11] The majority of the more educated women of the same generation remained unconvinced about the advantages of marrying later for a few more years of education.

The third generation, some still in their teens, is more literate than the first two generations. Several have completed either the first part or the full term at secondary school, while others have left school voluntarily because they did not wish to remain at school or because they had fallen in love and wanted to get married. Both saw marriage as a blessing and a way to freedom from education. Two girls in the group had been to university. They were both engaged to their cousins and waiting for their fiancés to find jobs so that they could get married. One had chosen not to work, and the other could not find a job in spite of her higher education.

Discussions with the parents about education indicated that the fathers saw their authority, hitherto unopposed, challenged by modernity and change, and they sensed the ground for their patriarchal authority beginning to shift. The gradual loss of power vis-à-vis the change and the challenge to their authority provokes two types of reactions among men in general. Fathers might allow their daughters a few extra years of education, even though most of them remain unconvinced of its advantages. In such cases, coercion shifts and appears in the form of a stricter control of the daily activities of their daughters or sisters and often by preventing them from pursuing their education even further. The boundaries of freedom for these girls are restricted to going to school for a few more years, but at all times accompanied by a male member of the family. A typical fourteen-year-old girl's time outside her school and homework is occasionally to go to a pizza restaurant with the family or, with the family present, watch local or even satellite television programs, to which a great majority of families now have access. Leisure and entertainment equals socializing within the kin group and an occasional pilgrimage to the Shrine of Imam Reza, the eighth Shia Imam, in Mashhad. Some of the younger generation of women recently had started going to the public swimming pool, but a gang of women had secretly filmed them in their swimsuits and sold the photographs. The predictable fury and loss of face for men led them to stop their wives and daughters from going to the pool. The paternal bargain, in most cases, stops at the end of secondary school, when the girl is either married or stays at home waiting to get married. In such cases, education, whether secondary or at a higher level, employment, or economic independence does not necessarily empower girls, as they effectively remain the property of their fathers and under their authority until they marry, at which point the responsibility is transferred to the husband (see Ebadi 2003a). The same argument applies to married women who have an income but have to hand their incomes to their husbands or families. Some of the women in this study earned a little from hairdressing but handed their earnings to their husbands, who controlled all expenditures, including everything needed for their hairdressing purposes. No financial decisions were made by these women. Neither education nor income earning made a dent in the patriarchal attitudes and behavior of the men in question (see also Afshar 1998).

The second type of reaction arising from modernity in relation to coerced marriages often occurs among less closely knit families. Evidence is abundant whereby the unity of family has been greatly affected by social transformations and the use of coercion and increased violence has become a substitute for the previously unquestioning paternal authority and a method of self-defense for men. In such cases, education and other empowering measures for women may well be a liberating force but also have led to adverse consequences. Girls' deviations that touch on their sexuality and the family's honor provoke fierce reactions by male members of the family and lead to violence and coercive measures. In its extreme form it can lead to honor killings. For example, the mobility created for young people in rural areas who have to go to school in a nearby town (since not every village has its own school) separates children from parents during the day and limits parental control of girls, giving the latter a certain degree of freedom and a resistance to total submission to their parents' will. The clash often leads to extreme violence. The suggestion by Kian-Thiébaut (2005) that patriarchal values are weakening and that Iranian society has become more child centered may be true in more liberal and educated urban families, but the weakening of parental, more specifically paternal, authority has not necessarily resulted in a child-centered society among the more conservative layers of the society, whether rural or urban. The result is shown in an increase in violence, suicide, running away from home (which often leads to prostitution and a life of crime), and setting fire to themselves to be freed from the tyranny of their dominant male members of the family. An example of this was widely reported in the media, when a young woman from Lorestan graduated from engineering studies and returned home to be controlled by her six-year-old brother in the absence of her father, which drove her to set fire to herself.

Attitudes toward Education and Marriage

Attitudes toward early or temporary marriage carried no stigma for women whose marriages were stable, and their main wish of sending their daughters to secondary school was to improve their chances of a marriage. However, they viewed a delay in the age of marriage as a mixed blessing, "seeing that girls who study further do not necessarily have a better life, we are not so sure now." Akram, who has two teenage daughters, said:

> Nowadays there is great pressure on our girls to continue their studies, and even our husbands have to submit to the pressure of letting the girls finish at least the secondary school. But the girls leave school and cannot find jobs, have no skills, have to sit at home, and can't find husbands either. In our community, no man who has a choice will marry an older girl who has passed her "desirable childbearing" age. So maybe it is better to marry the girls off if they have a good suitor than let them stay at school.

In their analysis, Abbasi-Shavazi, McDonald, and Hosseini-Chavoshi (2003: 18) also conclude that "the accepted pattern seems to be that it is good for girls to be educated, but so far the education has been mainly education for marriage and family rather than for employment." They continue that "education may have had an impact on the status of women within the marriage, but interestingly Yazd, a conservative province, maintains relatively conservative attitudes in this regard despite the fact that its education levels are actually higher than in any of the other four provinces" (see Abbasi-Shavazi, McDonald, and Hosseini-Chavoshi 2003: 18–19). However, as mentioned earlier, these attitudes are not unique to Yazd and persist in many other areas in Iran.

It was evident from the discussions that marriage remained ultimately the prime value for all the women in this study, and none of them could countenance a future without a husband. A woman can be a highly respected practicing medical doctor, but if she remains unmarried, she will live with her parents, since living alone for an unmarried woman usually is not an option; outside her professional life, her identity will remain uncertain, with people looking at her as an object of pity or wonder.

Although education is valued, none of the women viewed early marriage as a stigma or education as a barrier to marriage. One fourteen-year-old girl still in school mentioned that a few of her friends had already left school of their own choice to get married. She implied that she may do the same, since her father will not allow her higher education. On the subject of the continuation of early marriage, some mothers said they did not approve of the social pressure on girls not to marry young. Their reaction to the fact that early marriages lead to early pregnancies and might affect the health of women was that access to contraceptive facilities for married women can prevent unwanted pregnancies. The suggestion of "early" marriage was met with great amusement from most of the women interviewed. It was obvious that the first two generations of women had a clear idea about their future as wives and mothers and knew what to expect of marriage. When I asked an older woman who had married at the age of thirteen what marriage meant to her, she said, "Marriage to me meant the continuity of chores. I was working from the morning till the evening in my father's house. I moved next door to my husband's parents' house, and I continued to work from the morning till the evening." Her husband and mother-in-law, who were present in the room, nodded approvingly, as if this is how things should be. The younger generation, on the other hand, seemed more uncertain and confused about what they wanted from marriage. Similar to their mothers and grandmothers, marriage remained the ultimate aim and aspiration for the younger group. Husbands should be the breadwinners and responsible for maintaining the family. Young girls did not see their own level of education as a factor that might contribute to sharing the family's financial burdens.

I asked another woman to talk about her first memory of her marriage. She said that, curious to see her future husband, she went to the street where he lived and looked through his window. Her ten-year-old brother, who had followed her, felt his honor was offended and slapped her hard and took her back home. There was clear evidence that the sense of honor and duty to protect the female members of the family has not diminished among the younger generation of men, i.e., brothers and sons. They continue to consider themselves the custodians of the family's honor and are even more anxious than their fathers to protect it. While traditionally girls' chances of meeting boys were limited, more opportunities now exist for girls to meet boys, and young men are fully aware of the risks of letting their sisters out of sight. Among these families, at least one man in each family knew at all times where all the female members of the family were. Most families did not allow their women to leave the house without one of the *mahrams* (relatives who are not potential marriage partners—their fathers, husbands, brothers, or sons).

Identity and Marriage

For all the women in the study, marriage, motherhood, and identity remained closely linked. The identity of a married woman is clear at all times, unlike that of an unmarried woman, who is viewed as a failure and remains in limbo in her social interactions. Girls over the age of twenty are referred to as "gone sour" (*dokhtar-e-torshideh*). The length of time spent at school for girls in this study has no relation to their ultimate status. Beliefs such as "too much education jeopardizes the harmony of family life, since women will not submit to their husbands" or "younger women have healthier babies" seem to remain deeply anchored, especially among men and older women. However, higher education can work against girls, since many boys leave school to learn skills and earn money, and they do not wish to marry girls who are better educated than themselves. As a result, many girls who might have been married early but have attended secondary school remain unmarried, and the future identity they so badly seek remains uncertain. Although the ideals of motherhood strongly persist and retain their links with women's identity, they are no longer associated with having a large number of children.[12] While having too many children is no longer fashionable, infertility remains a stigma and a major cause of divorce and of conflicts between the families. Following the successful populating policies of the government, women are now able to yield some power and make joint decisions with their husbands on their reproductive decisions, and they tend to use this shift in the position to negotiate better deals, especially for their daughters, including their educations. Regardless, such power has its limitations, and once women have achieved the number of children they want, it ceases to be effective.

The Spinster

As discussed earlier, education per se and without further training has a limited scope for improving girls' prospect of employment. In general, working outside the home for a woman is still not viewed favorably in conservative communities. Occupations such as small-cottage industries, carpet making, hairdressing, and preparing food such as dried herbs is what many young girls do after their studies. But these often remain as sporadic pastimes. Sheeda was one such woman. She was thirty-two years old, had completed the first three years of secondary school, lived with her parents, had no skills, and had little hope of finding a husband. Her chances of finding a husband might have been improved by going to university or working in an office, but she had done neither. Due to her age, her social network was not making any effort to find a match for her; conservative neighbors did not approve of her "advanced" education and were reluctant to allow their sons to marry her. Although the rate of consanguine marriages is high, most of her cousins were married or younger, and the potential suitors' female relatives are on the lookout for much younger women. She regularly attends religious ceremonies and spends her time looking after her elderly parents, attending to her nieces and nephews when their parents are ill, and watching cooking television programs and foreign films. She is not judged young enough to bear children, and a likely possibility is to become a temporary wife to an older man or a second wife to a married man. Her mother, on the other hand, enjoys great power over the extended family, since her husband is old and incapacitated.

The Temporary Wife

Zhila, who is thirty years old and the youngest daughter in a family of nine children, completed her secondary education. While most of the women in her family married early, she missed her chances of marrying her cousins by attending school, after which she continued living with her mother. She found a job in an office as a secretary and came home every evening after work. One day, an acquaintance told Zhila's mother that Zhila was the temporary wife of her boss, who also has a first permanent wife. Unlike the case of temporary marriage for underage girls, Zhila's was a shameful one, since it had taken place purely for sexual purposes. When confronted, Zhila denied the story but under pressure admitted she had been married to the man for two years. The disgrace and loss of face for the family was beyond imagination. For a respectable family to have their unmarried young daughter secretly become the temporary wife of a married man is a true shame. No amount of pressure, however, convinced Zhila to leave her temporary husband, and when she said she loved him, the family's fury became even stronger. Letting down the family's honor for love was adding insult to injury. Finally, her brothers came over from another town, tied her up, and locked her in the cellar of the house until she consented to become the man's permanent second wife. Although her husband eventually divorced his first wife and married Zhila, her relatives treat her with contempt for having brought shame upon the family, and she is marginalized in social gatherings.

An increasing number of young girls are faced with the same predicament as Sheeda and Zhila and have to face the embarrassment of being a spinster, living a barren life, or becoming a temporary wife.

The Married Woman

As mentioned earlier, completing secondary education before marriage seems to have become the norm and an end in itself in Iran (Aghajanian and Mehryar 1999; Abbasi-Shavazi, McDonald, and Hosseini-Chavoshi 2003). Both Sheeda and Zhila had done so to no avail as far as their future was concerned. But Mahin, a twenty-year-old woman who had completed secondary school by the age of eighteen, married immediately after. Her father would have allowed her higher education if she had been admitted to Yazd University, but she did not get in and therefore had to give up her education. The anxiety about allowing their daughters to go to university outside Yazd is so great that some parents are even prepared to move to the town where their daughter has a place at university and stay there until she completes her studies.[13] Mahin had a baby, but her lifestyle is identical to that of her mother. She spends her days looking after her family, attending religious gatherings, and reading the Qur'an. She remains utterly financially dependent on her well-off husband, who would lose face if his wife had to work. She in no way could be considered "empowered" compared to her educated but unmarried friends and relatives. Her mother, however, enjoys great authority within the household, which Mahin may achieve in twenty years' time.

The Clerics

While the above reflects the new face of the families involved in early marriage and caught in conflicts resulting from the encounter between modernity and conservatism, the view of the religious authorities seems more definite and less paradoxical. Several of the senior clerics and, also, marriage registry clerks (who are also clerics) queried the definition of "early" marriage when I asked about it. One lecturer in divinity at the University of Yazd, an extremely elegantly dressed cleric with a matching green cloak and socks and a hairdo that obviously had been arranged to form curls around his turban, protested that "there is no such a thing as an early marriage. When a girl is ready for marriage it is not too early. It is the late marriage which is causing the most problems nowadays." He cited the Prophet as saying that "lucky is the girl who reaches puberty in her husband's house."

The marriage registry cleric agreed with this view. When I asked who decides whether a child is ready for marriage, he said, "I do," and when asked how he knows, he replied, "I ask them a few questions, and I know whether they are ready." When I advanced the idea that one of the most respected ayatollahs, Ayatollah Sanei, had set the age of puberty at thirteen and not nine for girls, the cleric became agitated and dismissed the Ayatollah's edict (*fatwa*) by saying that "his holiness is entitled to his views." When I asked the cleric about the rate of early marriages in Yazd, he looked disconcerted and said that the numbers have dropped drastically in the past few years and that only between 15 and 20 percent of girls are now married under the age of fifteen. Both clerics were emphatic that the rise in the age of marriage is the problem and not early marriage. It may be appropriate to mention that at the start of my interviews with the clerics, I was anxious to start the conversation on a friendly note and thus mentioned my respect for traditions and my desire to see them preserved whenever possible. The reply and body gesture was that of total dismissal, and the answer was, "most traditions are rubbish, and they must go. Islam is a modern religion and can accommodate modernity." A great deal of time was then spent explaining the application of the Islamic laws that had been devised to protect and empower women.

The Doctors

I also spoke with medical doctors who are natives of the villages around Yazd in which early marriage is practiced on a large scale. Two of them came from neighboring villages, and each denied that early marriage was practiced in his village, accusing the "people of low culture" in the next village for condoning the practice. While they showed their up-to-date knowledge by explaining in medical terms why early marriage involved risks, they refused to condemn it and cited some of its social and cultural advantages. One referred sarcastically to Ayatollah Sanei's *fatwa* and said, "*Ijtihad* [interpretation of the Qur'an][14] is a wonderful thing in Shia Islam. We interpret the Qur'an and come up with new ideas." It was clear that he did not approve of the Ayatollah's views on a later age of marriage for girls. Subsequently I found out that one of the doctors had married a thirteen-year-old girl from his village.

I also spoke with some of the health practitioners visiting Yazd from Tehran who were preaching the disadvantages of early marriage. It appeared that despite a general awareness that the practice of early marriage is undesirable from a health perspective, attitudes to these marriages have altered little, and different approaches to the issue live side by side without anybody paying much attention to the consequences of the paradoxes and the confusion that these conflicting messages are creating for young people and their identity.

Poverty

Finally, poverty is identified as one of the main reasons for the continuation of early marriage in the child rights literature. While this may be true in some contexts, it should not be taken as a universal reason, since poverty can also delay the age of marriage, as shown by a study from the Ministry of Crusade for Agriculture (2003) on the causes for the rise in the age of marriage among rural girls in the Province of Yazd. The findings of the study reveal that a considerable number of fathers prevent their daughters' marriage so that they can continue to contribute to the family's income, and as a result many girls remain unmarried. The link between poverty and early marriage also proved not to be the case among the closely knit community in this study. None of the families studied were rich, but they were not very poor either, and none of the girls had been married off because of their parents' poverty. They all had married men of their own social standing, and the marriage had not taken place with the prospect of improving the financial situation of the family; rather, the family bonds, obligations, and traditions were the driving force behind the choice of the marriage partner. I did, however, come across some cases of men who had married early because of their parents' poverty and because their uncles had persuaded their parents to coerce their sons into marrying their daughters who could not find husbands.

Several visits to the Yazd bazaar revealed that both the assumptions of poverty encouraging early marriage and the "small" scale of the practice of early marriage were not correct. There I found a considerable number of brides-to-be who had been brought to the bazaar to buy their wedding jewelry. As I was looking at them with great curiosity, a woman I had met earlier whispered with contempt, "The only way I can tell that these poor souls are very young is in their ignorance in choosing gold and good jewelry. The look of bewilderment in their faces gives it all away." The amount of jewelry purchased for the brides-to-be indicated that early marriage is not restricted to the poor.

Conclusion

In this chapter I have examined some of the global assumptions with regard to early marriage and the persistent belief that education is the most effective measure to prevent early marriage, which is largely driven by coercion and poverty. A conservative town in Iran with a high literacy rate and where early marriages continue to be practiced was selected to investigate these assumptions. The findings of the study demonstrated that progress in female education and employment may not necessarily lead to the empowerment of women and a decline in the practice of early marriage, and every success story appearing in the form of statistics and reports has another side.

The high level of literacy in Iran is shown not to have led automatically to the empowerment of women. Changes that have empowered women are often due to other factors, some of which leave a longer-lasting impact, while others are provisional. One such influence has been the impact of family planning, which gives women the power to negotiate their fertility but vanishes once reproductive activities are over. This is true even for illiterate women, albeit to a lesser degree. The reduction in the number of children also has adverse effects, as some men have resorted to second wives to have more children. I have argued that in the short term a few more years of education without a fundamental change in other aspects of their lives adds little value to their quality of life nor does it free them from their social bonds. Education has opened doors for girls from certain social and economic backgrounds, but at the same time it has also triggered, either directly or indirectly, inevitable reactions among the less-advantaged layers of society. As a result, those girls who do not have the protection of a closely knit social group find themselves in an increasingly vulnerable position. It remains to be seen whether the generally accepted assumptions about empowerment and education will prove correct in the long run in Iran.

From my study in Yazd, it can be seen that the ideals of marriage as the only route to acquiring an identity have remained unchanged among three generations of women, regardless of their level of education. Although early marriage continues at a relatively high rate, the age of marriage has gone up due to the girls completing secondary or higher education, although education without the additional skills has not added any apparent real value to their lives. In some instances, it has resulted in them missing their chances for marriage among their social equals. Education has been used as a bargaining chip, especially by mothers, with the idea of improving the chances for a better marriage for their daughters, but there was no evidence that girls had married up due to a higher level of education. The sanctity of family life has remained prevalent, but the expression of this sanctity differs greatly between the genders. While women's preferences are for smaller families and thus for providing better opportunities for their families, men continue to link the sanctity to creating larger family units.

Finally, to return to the question asked earlier: can we say that new rules are being established? At a microlevel there may be some consistencies in behavior in the short term, but there are also some indications of ongoing alterations and expectations, norms, and ideals. These rules may gradually shift from the patriarchal control of women to global and local influences, such as the question of women's and children's human rights and women's agency as choice makers and expecting to become central in such a process. The transformations in the patriarchy itself, which will be inevitable but unpredictable in their form and force, will shape the new perspectives on gender relations. Whatever the outcome of such interactions, there is hope that gender relations will find equilibrium, albeit via a bumpy road.

In the long run, several influences are all likely to impact young women's aspirations, e.g., a more open society in which a dialogue exists between young people, access to the outside world through, for example, television, and new values introduced through communication such as the internet. The diminishing importance of protecting the collective values and obligations toward the kin group following the drastic reduction in the size of the family; the development of a more individualistic personality among the young; the weakening of parental control; a shift in the way young people meet their future marriage partners; and also various legal changes giving women more equal rights with regard to marriage, all may help girls and young women have more freedom and a choice over marriage. The question remains whether this alternative will provide greater harmony and stability in the family.

Acknowledgments

This chapter was published originally as "Modernity and Early Marriage in Iran: A View from Within," *Journal of Middle East Women Studies* 2(1): 65–94, Indiana University Press (2006). I am grateful to Soheila Shahshahani and to Dr. Mojibian, Director of Mojibian Hospital, without whose generous help and insights the research could not have taken place.

Notes

1. This figure varies depending on the type of survey conducted. It also refers to the official rate of employment and does not include the contribution of women to the informal economy. The 2000 Iran Demographic Health Survey (IDHS 2000) gives the rate of employment for women as 10.5 for urban areas and as 19.5 for rural areas. On average, we can perhaps say that the rate of female employment is around 15 percent (personal communication with Abbasi-Shavazi, August 2005). For a detailed study of female employment in Iran, see Mansour Zarra-Nezhad (1998).
2. The Convention on the Rights of the Child (CRC) of 1988 defined anyone under the age of eighteen as a child.
3. This research is based on interviews with marriage counselors in Tehran and Ardebil and marriage registration offices in Tehran and Yazd.
4. For more details, see Zanan.co.ir/news/000129.html. (*Zanan* was a Persian women's magazine published in Iran. It has since been shut down and banned by the government.)
5. *Yas-e-No*, August 2004.
6. *Yas-e-No*, June 2003.
7. Various factors determine the level of female literacy, such as primary, secondary, or higher education. This figure is a general one for the total of the literate population.
8. Figures given by the Office of the President published on 12 May 2005 mention that Tehran, with an average of 15.6, and Yazd, with an average of 3.24, have the highest and lowest rates of divorce respectively.
9. See also DeJong et al. (2005: 52) on the high incidence of consanguine marriages.
10. This research is based on personal interviews with sociologists.
11. Confidential reports and personal interviews with academics and practitioners confirm this in several provinces.
12. The demographic transition in Iran has been discussed abundantly, and it is beyond the scope of this chapter to discuss this. For examples, see Abbasi-Shavazi, McDonald, and Hosseini-Chavoshi (2003), Mehryar (1998b), and Hoodfar (1995).

13. Some of the wealthy community leaders in Yazd have funded a girls' boarding house at Tehran University to secure their safety.
14. *Ijtihad* is unique to Shia Islam and allows changes to the original text.

References

Abbasi-Shavazi, Mohammad Jalal, and Abbas Askari-Nodoushan. 2005. *Changes in the Family and Fertility Reduction in Iran: A Case Study in Yazd Province*. University of Tehran.

Abbasi-Shavazi, Mohammad Jalal, Peter McDonald, and Meimanat Hosseini-Chavoshi. 2003. "Changes in Family, Fertility Behaviour and Attitudes in Iran." Working Paper in Demography 88. Demography and Sociology Program. The Australian National University.

Afshar, Haleh. 1993. *Women in the Middle East: Perceptions, Realities, and Struggles for Liberation*. London: MacMillan.

———. 1998. *Islam and Feminism: An Iranian Case Study*. New York: MacMillan.

Aghajanian, Akbar, and Amir H. Mehryar. 1999. "Fertility Transition in the Islamic Republic of Iran: 1976–1996." *Asia-Pacific Population Journal* 14(1): 21–42.

DeJong, Jocelyn, Rana Jawad, Iman Mortagy, and Bonnie Shepard. 2005. "The Sexual and Reproductive Health of Young People in the Arab Countries and Iran." *The Journal of Reproductive Health Matters* 13(25): 49–59.

Ebadi, Shirin. 2002. "Serious Steps Taken to Enforce Children's Rights Convention." Iranian News Agency, 26 May.

———. 2003a. *Women's Rights in the Laws of the Islamic Republic of Iran*. In Persian. Tehran: Ganje Danesh.

———. 2003b. Interview with *Yas-e-No*. In Persian. 10 October.

Fargues, Philippe. 2003. "Terminating Marriage." In *The New Arab Family*, ed. Nicholas S. Hopkins. Cairo Papers in Social Science 24 (1–2). The American University in Cairo Press.

Forum on Marriage and the Rights of Women and Girls. 2000. EENET, School of Education, May. The University of Manchester.

Haeri, Shahla. 1989. *Law of Desire: Temporary Marriage in Iran*. London: I.B. Tauris.

Hamamsy, Laila. 1994. *Early Marriage and Reproduction in Two Egyptian Villages*. Cairo: Population Council/UNFPA Occasional Paper.

Hoodfar, Homa. 1995. "Population Policy and Gender Equity in Post-Revolutionary Iran." In *Family, Gender and Population in the Middle East: Policies in Context*, ed. Carla Makhlouf Obermeyer, 105–135. Cairo: American University of Cairo Press.

Hopkins, Nicholas S., ed. 2003. *The New Arab Family*. Cairo Papers in Social Science 24(1–2). Cairo American University.

IDHS (Iran Demographic Health Survey). 2000. http://ghdx.healthdata.org/record/iran-demographic-and-health-survey-2000.

International Center for Research on Women. 2003. *Too Young to Wed: The Lives, Rights, and Health of Young Married Girls*. International Center for Research on Women.

Kabeer, Naila. 2005. "Gender Equality and Women's Empowerment: A Critical Analysis of the Third Millennium Development Goals." *Oxfam* 13(1): 13–24.

Kian-Thiébaut, Azadeh. 2005. "From Motherhood to Equal Rights Advocates: The Weakening of Patriarchal Order." *Iranian Studies* 38(1): 45–66.

Locke, Catherine, and Heather Xiaoquan Zhang. 2004. "Social Analysis and Selective Inclusion in Rights-Based Approaches to Reproductive Health." Special Issue on Fertility and Reproduction, Guest ed. Soraya Tremayne. *Journal of the Anthropological Society of Oxford* VXXXI(1): 88–100.

Mehryar, Amir. 1998a. *Country Population Assessment Report*. Plan Organization of Islamic Republic of Iran, unpublished draft with limited circulation.

———. 1998b. *Evolution and Attainment of the Family Planning Programme in the Islamic Republic of Iran*. Tehran: Institute of Research on Planning and Development.

Mehryar, Amir, and F. Tajdini. 1998. *Population and Development in the Islamic Republic of Iran: A Review of the Main Findings of the 1996 Census and Other Sources of Data*. Tehran: Institute for Research on Planning and Development.

Ministry of Crusade for Agriculture. 2003. "Reasons for the Rise in the Age of Marriage among Girls in Rural Areas with Regard to Employment." Ministry of Crusade for Agriculture.

Moghadam, Valentine, ed. 1993. *Modernizing Women: Gender and Social Change in the Middle East*. Boulder, CO: Lynne Rienner.

Petchesky, Rosalind P., and Karen Judd. 1998. *Negotiating Reproductive Rights: Women's Perspectives across Countries and Cultures*. London and New York: Zed Books.

Singerman, Diane, and Homa Hoodfar, eds. 1996. *Development, Change, and Gender in Cairo: A View from the Household*. Bloomington: Indiana University Press.

Statistical Center of Iran. 2000. *Statistical Yearbook of Iran*. Tehran: SCI Publications.

Tremayne, Soraya, ed. 2001. *Managing Reproductive Life: Cross-Cultural Themes in Fertility and Sexuality*. Oxford and New York: Berghahn Books.

Tremayne, Soraya. 2004. "'And Never Shall the Twain Meet': Reproductive Health Policies in the Islamic Republic of Iran." In *Reproductive Agency, Medicine and the State: Cultural Transformations in Childbearing*, ed. Maya Unnithan-Kumar, 297–327. Oxford and New York: Berghahn Books.

Tucker, Judith, ed. 1993. *Arab Women: Old Boundaries, New Frontiers*. Bloomington: Indiana University Press.

UNICEF. 2001. *Early Marriage: Child Spouses*. Innocenti Digest no. 7. Florence: Innocenti Research Center.

Zarra-Nezhad, Mansour. 1998. "Employment of Women in Iran." *SOAS University of London Economic Digest*, December 2(2).

Chapter 3

THE FOUR FACES OF IRANIAN FATHERHOOD

Introduction

The impact of globalization on fatherhood in Iran can best be understood in the context of the major social and political changes that have taken place since the Islamic Revolution of 1979.[1] The establishment of an Islamic state initially meant the resurgence of conservative values and norms, which were undermined and threatened by the previous regime's modernizing reforms. Such a revival and its associated practices became so prominent that they gave the outside world the impression that Iran was an insular and fanatical country. On one level, Iran became a closed society, protecting conservative and conformist values and practices and rejecting what it saw as imported corrupt Western values; but on another level, the country has never closed its doors to change and has adopted many innovations offered by globalization with open arms (Tremayne 2006a). However, an assumption that such a dichotomy has resulted in a polarization of the society into the conservative versus liberal groups, or an attempt to identify and define clear-cut social and ideological categories, would be misleading and simplistic. The ongoing intermingling of old norms and values with modernity and global practices results in the emergence of complex and varied, or even paradoxical, responses among different groups in society. Inevitably, such diversity affects the core values attached to fatherhood and has transformed the relationship between fathers and their globalized children. The questions, therefore, are not whether but how and to what extent the changes brought about by globalization have altered the ingrained cultural understanding of what constitutes fatherhood. The fact that global trends, on reaching various cultures, are interpreted by their local recipients to make them fit into their own cultural molds is by now well-trodden ground and has been addressed by various scholars from different disciplines.[2] This chapter therefore focuses on the specific cultural responses of Iranian fathers in this study, and the strategies they adopt to maintain their position vis-à-vis their children, to realize their vision of fatherhood. I argue that, faced with the threat of losing their position, fathers strive to remain in control of their children and resort to a variety of tactics to secure their authority over them.

This chapter opens with a brief explanation of what fatherhood means in Iranian culture in light of the fact that, historically, controlling the family has been an inextricable part of fathering. Through analysis of the data in this study, I conclude that Iranian fathers, faced with the changes in the behavior of their globalized children, have been forced to give fatherhood new guises in order to remain in control and to avoid losing "face" for failing to maintain their authority. In examining the global factors as agents of change, I consider the outcome of two areas of reform: population policies and literacy campaigns. These initiatives aimed at modernizing the country and, by implication, improving the relationship within the family; both proved highly successful.

Methodology

The data presented in this chapter include 120 case studies of fathers and their families in three different locations. The study in Tehran includes two groups of fathers: one of highly educated, economically well-off fathers of liberal and secular backgrounds, and another of fathers from predominantly—although not necessarily—religious and/or conservative backgrounds of varying levels of education and income. The second site of study is Yazd in central Iran. Here almost all of the fathers are less educated, with no more than a high school education. They come from low-income, religious, and conservative homes. The third site is a group of Iranian refugees in the United Kingdom, who are predominately religious and conservative and come from the middle or lower strata of Iranian society. The main method used in all three sites was that of participant observation and in-depth interviews, conducted in Persian. In addition, the findings of this study rely on data from two separate studies (Tremayne 2006b, 2009), as well as on research on runaway and street children carried out from 2000 to 2004.

Fatherhood and Patriarchy

Iranian culture is predominantly patriarchal, and although modernity and globalization visibly affect the role and position of fathers vis-à-vis their families, their impact is not yet profound enough to dislodge the deep-seated values attached to fatherhood. The reinforcement of *sharia*, which has been the basis for the country's legal code since the 1979 Islamic Revolution, further supports and lends legitimacy to patriarchal practices. According to *sharia*, the father owns the child, and the mother is considered a caretaker, not an owner (Ebadi 2002; Mir-Hosseini 1993).[3] Fatherhood, therefore, symbolizes an overall figure of control and authority, whose powers over his family are unlimited and assumed. However, the social, cultural, and legal recognition of fathers' overall authority and right to control should not be interpreted only as legitimizing the use of physical force and violence. Instead, such authority can be exercised and demonstrated in a variety of ways, including through the expression of genuine love and affection, and when necessary through violence and aggression. "Patriarchal connectivity," a term coined by Suad Joseph (1999) to define the structure of the Arab family, provides the key to understanding the subtle and often invisible aspects of the multifaceted and complex relationships that underlie the patriarchal systems of Arab—and Persian—societies. As Joseph explains, the relationships in patriarchal systems are not just about control, authority, and violence; they also include emotions, affection, tolerance, and many other forms of articulating connections, which are called upon to ensure the survival of the system. In Joseph's (1999: 11–13) words, "By connectivity I mean relationships in which persons' boundaries are relatively fluid so that persons feel a part of significant others. Persons do not experience themselves as bounded, separate, or autonomous." Such connectivity means that the children are considered inseparable parts of the father and that their actions reflect those of the father. A child's deviation is, therefore, interpreted as that of the father, and this is what gives meaning to and justifies the exercise of control of children by the patriarch. Following Joseph's work, Marcia C. Inhorn (2012), in her study on "the new Arab man," also offers a new understanding of patriarchy in its globalized context by challenging the stereotypes of Arab men in patriarchal societies as controlling, aggressive, and brutal and as oppressors of women and children (see also Inhorn 2014). Inhorn's (2012) new Arab man is "self-consciously rethinking the patriarchal masculinity of his forefathers and unseating received wisdom." In Inhorn's words, "he is loving, caring and committed" and he is "seriously re-thinking marriage, family life, and what it means to be a man in the twenty-first century" (158). Both Joseph's and Inhorn's groundbreaking work on the Arab world strikes chords with evolving forms of patriarchal practices in Iran. Research on the modern Iranian family demonstrates that it is closely knit and that the relationship between its members remains unaffected, in spite of the considerable changes in its structure. For example, in his article on love for children, Mohammad Taghi Sheykhi (2009) argues that children are a source of happiness in Iranian culture. Massoume Price (2006) and Elton L. Daniel and Ali Akbar Mahdi (2006) emphasize the persistence of warmth and affection between family members. However, such warmth and closeness, or any other forms of connectivity fathers may have with their children, are increasingly affected by modernity and globalization, and the fathers' perceptions of the real or imaginary threats posed by globalization are forcing them to rethink their relationships with their children and to reposition themselves to counteract such threats, as demonstrated in the following examples.

Massoud is a successful surgeon and a gentle and mild-mannered man. He is devoted to his family, and his love for and closeness to his four children are exemplary. Massoud's children were educated in the West and, despite the freedom of choice and the financial ability to remain abroad, they were tempted to return to Iran by their father's promise to provide them with the familiar and generous comforts of home. However, even within such a harmonious and happy family, the father's authority remains incontestable. The mother presents the important decisions as that of "your father thinks" to the children, who would not even conceive the idea of going against their father's will. During one of his more relaxed moments, Massoud confided in me:

> Frankly, there are times when I grind my teeth and stop myself from shouting and asking the children to move away and have their own independent lives. But, I know that unless I keep my smile and continue to be generous with them, I shall lose my authority over them. I will no longer know what they are doing and who their friends are,

> whereas by letting them think that they are welcome at home, I can keep better control over them.

Although Massoud loves his children, he worries about losing control over them. This separation of emotions from authority is confirmed by various other studies. For example, in her study of Iranian mothers, Mahnaz Kousha (2002) shows that even the most sensible and gentle fathers behave irrationally when their children challenge their authority. In one case when the husband lost his temper with his children, the mother explained, "My husband is a good man and makes rational choices but when it comes to children and their emotional matters he is at a loss" (Kousha 2002: 211). Another study by Behnaz Jalali (2005) describes how mothers mediated between fathers and their children, especially their sons. She argues that the relationship between fathers and sons is more difficult and that mothers constantly act as go-betweens to establish peace between the two sides. "Wait till your father comes home" was one of the most frequently heard sentences in many households and was meant as a threat by mothers, who were unable to control the children, especially the boys. In such cases it was not just the father's physical presence that made the children comply, but the awesome force of his omnipresence, which created an aura of self-control and haunted the children long into adulthood, if not for the rest of their lives.

Marjan is an architect and a Western-educated woman whose husband is infertile. When they decided to use donor sperm to have a baby, Marjan's only and real concern was that this should be kept a secret from her father. She said:

> If my father finds out, all hell will break loose and the world will come to an end as far as he is concerned. For him, using another man's sperm means that I have committed adultery. The thought of his son-in-law being infertile and his grandchild being a "bastard" is a complete blow to his manhood and too shameful to be able to face.

In general, the fathers' treatment of their children is guided more often by their concern to protect and reinforce their status as worthy fathers. The loss of authority and control of their children means a loss of "face," in all its social implications, for fathers. As I have discussed elsewhere, one of the manifestations of the deep-rooted values that determine the form and extent of acceptance of modernity is the consideration of one's "face" (*aberu* in Persian) in public (Tremayne 2006a). Face acts as a regulating agent directing the choices people make vis-à-vis societal change. In a society such as that of Iran, which is constantly in flux, people do not remain passive. In making decisions about where and how to adapt to change, face plays an important part in checking and shaping cultural responses. Face is one of the manifestations of Iranian culture that has not been weakened by the challenges of modernity and the introduction of new elements in society. Whereas the concept and definition of face exists in every culture, its meaning can be more critical and extensive in some cultures than others. While the loss of face in Western cultures may mean embarrassment, it often means much more than this in Middle Eastern cultures. There, the loss of face implies a failure to meet expectations and often causes loss of honor and a deep humiliation, which in turn can lead to loss of credibility and entail other social and economic consequences. In extreme cases, it can provoke strong reactions, violence, and even blood feud. Awareness of one's social position and of appropriate related behavior is imperative in all social interactions. Therefore, any decision must consider these social consequences, as far as the status and respectability of the family are concerned. Face controls the actions and decisions taken by individuals in the public aspects of their lives, regardless of class, age, ethnicity, or gender. It follows that loss of control over one's children is not an option for fathers, and the underlying reason for their willingness to make unexpected and surprising compromises is to control, or to be seen to control, their children, as the following case illustrates.

Karim is a money exchanger who runs a profitable business in Tehran. When his twelve-year-old son started secondary school and became involved in an unsavory social circle, he became unruly and no longer obeyed Karim. No amount of counseling by other relatives had any effect on him, and the inevitable involvement of relatives meant that rumors began to circulate about Karim's inability to bring this young boy under control. Karim said, "To regain control of my son and save face, I was left with no choice but to uproot the family and start a new life in a different country, Dubai, where I have opened a new branch of my business, and hope that my son will behave better there." Since moving to Dubai, Karim's esteem among his relatives has risen, and his brother-in-law proudly announced, "Karim has proved that he is a real man and a very good father, who does not easily give into his children's unruly behavior." The drive to control one's children is also shown in the example of fathers from Yazd, whose daughters had been admitted to university in Tehran. Not wishing to deny their daughters the benefits of higher education, fathers asked their wives to move to Tehran to stay with them for the duration of their studies. Such upheavals seem a small sacrifice on the part of fathers in exchange for making sure that their children behave as the fathers think fit.

The Small-Sized Family and the Value of Children

Karim's situation, similar to those of other Iranian fathers, is largely the inevitable consequence of two major policies that have altered the structure of the Iranian family and the gender and intergenerational relationships in society. Beginning in 1986, Iran initiated a public awareness campaign to educate people about the advantages of having smaller families, arguing that having fewer children would result in more responsible parenthood, better health, better education, and better life conditions for their children. The policies assumed that having fewer children meant that the children would be more cherished and valued by their parents. These policies were so successful that the rate of population growth dropped from 3.8 percent per annum in 1986 to around 2 percent in 1996 and 1.3 percent in 2011, with variations among the rural and urban areas (United Nations Population Fund 2011). This outstanding achievement, which won Iran the United Nations Award for Population Policies in 1999, led to a major reduction in family size at the national level. However, this attempt to improve the status of children in smaller families was not universally successful. Educated and more secular layers in society, who lived in urban areas and had started reducing their family size before the policies were introduced, were familiar with these arguments. They treated their children with more care and valued them already, to the point that some researchers argued that the Iranian society had become a child-centered society and that the patriarchal values had weakened (Kian-Thiébault 2005: 52).[4] A study by Marie Ladier-Fouladi (2002: 369) also points out that the relationship between members of the smaller families has been altered and that the Iranian urban family is now nuclear, relationships are more egalitarian, and family solidarity is based on emotional affinities.

While these studies reflect some of the changes among certain groups in society, they do not address the widespread violence inflicted on children by parents who refuse to adapt to modernity. As evidence shows, a reduction in the size of the family or an increase in the level of education of children bears little relation to the behavior of fathers and the traditional values attached to fatherhood. For example, a recent article by Rob Stephenson et al. (2006), on the maltreatment of school children in Kordestan in western Iran, reports on the extent of both physical and psychological violence inflicted on children, as do regular reports by international agencies. Similar behavior can be seen in cases of refugee children or young people who have run away from parental physical and/or psychological abuse and violence. Even then, those cases that come to public attention are only the tip of the iceberg; the majority of cases go unreported or are ignored by the authorities, who reckon that such matters are for the family and do not require police involvement. The following examples illustrate the extent of the Iranian father's power and authority, which is exercised through persistent physical and psychological violence, or the threat of it.

Mina is a 35-year-old woman from Yazd who had been forced to marry her husband at the age of fifteen. When the Welfare Organization opened an office in Yazd, she went to its director for help and told him, "I hated my husband from the first day of marriage and wanted to divorce him. I cringe at the thought of him approaching me. But I am afraid of my father and the likelihood that he will harm me because I have put him to shame by going over his decision of having chosen this man for me." The Welfare Office summoned Mina's father and asked him about his views on his son-in-law. He said that he found him quite revolting and could not stand him, but, he added, "My daughter is not allowed to divorce him, or I shall kill her." Mina remains married to her husband to date.

Unlike Mina, Fatemeh, who is in her late twenties, had secretly entered into temporary marriage with a married man, whom she had met on the Internet, and had a child by him. When her father found out, he asked her not to renew her marriage contract, but she refused.[5] The father then called his two sons from another town, and together they locked Fatemeh up in the basement for days and beat her until she conceded to break up her marriage. While imprisoned, her temporary marriage had expired, and the husband did not renew it. Fatemeh's marriage without her father's permission was bad enough to make the father lose face among his equals. Having his daughter being married as a temporary wife and to a married man was even more insulting. Because no respectable girl would enter into temporary marriage, this meant that Fatemeh was unfit to be married as a permanent wife. Fatemeh's actions proved too humiliating for the father to bear and, with the mother's intervention, she was allowed to stay at home, but neither she nor her child are accepted as equals at home or among her wide network of relatives. She has to endure this shame, which will not abate as long as she lives in the same town.

Amir is a 25-year-old man who has finished secondary school and lives with his illiterate parents. When he met and fell in love with a young woman and wanted to marry her, he was told by his father that he was not allowed to do so because the father had decided already who Amir's wife should be. Amir's father forbade him the marriage of his choice. When Amir protested, his father, with help from his brothers and other sons, tied Amir up, locked him in the basement, whipped him twice per day, and denied him food until he submitted to his father's will.

Not all fathers exercise such violence, and any generalization about fathers, the family, and the relationship between family members could be misleading. As Sheykhi (2009: 526) explains:

> Living in harmony within family depends on the quality and quantity of children in Iran as in any other developing country. It is argued that we need to consider the family as a controversial issue because of the differences between ideology of the family and the reality of the variety of various ways in which men, women, boys and girls, live together and interact.

However, what is viewed as a weakening of patriarchy can be a misinterpretation of what are often conciliatory and negotiating tactics, used by fathers to ensure their connectivity with their children. Such a soft approach does not necessarily imply an absence of authority and control and is likely to be more of a veneer than a profound uprooting of their cultural norms and values, as the following cases show.

Ahmad lives in Yazd and is a clerk in a brick distribution business. He has a modest income and a lower secondary-level education. He is moderately religious but is conservative to the extreme. He has two daughters ages ten and fourteen and keeps the women in his household under strict control. They are not allowed to go out of the house without a man accompanying them. Although the family struggles financially, it has a satellite television and a computer and all the family members have mobile phones. Most evenings, Ahmad puts his ten-year-old daughter on his knees, and the entire family watches a variety of television shows, indiscriminately. These range from the erotic, touching on pornography, to horror or violent shows, to soccer matches. They can be Western, Indian, or Turkish films. Ahmad sees nothing wrong with letting his women watch these potentially inappropriate films, because "[his] women are completely free to do what they like, as long as this takes place in the house and under [his] watch." While there were only two books in the house, the Qur'an and another religious book, the family had stacks of videos and other audiovisual gadgets. When I gave the ten-year-old girl a translated copy of *Harry Potter*, a popular book for children in the West, she said that her father had bought her the DVD and that she does not need to read the book. Ahmad's two daughters are confused as to which values are the right ones to follow because, although they were allowed to watch television and use the Internet, their father forbade them to mention the television at school or discuss it outside the house.

Ahmad's brother, who also has a satellite television, is stricter with his children. He mentioned that he would never allow his child to marry someone from a family that has a satellite television. Both brothers allow their daughters the use of the latest global technologies but under strict control. Similar to Ahmad, Ali lives in Tehran and is illiterate and highly conservative, with limited religious beliefs. For most of his life he has treated his five children in an autocratic and loveless manner. Four of the children, now adults, live with their parents and earn good salaries, but none of them contributes to the housekeeping. Ali, in his mid-sixties, continues to work until late at night to provide for his family. Ali has no authority over his children and even receives some criticism from them. He could throw them out of his home but refrains from doing so. Ali is only too aware that there is a price to be paid for such an act and that is his loss of face for being defeated by his children. By letting them stay, Ali claims that his children still need him and are dependent on him. Oblivious to his harsh treatment at the hands of his children, the outside world views him as a devoted father. He has gained the admiration of his relatives and has become a greatly respected public figure in his neighborhood. As discussed earlier, traditionally, obedience, fear, and respect have been some of the most effective pillars of patriarchal structures in upholding the paternal authority. However, while these factors seem to have weakened, respect, bashfulness, and modesty have not, and they remain determining factors cementing the relationship between fathers and their children and preventing children from serious confrontation with their fathers. However, even when asking for the children's respect, as witnessed in Ali's case, parents have to make compromises. Ever-married women in Ladier-Fouladi's (2002: 367) interviews felt that children should respect their parents as long as parents' demands were "reasonable."[6]

Education

One of the main factors responsible for the gradual weakening of obedience and fear of fathers is the literacy campaign. On implementing the literacy campaign, policymakers argued that by having a well-educated young generation as potential future parents, the nation will be better equipped to cope with raising children to succeed in a modern and globalized world. Soon after the Islamic Revolution of 1979, massive resources were allocated to the literacy campaign, which proved greatly successful. One significant factor in this success was the introduction of sex segregation at schools, which led to the conservative parents' approval to send their daughters to school.[7] By 2010, the literacy rate stood at 90.5 for men and 87.5 for women,[8] and research shows that not only do fathers no longer object to their daughters going to school, but they insist on their daughters completing their secondary education, too.[9] However, a series of research projects carried out in earlier decades of the literacy campaign showed that the impact of education on the relationship between the generation of parents and their children had not yielded the anticipated results. For example, a study carried out by the Family Planning Association of the Islamic Republic of Iran (1998: 23), which included a substantial qualitative survey and focus group discussion on reproductive health of twelve- to nineteen-year-old adolescent boys, concluded that:

> The knowledge of 15–19 years old boys—the future fathers—in the city of Tehran on matters of puberty, marriage, family planning, and venereal disease is very low. In most cases half of the group is totally ignorant . . . considering that their present attitude and future practice will be a direct consequence of their knowledge and that their knowledge is relatively better than that of the corresponding age/sex group in other cities, it seems there exists a real problem.

Follow-up surveys in 2006 and 2007 confirmed that little had changed during this decade and concluded that the relationship between the fathers and their children remains by and large unchanged and that communication and relationships between fathers and their children remain poor, in general.[10] But, as more recent studies indicate, with the generation of the more educated post-revolutionary men becoming fathers, and with the spread of global media technologies, relationships between the educated children and their less educated fathers are changing, as Ladier-Fouladi's (2002) study confirms. As a result, the one-way pattern of respect for the older generation is also undergoing changes and, in some instances, young people's high level of education and knowledge of modern means of communication have gained them a special place among their elders' kin group and their community. This is especially true in the rural areas, where few people have the knowledge of or access to media technologies. However, this reversal is thus limited and is true of only certain groups in society, with particular levels of education and lifestyles.

Global Technologies and Fatherhood

Beyond the consequences of the demographic changes and the rise in literacy, other global factors, such as the prevalence of satellite television, mobile phones, and the Internet, have had an unanticipated impact on the relationship between fathers and their children. While fathers neither wish to nor are able to prevent their children from accessing these technologies, they remain anxious to retain some control over their children's use of them. To do so, some educated fathers have developed a closer relationship with their children, trying to familiarize themselves with these technologies, with help from their children. Even in such cases, these liberal fathers check their children's computers regularly and secretly to monitor their activity.[11] Other fathers, who are unable to master these technologies, especially the Internet, have become alienated from their children; their frustration is shown in either withdrawing from all activities within the family, or adopting an even more controlling attitude toward their children.

Moving beyond these cases, there are also examples of fathers in their most modern and accommodating, but, in fact, most controlling guise. For example, a few years ago, fathers from Yazd raised funds and built a boarding house in Tehran for their daughters who had been admitted to the university there so that the girls' movements could be controlled. Eric Hoogland's (2007) longitudinal studies of some villages in Fars Province in the central south of Iran refer to fathers who insist on their daughters completing their secondary education, which was initially interpreted as a sign of fathers being modern and enlightened. However, findings of this research show a different side to such fathers' liberal decisions, revealing that it is the fathers' wish to improve their daughters' chances of marriage that drives these decisions. Literature is abundant on how every aspect of both young girls' and boys' lives are controlled by their fathers, regardless of the young people's degree of education.

Finally, any attempt to define fatherhood by situating fathers into well-defined categories could lead to confusion, contradiction, and misrepresentation. As is the case elsewhere, Iranian fathers come from a variety of social and cultural backgrounds and are not unanimous in their responses to change. The case studies presented in this chapter illustrate how the fathers' reactions to globalization often turn out to be the opposite of what one might expect of men of their particular backgrounds. For example, the two following cases, of two highly educated fathers from very different social and economic backgrounds, are surprisingly similar.

Mansour is seventy years old and is highly religious, to the point of being fanatical. He has a PhD in economics from a university in the United States and has held high office in the government since the revolution in 1979. His two sons and one daughter were brought up according to the strictest Islamic values and practices until they went to university. Once they graduated from college, they rebelled and started breaking every rule set by their father. The sons started going out with girls, drinking, breaking their religious fast, and gambling. They became contemptuous of their father's "backward" ideas and called him "moron" behind his back. The daughter took to blogging and found new friends on the Internet, much to her father's horror. When Mansour realized that they were a lost cause and were unlikely to revert to their original upbringing, he first asked them to leave the house, which they refused to do. Like Ali, Mansour was aware that throwing his children out was not a real option, as this would mean a total loss of face and admission to failure as a father. To everyone's surprise, he did not use violence to impose his will on his children. Instead, he let them stay and live the lives they wanted but withdrew from any communication with his family and lived a solitary life. He even refused to attend his son's wedding. He is totally alienated and has lost all connectivity with his family. What is left for him is that, to the outside world, he is still seen as the head of his family.

Mohsen shares Mansour's alienation, albeit in a different way and to a different degree. Mohsen is a secular man from a liberal family. He possesses a degree in engineering and is self-employed and financially successful. Soon after the Islamic Revolution, Mohsen brought his young children to America because he could not tolerate the "controlling" and "suffocating" atmosphere created by the regime. When his daughter grew up and chose to go to a university outside the town where they lived, Mohsen objected and refused to pay for her education. The mother sided with her daughter and eventually the fights became so intolerable that the family broke up, and his wife and daughter left him. He returned to Iran feeling humiliated and disconnected, until his son, who is a mild-mannered young man, joined him to work under his supervision. Even though Mohsen feels that his status as a father has been restored once more, he has withdrawn from socializing with his large group of relatives as he has not recovered from the humiliation and loss of face he suffered due to his own lack of ability to control his daughter.

The Four Faces of Controlling Fathers

Fathers in this study can be classified into four broad categories. The first category is comprised of resourceful fathers, who foresee and preempt potential disobedience from their children or who, faced with it, go to any length to diffuse the children's rebellion by seeking new solutions. Both Massoud and Karim fall into this group: Massoud pampered his children and bought their respect and compliance through love and affection. Karim realized that the use of force against his disobedient son would only make matters worse; ultimately, he changed his life altogether and left Iran.

The second category includes resilient fathers, whose authority is challenged by globalization but who show flexibility and adjust their approaches to retain a degree of control and to ensure their connectivity with their children. Ahmad and Ali are examples of resilient fathers: Ali has no authority over his children but is still able to retain his position as the father figure. Ahmad yields to his children's demands and goes as far as allowing his daughters unlimited access to modern technologies, as long as he can maintain control of the situation. There are similar examples among other patriarchal cultures, whereby fathers, in order to impose their decisions, make surprising compromises. An interesting case was recounted by two British Pakistani men, who were critical of Pakistani fathers' authority and control, on the topic of forced marriage among the Pakistani community in the United Kingdom. They reported that a Pakistani family, in trying to force their son to marry a girl from Pakistan and faced with his objection, made a deal with him that if he agreed to marry the girl they wanted, they would let him marry the girl he wanted, as his second wife.[12]

The third category is comprised of alienated fathers, who refuse to accept their children's aspirations to modernity but do not resort to violence. These fathers become isolated and lose all connectivity with their families, even though some continue to live with their families in the same house. Mansour and Mohsen are two such examples.

Finally, the fourth category comprises violent fathers, for whom physical violence is the only way to counteract any form of disobedience. Mina's, Fatemeh's, and Amir's fathers fall into this category. These cases are not extreme in comparison to tens of others, whose stories are reported regularly by the media, by the authorities themselves, and through the work of charitable organizations. Faced with extreme paternal violence, the children are left with no choice but to run away from home and live on the street, a life that some believe to be better than what they experience back at home. Their stories are echoed in Rachel Baker and Catherine Panter-Brick's (2000) study of street children and the hardship and occasional abuse they encounter while living on the streets, which nevertheless proves safer than living at home and being exposed to systematic abuse by family members. A visit to various charities' websites in Iran also reveals the extent of violence some families inflict on their children.[13] The following examples are typical of the violence that Iranian fathers inflict on their disobedient children and represent a widespread problem. In one case, described in a confidential report by one of the child protection agencies, a runaway boy was so frightened of his father after having been late attending school that he left home. In another case, a girl fled a forced marriage, ended up in prostitution, and was eventually murdered. During the court trials the father accepted the blood money offered by the murderer and forgave him. But, as he was leaving the court, the judge mentioned that the girl had been raped before being murdered. The loss of his honor proved such a serious blow that the father changed his decision and asked the judge to sentence the man to death. Finally, there is the case of a girl who ran away from domestic violence and took refuge in one of the shelters in Tehran. When the police contacted her father and asked him to collect his daughter, he turned up with a butcher's knife to "wash this stain of shame" for dishonoring the family.

Conclusion

To examine the impact of globalization on fatherhood in Iran's predominantly patriarchal culture, an in-depth study of fathers in three locations was carried out. The findings of the study show that, for men, fatherhood remains the culmination of their personhood and identity, from manhood to masculinity and sexuality (Inhorn 2012, 2014; Inhorn et al. 2009). The findings also reveal that globalization has not dislodged these core cultural values attached to fatherhood and that men's lives are shaped by and become meaningful in their role as fathers and as the custodians of the family and its honor. Losing control over one's children is therefore not an option and equals a total failure for fathers. Furthermore, faced with globalization, fathers are shown not to be averse to what modernity has to offer, as long as this does not pose a threat to their authority or disrupt their connectivity with their children. To this end, fathers adopt new strategies to diffuse any potential threats and adjust their behavior toward their children in a variety of ways. However, a close examination of these changes shows that they are not fundamental transformations of the ideals of fatherhood, but mere strategic adjustments, carried out in self-preservation. Furthermore, in spite of these variations and against their diverse sociocultural, political, educational, and religious backgrounds, these fathers share a fundamental interest in retaining control over their children.

In trying to meet their children's aspiration for modernity, fathers respond in unconventional and unexpected ways that do not fit certain stereotypes, such as conservative fathers resisting change and liberal fathers embracing it. In some cases, the religious and/or conservative fathers show incredible tolerance in meeting the aspirations of their children, and the secular and educated ones lack flexibility, resisting their children's most basic demands. The responses of fathers fall into four categories: the resourceful father finds new solutions to ensure his authority; the resilient father accommodates his children's demands to a certain extent; the alienated father lacks flexibility, saving face but losing connectivity with his children; finally, the violent father resists change completely and resorts to physical abuse. Furthermore, fathers who accommodate their children's demands are shown to retain control more successfully than those who refuse to adjust. For these inflexible fathers, isolation is the price to pay for saving face, and fatherhood for them is just an empty shell. Regardless, the father figure remains an omnipresent force for the children. Although the fear and obedience that fathers commanded, traditionally, are gradually receding, children's respect for their fathers remains intact and prevents children from confronting their fathers.

However, as young people's aspirations continue to move toward a more globalized lifestyle, the boundaries of the relationship between fathers and their children are likely to shift and require renegotiation. Further research is needed to discover whether the future generation of fathers will be fundamentally different and will forgo this strong desire to control and exercise authority over their children.

Acknowledgments

This chapter was published originally as "The Four Faces of Iranian Fatherhood." In *Globalized Fatherhood*, ed. Marcia C. Inhorn, Wendy Chavkin, and José-Alberto Navarro, 336–355. New York and Oxford: Berghahn Books (2014).

Notes

1. For more details see Abbasi-Shavazi (2001) and Tremayne (2004).
2. For example, see Miller and Horst (2006) on digital and mobile technologies, Unnithan-Kumar (2010) and Tremayne (2012) on reproductive technologies, and Parkin and Wilker (2012).
3. As Ebadi (2004: 79) explains, if a father or paternal grandfather kills his child, he can only pay the blood money. The mother has no right to take him to court and must be content with this blood money. This biased law applies only to the father and grandfather but not the mother. If the mother kills her child, the father can request her death sentence. Ziba Mir-Hosseini (1993) also discusses the fact that in Shia Islam, although a child takes his filiation and parentage from both the father and mother, it is the paternal side that has ascendancy over the maternal. The father is, therefore, the central figure, and the children are considered his property. In Mir-Hosseini's (1993: 136) words, "In all schools of Islamic law the primary significance of filiation and parentage is that of paternity, closely tied to legitimacy, through which

a child acquires its legal identity and its religion." The Iranian Civil Code (Article 1170) further confirms that mothers' access to children in the case of divorce and custody is severely restricted. The following website also highlights fathers' uncontested rights over their children, through the lens of runaway children: http://childrenofiran.wordpress.com/about/orphans-vulnerable-children/. However, despite Iran being a signatory to the Convention on the Rights of the Child, children do not in reality have any rights in Iran: the rights of a child are given to his or her parents. If a child is being abused by anyone, it is rare to get attention unless the parents claim that someone is abusing the child. If a parent is abusive, there are simply no laws to protect the child against the parent. Many children die each year in Iran because of the abuse of their parents. What makes the situation worse is the fact that women do not have any rights to defend their children or themselves against abusive fathers and in many cases against other abusers.

4. However, in one of her more recent studies, Azadeh Kian-Thiébault (2012) revised her statements about the weakening of patriarchy.
5. Temporary marriage bears a time limit; when this time expires, the marriage automatically becomes null.
6. The importance of respect was also emphasized by anthropologist Soheila Shahshahani during a recent conversation in September 2012.
7. For more details of the education campaign, see Mehran (2003/4) and Mehryar (1998).
8. The exact literacy rate varies depending on how it is measured, but these are general figures according to United Nations Educational, Scientific, and Cultural Organization records: http://www.accu.or.jp/litdbase/policy/irn/index.htm.
9. See, for example, Hoogland (2007).
10. See, for example, the reports available at: http://www.who.int/reproductivehealth/publications/adolescence/boys_iran.pdf and http://www.prb.org/pdf07/menayouthreproductivehealth.pdf.
11. A lecture given by Nadia Aghtai, at Women's Rights in the Middle East Seminars, St. Antony's College, University of Oxford, in February 2012, confirmed similar reactions by husbands in Iran, who secretly check their wives' computers to find out who they are in touch with via the Internet.
12. Interview with a Pakistani lawyer with BBC's Radio 4, 13 August 2012.
13. For example, among tens of similar charities, see Omid-Mehr's, a charity that houses tens of runaway girls, most of whom fled abuse from family members, predominantly fathers: http://www.omid-e-mehr.org/.

References

Abbasi-Shavazi, Mohammad Jalal. 2001. "La Fécondité en Iran: L'autre Revolution" [Fertility in Iran: The other revolution]. *Population et Societé* 373.

Baker, Rachel, and Catherine Panter-Brick. 2000. "A Comparative Perspective on Children's 'Careers' and Abandonment in Nepal." In *Abandoned Children*, ed. Catherine Panter-Brick and Malcolm T. Smith. Cambridge: Cambridge University Press.

Daniel, Elton L., and Ali Akbar Mahdi. 2006. *Culture and Customs of Iran*. Westport and London: Greenwood Press.

Ebadi, Shirin. 2002. "Serious Steps Taken to Enforce Children's Rights Convention." Iranian News Agency, 26 May.

———. 2004. *History and Documentation of Human Rights in Iran*. Tehran: Roshangaran and Women's Studies Publishing.

Family Planning Association of the Islamic Republic of Iran. 1998. *Reproductive Health Needs Assessment of Adolescent Boys*.

Hoogland, Eric. 2007. "Changes in an Iranian Village, Aliabad." Conference on Iran on the Move, Leiden University.

Inhorn, Marcia C. 2012. *The New Arab Man: Emergent Masculinities, Technologies, and Islam in the Middle East*. Princeton: Princeton University Press.

———. 2014. "New Arab Fatherhood: Emergent Masculinities and Assisted Reproduction." In *Globalized Fatherhood*, ed. Marcia C. Inhorn, Wendy Chavkin, and José-Alberto Navarro, 243–263. New York and Oxford: Berghahn Books.

Inhorn, Marcia C., Tine Tjørnhøj-Thomsen, Helene Goldberg, and Maruska la Cour Mosegaard, eds. 2009. *Reconceiving the Second Sex: Men, Masculinity, and Reproduction*. New York and Oxford: Berghahn Books.

Jalali, Behnaz. 2005. "Iranian Families." In *Ethnicity & Family Therapy*, ed. Monica McGoldrick, Joe Giordano, and Nydia Garcia-Preto. New York: Guilford Press.

Joseph, Suad, ed. 1999. *Intimate Selving in Arab Families: Gender, Self, and Identity*. Syracuse: Syracuse University Press.

Kian-Thiébault, Azadeh. 2005. "From Motherhood to Equal Rights Advocates: The Weakening of Patriarchal Order." *Iranian Studies* 38(1): 45–66.

———. 2012. "Gendered Citizenship and the Women's Movement in Iran." In *Iran: A Revolutionary Republic in Transition*, ed. Farideh Farhi, Azadeh Kian, Rouzbeh Parsi, Evaleila Pesaran, and Paola Rivetti. European Union Institute for Security Studies.

Kousha, Mahnaz. 2002. *Voices from Iran. The Changing Lives of Iranian Women*. Syracuse: Syracuse University Press.

Ladier-Fouladi, Marie. 2002. "Iranian Families between Demographic Change and the Birth of the Welfare State." *Population* 57(2): 361–370.

Mehran, Golnar. 2003/4. "Gender and Education in Iran." Paper commissioned for the EFA Global Monitoring Report, *Gender and Education for*

All: The Leap to Equality. Retrieved 19 September 2021 from http://unesdoc.unesco.org/images/0014/001468/146809e.pdf.

Mehryar, Amir. 1998. "Draft Country Population Assessment Report." Plan Organization of Iran, unpublished and with limited circulation.

Miller, Danny, and Heather Horst. 2006. *The Cell Phone: An Anthropology of Communication*. Oxford: Berg.

Mir-Hosseini, Ziba. 1993. *Marriage on Trial: A Study of Islamic Family Law*. London: I.B. Tauris.

Parkin, Robert, and James Wilker, eds. 2012. *Modalities of Change: The Interface of Tradition and Modernity in East Asia*. New York; Oxford: Berghahn Books.

Price, Massoume. 2006. "Patriarchy and Parental Control in Iran." Iran Chamber Society.

Sheykhi, Mohammad Taghi. 2009. "Children as a Source of Happiness within the Iranian Families: Profiles and Challenges." *African Journal of Political Science and International Relations* 3(11): 526–531.

Stephenson, Rob, Payam Sheikhattari, Nazilla Assasi, Hassan Eftekhar, Qasem Zamani, Bahram Maleki, and Hamid Kiabayan. 2006. "Child Maltreatment among School Children in the Kurdistan Province, Iran." *Child Abuse & Neglect* 30(3): 231–245.

Tremayne, Soraya. 2004. "'And Never the Twain Shall Meet': Reproductive Health Policies in the Islamic Republic of Iran." In *Reproductive Agency, Medicine and the State: Cultural Transformations in Childbearing*, ed. Maya Unnithan-Kumar, 181–202. New York and Oxford: Berghahn Books.

———. 2006a. "Change and 'Face' in Modern Iran." *Journal of the Anthropology of the Middle East* 1(1): 25–41.

———. 2006b. "Modernity and Early Marriage in Iran: A View from Within." *Journal of Middle East Women Studies* 2(1): 65–94.

———. 2009. "Law, Ethics, and Donor Technologies in Shia Iran." In *Assisting Reproduction, Testing Genes: Global Encounters with New Biotechnologies*, ed. Daphna Birenbaum-Carmeli and Marcia C. Inhorn, 144–163. New York and Oxford: Berghahn Books.

———. 2012. "The 'Down Side' of Gamete Donation: Challenging 'Happy Family' Rhetoric in Iran." In *Islam and Assisted Reproductive Technologies: Sunni and Shia Perspectives*, ed. Marcia C. Inhorn and Soraya Tremayne, 130–156. New York and Oxford: Berghahn Books.

United Nations Population Fund. 2011. "Country Report."

Unnithan-Kumar, Maya, ed. 2004. *Reproductive Agency, Medicine and the State: Cultural Transformations in Childbearing*. New York and Oxford: Berghahn Books.

———. 2010. "Learning from Infertility: Gender, Health Inequities and Faith Healers in Women's Experiences of Disrupted Reproduction in Rajasthan." *South Asian History and Culture* 1(2): 315–267.

Part II

Population, Reproduction, Politics

Chapter 4

"And Never the Twain Shall Meet"

Reproductive Health Policies in the Islamic Republic of Iran

Throughout the world one of the key areas in development planning over the past four decades has been that of population regulation. Most governments have adopted some form of policy to deal with their population size, to either increase or, in the majority of cases, reduce population growth. To achieve this, the state plays an increasingly active role in the reproductive life of its citizens, intervening in various ways, directly or indirectly. Some three decades after the first World Population Conference in Bucharest (1974), trial and error, together with a considerable accumulation of new facts emerging from research at an international level, have led to a move away from treating the issue of population from a demographic perspective. The recent paradigm shift from the term reproduction to "reproductive health" and "reproductive rights" is the result of this awareness. Human reproduction is no longer treated as an isolated aspect of human life more concerned with numbers and mere economic facts but is instead placed in its broader sociocultural context. There is today universal recognition among policymakers that human reproduction is a complex and intricate process determined by a combination of biological, social, economic, and political factors, and that the dynamics of reproduction are unique in each case. At a rhetorical level, planners appear to be aware of the need to understand the underlying cultural factors which determine reproductive behavior. In practice, however, the gap between rhetoric and reality remains wide. The frequent discordance between the policies devised by health planners and realities at the grassroots level is well documented. In many cases, policies are still more concerned to educate people into their objectives, than to first gain an in-depth awareness of lived experiences on the ground. Furthermore, in many parts of the world, the traditional cultural ideologies are in conflict and compete with the modern rationalities adopted by health policymakers and planners on the basis of international agreements and guidelines. Attempts to accommodate these two worldviews often lead to the adoption of top-down policies, which in turn create further complications and discrepancies in health policies. In this chapter I will illustrate these points by examining the population policies of the Islamic Republic of Iran concerning the reproductive health of adolescents, the compromises which have made their implementation possible, and the result so far. This is not a straight case of modern health policies versus people's traditional values. The situation in Iran is further complicated by the fact that many of the traditional practices and values attached to fertility and reproduction, such as early marriage and high fertility, are encouraged by the jurisprudence (*sharia*)[1] of Islam and the Civil Code adopted by Iran (Mehryar 1998: 40). Both promote values that are in direct contradiction to those adopted by modern health policies. The chapter is divided into two parts. The first part provides a brief background of Iran's Population and Family Planning Program and its implementation. In the second part I examine the policies adopted in one of the high-priority areas of that, namely adolescents' reproductive health. The chapter will consider the three main parties involved in this process—the conservative authorities who act as the custodians of religious and traditional values, the modernizing health policymakers, and the young people who are the recipients of both ideologies. Since the focus of policies is on the reproductive health and activities of adolescents within the sanctioned rules of the society, the chapter will refer only to those areas which concern the "legitimate" and endorsed reproductive behavior and activities of young people. References to Islamic practices in this chapter are to *sharia*, which is universal and followed by all Muslims. It does not examine or compare the differences between the Shia and other Muslim sects.

The Background to the Population Policies

Iran's population policies won international acclaim for their success in reducing population growth in a dramatic fashion within a ten-year period, from 1986 to 1996. Iran received the UN Population Award for its achievement in 1998. Through the Population and Family Planning Program, according to the Statistical Center of Iran (SCI), the population growth rate, which was 3.8 in 1986, was reduced to 2.5 in 1991 and to 1.5 in 1996.[2] Following this success, the Iranian government gave high priority to reproductive health in its family planning programs and has steadily increased its budget from $US2.2 million in 1991 to $US10.7 million in 1996 (Country Report on Population, Reproductive Health, and Family Planning Program of the Islamic Republic of Iran 1998). The program's achievement is thus considered to be well ahead of the target set in the Second National Five-Year Development Plan.

Iran's family planning program was exemplary from its start in that the policies paid special attention to the cultural characteristics of the country and were carefully tailored to social, political, and religious rules, including the special requirements of the country's constitution based on *sharia* and religious teachings. By the time the International Conference on Population and Development (ICPD) took place in Cairo in 1994, the Government of Iran had already addressed and integrated the family planning program into the broader concept of reproductive health and reproductive rights. This was a remarkable achievement, and it clearly demonstrated the awareness of the health policymakers of the intricacies of human reproduction and its interaction with other social institutions.[3]

The Iranian delegation to the ICPD also played an active part in redefining the Program of Action adopted at that conference. However, it did not endorse all the topics included in its agenda. For example, while it agreed with the basic ideals of reproductive health, particularly those concerning the health of women and their right to use contraception for pregnancy prevention, it expressed reservations on some of the topics, inter alia "the redefinition of the concept of 'family' to accommodate non-marital unions," and the "recommendation of the universal exposure of all children to 'sex education' programs at an early age, as contrasted with 'an appropriate age'" (Mehryar 1998: 3). Also, in spite of the general agreement with the ICPD's Program of Action, and in spite of the fact that Iran had in theory adopted a model of reproductive health which covered the whole life span extending from birth to old age, Iran concentrated its efforts in certain areas of reproductive health only. The Draft Country Population Assessment Report mentions that "for practical reasons, including lack of resources, all areas and problems of reproductive health are not regarded as of equal concern . . . those concerning the health of mothers and children and the provision of contraceptive supplies and services have received much more attention than others" (Mehryar 1998: 4). Other areas of priority included: family planning aimed at enabling couples to make informed decisions about the number of children they wish to have; treatment of disorder resulting from unwanted pregnancies; the promotion of the reproductive health of adolescents, particularly adolescent girls, through education, information, and premarital counseling; and the promotion of healthy sexual relations within marital unions.

The Population Policies of the Islamic Republic of Iran

In general, the open-mindedness with which the Iranian government approached the family planning program was admirable. As Hoodfar (1995: 105) puts it:

> The development of population policy in the Islamic Republic of Iran provides fertile ground for re-examining the widely-held assumptions that Islamic ideology is the antithesis of modernity and incompatible with feminism. By analyzing the strategies the Islamic Republic has adopted, in order to build public consensus on the necessity of birth control and family planning, this paper [Hoodfar's] draws attention to the flexibility and adaptability of Islamic ideology to political and economic realities.

After the downfall of the Shah and the establishment of the Islamic Republic in 1979, the family planning program of the previous regime fell into disarray. The new regime did not formulate an explicit policy, and the religious authorities maintained that controlling population growth was a plot by Western powers to subjugate oppressed nations and limit the number of Muslims. High population was viewed as the sign of a strong nation and family planning clinics were dismantled. The Iran–Iraq War, which resulted in the heavy loss of approximately one million people, became an important additional reason for the justification of a pronatalist policy by the government and the religious leaders. The supreme leader of the Islamic Revolution, Ayatollah Khomeini, in his public speeches encouraged people to have large families to replace the "army of 20 million." The new regime also adopted a policy of lowering the legal age of marriage to nine years for girls and fourteen years for boys, according to Islamic teaching.[4] The above were some of the contributory factors for the rise in population growth, which became apparent in the National Census of 1986.

The National Census of 1986, which estimated the population at over fifty million, made the authorities realize the enormity of the problem they faced. The population, estimated at 25.7 million in 1966, had almost doubled in the space of two decades. In the light of massive urbanization, a depressed economy, and the demand for jobs and amenities, the high birth rate posed a palpable threat. The Islamic regime had committed itself to the protection of the oppressed and the powerless both ideologically and constitutionally and, unless it could meet some of these undertakings, it would encounter political unrest. It seemed that the government, which was predominantly formed of the clergy, had no choice but to introduce a population control policy, albeit within an Islamic framework. After lengthy negotiations between the religious leaders and planners and policymakers, such a policy was understood and endorsed by a number of the more enlightened religious leaders, who agreed to address the question of overpopulation and its dangers publicly. Ayatollah Khomeini himself discussed the necessity of family planning in Friday sermons, as did the imams of each major city in Iran. By 1988, the Board of Family Planning, with full support from the highest-ranking clergy, had begun work under the control of the Ministry of Health which launched a coordinated campaign aimed at reducing population growth.

In her analysis, Hoodfar (1995) relates the success of the campaign to two factors: first, the effort to convince the population of the necessity of family planning, and the launch of a powerful campaign to build consensus; second, the establishment of an effective network to implement the policy of educating the population, especially women, and to provide facilities such as free contraceptives. She distinguishes three broad overlapping themes in the campaign. The first was the international dimension, which addressed the consequences of increased population and argued that high population results in the dependency of the poorer nations on the rich ones. Against this background the clergy (*ulama*) allowed that Muslims could practice contraception in times of economic hardship, which Iran was now facing due to a revolution, economic sanctions imposed by the outside world, and several years of war with Iraq. The clergy even emphasized the practice of contraception as desirable/prescribed in such circumstances.

The second theme was that of family planning based on reciprocity between the government and people. The campaign pointed out that while no government could legitimately ask individuals not to have any children at all, in exchange families could not have as many children as they wanted since this would put pressure on the government and resources. If Iranians were to build a healthy, educated, and able Muslim nation, they must find a balance between their individual desires and what the nation could afford. Also, in advocating the methods of contraception, the religious authorities argued that all measures which were temporary and could be reversed (such as pills, intra-uterine devices, tubal legation) were permitted. But those which led to permanent infertility remained forbidden. Abortion, however, remained officially illegal unless the life of the mother was in danger.

The third feature of the campaign was the emphasis on the health of mothers and children. Too many children too closely spaced were considered undesirable for the mother, and the right of children to two years of breastfeeding was highlighted.

In its awareness-raising campaign, the government made funds available for research into Islamic texts to provide proof that family planning had been a concern of Islamic societies in the medieval times and long before the West started thinking about it.[5] The history of Islamic family planning was included in the national curriculum at schools, in adult literacy classes, and in local mosques. Special family planning sessions were organized for girls, for male and female workers at the industrial establishments and at urban health clinics. In rural areas, health centers and local mosques were used as a forum for family planning discussions and the media, especially women's magazines, played an important role. Contraceptives such as pills, condoms, IUDs, and injections were distributed either free or heavily subsidized. Vasectomy and tubal legations were legalized, although in practice a shortage of trained personnel meant that the latter were not always carried out and the pill became the main method of contraception. The existing health network was strengthened and included health units throughout the country both in rural and urban areas. The health workers, trained especially to work in these units, played a significant part, especially in the rural areas, in the implementation of the family planning program.

Although the sharp decline in fertility rates was considered to be the result of this well-coordinated campaign, and the Islamic Republic took credit for it, there are other views on the factors responsible for the decline. For example, Abbasi-Shavazi (2001) argues that the decline in fertility in Iran started in 1984, when the government was still in the middle of its pronatal campaign and before the official family planning program was launched in 1989.[6] In his view, the decline was not the result of the family planning campaign, although without doubt it benefited from the government's capacity to mobilize various organizations and networks and the mass media. Unlike the first pre-Revolutionary campaign launched in 1967, the 1989 campaign was implemented under conditions which were socially, culturally, and economically ready to receive it. Moreover, unlike the first program sponsored by the Shah's regime, the second had the approval and strong commitment of the clergy. The improvement of life conditions, the modernization of the infrastructure, and increased education (especially that of girls) all contributed to the fall in fertility rates. Abbasi-Shavazi (2001) argues further that the reduction of infant mortality and the possibility of a better lifestyle for their children encouraged parents to reduce the number of their children. More research is needed to confirm these theories. For example, anecdotal evidence tends to support the view that during the Iran–Iraq War years birth rates increased at all levels, including among some groups of middle-income educated people, as well as the more deprived layers of society.[7]

Whatever the reasons behind the remarkable success of the family planning program, high population growth during the years preceding its implementation in 1986 meant that the 1996 Census population pyramid showed that over 50 percent of the total population of over sixty million was under twenty years of age, and around 43 percent of this group were under fifteen years of age. It also revealed that ten- to fourteen-year-olds form the largest age group in the country, with the second largest age group, the five- to nine-year-olds, coming up right behind them (Country Report on Population, Reproductive Health, and Family Planning Program of the Islamic Republic of Iran 1998; see Figure 4.1). The same findings draw attention to the fact that the country should expect a dramatic increase in population in the coming decade when those children, born in the baby boom years of the early 1980s, reach fertility. Some other critical unresolved areas include: the high population growth in rural areas; the unsatisfactory participation of men in reproductive health and family planning programs; misconceptions about the most effective contraceptive measures such as the pill, IUD, vasectomy, and tubal legation; and finally the high

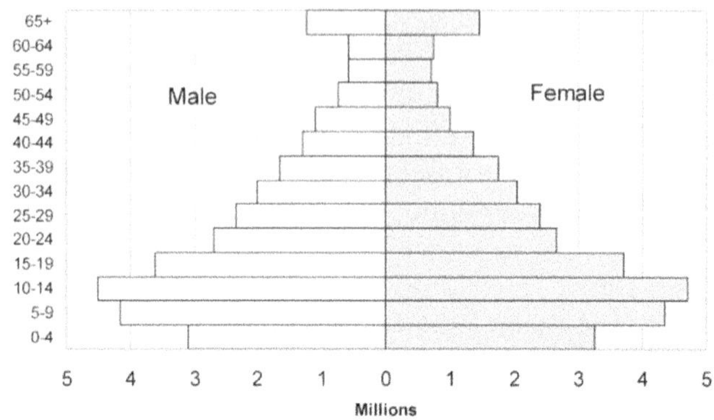

FIGURE 4.1. Population Pyramid Based on the 1996 Census. Source: Iranian Center for Statistics, also cited in Mehryar (1998)

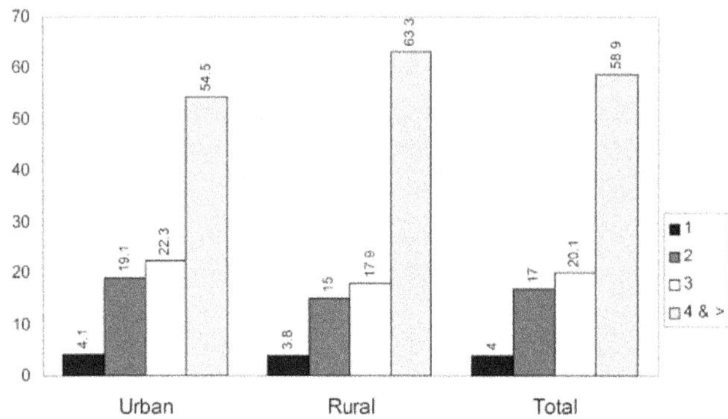

FIGURE 4.2. Distribution of Unplanned Pregnancy by Parity in 1996. Source: Family Health Department, Ministry of Health, Statistics Unit, Iran

percentage of unwanted pregnancies (see Figure 4.2). Future population estimates in 1997 were that the total population of Iran in 2001 would be 65.7 million and is expected to exceed 90 million by the year 2021, although the growth rate of population will decline but only modestly until 2016–21, during which period it is estimated that the birth rate will average around 1.4 percent per year. The population will therefore stay young for the foreseeable future.

The Modernizing Health Policies

In Iran, young people are a dynamic force whose well-being and problems present a formidable challenge to the society as a whole. The authorities are well aware that, unless they can stem population growth, they will have to face major socioeconomic and political problems, and that to control growth they must address the young people's reproductive health. Young people's reproductive health is therefore one of the most important aspects of health planning, and at the ICPD the Islamic Republic undertook the "Promotion of the reproductive health of adolescents, particularly adolescent girls, through education, information and premarital counseling, and promotion of healthy sexual relations within marital unions." The concern for "adolescents" is evident in every official document produced by the government. Various strategies have been developed to address the question of reproductive health among young people, and coordinated efforts are made between the ministries of Health, Education, the Family Planning Association and others[8] to understand and improve their sexual and reproductive health and behavior. These efforts can be summarized as follows.

Publications: A series of educational textbooks on reproductive health have been prepared for young people by Iran's Family Planning Association. These are written for ten- to fourteen- and fifteen- to nineteen-year-old girls, and fifteen- to nineteen-year-old boys, presumably on the assumption that boys under the age of fifteen years do not need to be familiarized with reproductive health matters. There are also training manuals and guidebooks for parents, teachers, and other trainers to familiarize them with the biological and psychological facts concerning the reproductive health of adolescents. Most of the literature is based on books prepared by international organizations concerned with population and reproductive health matters, including the International Planned Parenthood Federation. These texts are translated and adapted to the requirements of the Islamic Republic by the Family Planning Association of Iran (FPA).[9] The booklets have been issued at schools and other educational institutions. They have also been distributed on a door-to-door basis in various areas of Tehran. To the surprise of the official in charge of the project, the books were better received by people living in the poorer areas, and possibly with less education, than in the wealthier areas where more modern and better-educated people live. He interpreted this reaction as "people from more modest backgrounds respect authority and respond to anybody in an official capacity. They also look up to authorities and are willing to learn from them." He added that "people, especially mothers, from the more educated middle classes and from the better off layers of society were reluctant to accept the booklets and said that their children, especially daughters, were already out of control, and they did not want to encourage them to learn more on matters of sex and reproduction."

Research: A series of research projects have been carried out by the FPA. A substantial qualitative survey (focus group discussion) on the reproductive health needs of twelve- to nineteen-year-old adolescents was carried out in 1998 among boys and girls in Tehran. The conclusion in the survey on boys point out that

> the knowledge of fifteen- to nineteen-year-old boys—the future fathers—in the city of Tehran on matters of puberty, marriage, family planning and venereal disease is very low. In most cases half of the group is totally ignorant. . . . Considering that their present attitude and future practice will be a direct consequence of their knowledge and that their knowledge is relatively better than that of the corresponding age/sex group in other cities, it seems there exists a real problem. (Reproductive Health Needs Assessment of Adolescent Boys 1998: 23)

A second project was carried out in some of the northern cities of Iran among ten- to fourteen-year-olds, based on focus group discussions. This included parents and teachers as well. The aim was to find out the extent of knowledge among this age group of certain aspects of reproductive health, such as puberty, and also to explore the most suitable channels of communication with young people: whom they trust, with whom they talk, and from where they get their information. The survey was ongoing in 2000, and the results not published. The plan was to extend this kind of research to other provinces.

The outcome and recommendations of the existing surveys invariably point to the need to produce more training manuals and books and some counseling for all concerned. The survey samples also seem to be confined to students from schools and other formal teaching organizations. There are no references, for example, to young people at rehabilitation institutions, centers for runaway children, prisons, or counseling committees advising young people on marriage or divorce matters. Furthermore, the surveys are limited to certain aspects of reproductive health and do not provide a full picture of the reproductive activities of young people.

Health Records: The Educational Division of the Ministry of Health has initiated a new project to establish a baseline on all aspects of the health, both biological and psychological, of children at school. This is a kind of health log book, which will register children's existing state of health, and monitor their progress throughout their school years. The official view is that this method will allow the ministry to obtain valuable information on all aspects of health, including reproductive health of children. In the summer of 2000, the project was still at an experimental stage and the results had not been analyzed.

From the above it can be seen that the main focus of health policies is on educating the young. Implicit in this approach is the assumption that education is the best, or perhaps the only, way to help the young improve their knowledge of reproductive health matters, and that in the long run this will protect them against the hazards arising from their sexual and reproductive behavior and hopefully also reduce the fertility rates. What is missing from this equation is the recognition that the target group—twelve- to nineteen-year-olds—might already be sexually active within (or outside) wedlock. No official records refer to reproductive activities in the under-fifteen age group which take place within marriage and the approved rules of society and with the positive encouragement of the *sharia*. The 1996 Census does not include data on early marriages, pregnancies, or mother and child mortality and morbidity for this age group (Mehryar 1998),[10] although other official documents make several references to their existence. Reference in official surveys is for women over sixteen years of age. The more sensitive areas of reproductive health, such as early pregnancies among schoolgirls, HIV/AIDS, sexually transmitted diseases (STDs), abortions, and other sexual activities, such as homosexuality and prostitution, are deemed sensitive and are, understandably, missing.[11] This is not unique to Iran; the majority of states prefer not to release information on these issues.

Legitimate but Absent Reproductive Practices

We mentioned earlier that the ungrudging support of religious leaders gave legitimacy to various methods of family planning, and the condition of this consent was that the program should act within an Islamic framework. Here we examine the traditional and religious understanding of reproductive health and the boundaries the health policies are permitted in their planning in this area. When the policies refer to the reproductive health of adolescents, apart from designing schemes for educating them, they invariably raise the issue of early marriages as the only existing form of reproductive activity for this age group as if no other activity of this kind exists or is recognized and accepted. For example, according to the Draft Country Population Assessment Report (Mehryar 1998: 40), "as part of the genuine commitment to improving the reproductive health of young people, especially girls, the Civil Code in recent years has raised the age of marriage to fifteen and eighteen for girls and boys respectively." In practice however, there is to date no definite lower limit for the age of marriage other than that prescribed by Islam, and the efforts of Islamist female members of parliament to raise the age of marriage have met with strong resistance, mainly from the conservative male members, according to debates in the Iranian parliament of October 2000. The existence of early marriages is also openly acknowledged: "Because of the emphasis of Islam on early marriage and the large number of adolescent brides and grooms, the reproductive health needs of young married couples requires serious attention by the family and health system. Over the past few years, a number of steps have been taken to address these particular needs of youngsters intending to get married" (Mehryar 1998: 44). To achieve this, premarital counseling committees have been formed by the government to advise young couples on reproductive health matters, family planning, and child spacing. Although the original aim was to try and delay early marriages through counseling, in practice, and ironically, some of these committees are used as advisory committees by people who intend to marry their young children (both boys and girls). Counselors in some of the more conservative areas of the country find themselves faced with having to advise ten- to twelve-year-olds brought to them for marriage counseling.[12] This is further illustrated by the activities of various traditional and/or religious organizations aimed at encouraging traditional practices such as early marriage. For example, the charity organization known as the "Imam's Relief Committee," which periodically organizes mass marriage ceremonies for the economically deprived youth under its care, has established a premarital family planning education and counseling service for these young couples.

As well as the official sources which acknowledge the existence of early marriages, there is abundant evidence of them in the daily papers. One such report, by no means rare, recounts a case referred to the police of a ten-year-old girl and her mother beaten up by the girl's husband for refusing to do the housework because the girl wanted to play with her dolls.[13] A further confirmation of the existence of early marriages, which is also given as proof of the commitment to the education of women, is that the National Education Policy mandates schooling for married pregnant girls.

Official records exist for marriages of sixteen-year-olds and above, but no specific data exist for the age group below. Nevertheless, the indications are that not only do early marriages exist, they may even be on the increase, as is the case in the rest of the region (UNICEF 2001). A United Nations Population Fund report, for example, draws attention to the fact that statistics showing that the age of marriage is on the rise may disguise the continued practice of early marriage in certain areas or among certain population groups (Sadik 2001: 18–19). According to this report, early marriage is apparently increasing among populations under severe stress—in conflict situations, confronted by the HIV/AIDS epidemics, or facing extreme poverty. In Iran the age of marriage has gone up considerably in many areas, but the extent of the practice of early marriage varies in different provinces and among different ethnic groups. In spite of the lack of data on early marriages, it would perhaps be a safe guess that in those areas where they were traditionally practiced extensively—in the less developed and more conservative parts, and where there is perhaps more continuity than change as far as family values and fertility and reproductive practices are concerned—they still exist to a considerable extent.[14]

Ethnographic research carried out before the 1979 Revolution includes a wealth of information on early marriages. To mention one such study, research among the Bahmei tribes of Kohkiloye (a province in central southwest Iran) revealed that from a sample of 372 women interviewed, 75 percent had married before they were fifteen years old (Restrepo-Afshar 1975).[15] Kohkiloye was thought of as one of the most remote areas of Iran in the 1970s, and the existing socioeconomic indicators show that it remains one of the least developed and most conservative and traditional parts of the country. The consistency of the socioeconomic indicators between past and present may be one indication that reproductive health practices also remain consistent. This view is further substantiated by the Country Population Assessment Report (Mehryar 1998: 38), which mentions the considerable gaps that exist in the rates of maternal mortality and morbidity between different provinces. The report gives details of prevalence and cites as an example the percentage of births unattended by trained personnel in some rural areas such as Sistan and Baluchestan (80 percent), Kohkiloye and Boyerahmadi (61 percent), and Hormozgan (56 percent). A final insight into the prevalence of traditional family structures comes from research on female suicide (usually by self-immolation) in Kohkiloye, where the rate is among the highest in the country. The persistence of strong patriarchal values, and their clash with the changes (albeit limited) brought about by development, are cited by some as the causes of these suicides.[16] Similar observations could be extended to some other provinces such as Ilam and Kordestan.

In spite of the absence of reliable data, all the indications point to the practice of early marriages, and an in-depth investigation of the extent as well as the context in which they happen is crucial to throw new light and open new avenues for health policies.

The Adolescents

The agenda of health policymakers is to modernize societies with the general well-being and "improvement" of life conditions in mind. Opposition to modernization and development usually comes from the conservative forces in society. These too have the "well-being" of people in mind and are anxious to achieve it by trying to preserve the continuity of traditional cultural practices. In the case of population and health planning in Iran, the clash between tradition and modernity does not begin or end with planners versus people, on a straight line with two forces pulling in two different directions. There is a third force, namely the massive group of adolescents, the recipients of both ideologies, which is changing the shape of the confrontation into a triangle.

The young form a formidable and dynamic force in Iran, with 50 percent under twenty years of age, 43 percent of these under fifteen years of age, and 27 percent (nearly sixteen million) in the ten- to nineteen-year-old age range. Overlooking the importance of in-depth research on the social and cultural factors which determine sexual and reproductive practices can but contribute toward their perpetuation. Devising policies on the assumption that adolescents are passive consumers of policies and hoping that through coercion (by the conservative forces) or education (by the health planners) only, the aims of health policies will be achieved goes beyond the bounds of optimism and any vision these ideologies may have for resolving the question of high fertility growth. Their project, in other words, becomes utopian.

Notwithstanding socioeconomic and cultural differences, and ethnic and regional variations, this massive group of young people has one thing in common: its exposure to the outside world through education, urbanization, the media, and the general process of globalization, which have created certain common values and aspirations among them. Young people play an active role both in reconstituting the traditions they inherit and in negotiating the modern values that are imposed on them. They react in a variety of ways to both ideologies, if these do not fit in with their own social realities and ideals. Even though they may not always have the power to fully control their lives, they use whatever means are available to them to find ways of reshaping them. Their reactions vary and can generate a range of responses from inventiveness and imagination to resourcefulness and adaptation. There is abundant evidence that in Iran the social world of young people does not necessarily match that of either authorities, and this is reflected in a variety of ways. It is, however, beyond the scope of this chapter to elaborate on this fascinating issue. In what follows I shall concentrate on the fundamental cause of the polarity of reproductive ideologies that has resulted in a widespread malaise among all concerned.

Age Categories and Gender Roles

The persistence of traditional reproductive practices, and the obvious reluctance of policymakers to admit that there are "children" who are married and have children, and/or are, "legitimately" or "illegitimately," sexually active, is not just a matter of the dichotomy arising from the struggle between the traditional values and modern practices. Society has its own understanding of the concept of age, and of gender roles within this. Age categories and gender relations are closely intertwined, and both reflect and determine the ideology a community holds of its identity and reproduction.

The understanding and interpretation of age categories vary greatly across cultures and remain a universal dilemma for policymakers. The rapid changes in transitional societies have created an inevitable clash between the modern and the traditional worldviews. Factors referred to earlier such as urbanization, globalization, the influence of the media, and the increase in consumerism, combined with better access to education, and improvement in some aspects of health, have created similar trends worldwide. The apparent similarity of these trends has been taken as a cue by policymakers to search for universal solutions. In an effort to respond to the needs of different groups, universal age categories such as "children," "young people," "adolescents," "youth," and "young adults," have been identified, without differentiating the specific social and cultural contexts which determine these categories. The discrepancies which exist between the international definitions of children, young people, teenagers, and other age categories on the one hand, and local practices and values as far as life trajectories are concerned on the other hand, are creating constraints at several levels. What definitions of this kind do not take into account is the extent to which such terms are social and cultural constructs grounded in their unique historical and economic settings (Harcourt 1997: 11). For example, while according to the Convention on the Rights of the Child, anyone under the age of eighteen is a child, in many developing countries married twelve-year-old girls are considered adults, while a seventeen-year-old boy at school is considered a child.[17] Likewise, the concept of adolescence needs clarification in its specific context. Indeed, it is a relatively new one in most cultures. Even in the West it has a history of a hundred years or so and has been introduced to non-Western cultures exposed to development through the process of modernity (Harcourt 1997: 12).

The 1989 Convention on the Rights of the Child defines a child as anybody under the age of eighteen. Although Iran is a signatory to this convention, it has reserved the right not to apply some of the clauses if they contradict Islamic standards and internal laws and practices of the country. For example, the Iranian delegation to the convention maintained that *sharia* provides clear instructions for the responsibilities and conduct of people, and in some instances these do not accord with international agreements. A review of the Iranian laws concerning children reveals that there is no clear definition of the end of childhood; a child can be considered a child in one context and an adult in another. For example, a ten-year-old girl is considered to have reached puberty (according to Islam) and therefore to be eligible for marriage and commercial transaction. However, the same girl cannot be employed according to the labor law, which stipulates a minimum age of fifteen, or obtain a passport or driving license. Although a nine-year-old girl can get married and have children, she is not eligible to vote (the age of voting is currently set at fifteen), in spite of the fact that she has the status of a full adult. In the area of criminal law, a ten-year-old girl and a fifteen-year-old boy are liable to sentences similar to a full adult. In theory they can be sentenced to death, although in practice such a sentence has not happened. In a case of theft, a nine-year-old girl and fifteen-year-old boy can be sentenced in the same way as a forty-year-old man. A recent report from UNICEF (1998) mentions that the minimum age for sentencing children has now been raised to fifteen.

Adjusting the Islamic worldview of age to recent changes in the position and status of children is a difficult process and it will take some time for these to filter down into the traditional and conservative values and alter them. The obvious conflict between the two sets of values is summarized in the findings of the survey on Reproductive Health Needs Assessment of Adolescent Boys (1998), which reveals the resentment of young people about their confused status in society: the young lamented that "generally there is a lack of respect for young people from parents and teachers in the society"; that "adults don't pay enough attention to our ideas"; that "there is a lack freedom, especially for girls, and restrictions in making contact with the opposite sex."

Gender

Concepts of gender and gender roles are closely linked to age, universally. Islamic scholars have debated the issues of gender and Islam exhaustively, and I shall not elaborate in detail on them. In summary, in Islam, women are viewed as responsible for the protection of family and the preservation of its rules. The traditional view of marriage is directly linked to the formation of family; the desirable age of marriage and the way in which a spouse is selected depend on a society's view of the family, its role, structure, pattern of life, and the individual and collective responsibilities of its members. The idea and function of "family" varies across the world and is in a state of constant evolution. Traditionally, marriage and the formation of marital unions in the patriarchal Muslim societies were viewed as transactions, with female sexuality as a commodity traded by men. In an essay on female sexuality, Moghadam (1994) addresses the issue of its ownership and argues that the legal commoditization of female sexuality should be incorporated into the analysis of gender economics in Muslim societies.[18] Moghadam

(1994: 83) defines the concept of commodity as follows: "an object that is voluntarily bought and sold at an agreed price is a commodity. Once the sale transaction is completed, the original owner loses ownership, and the buyer becomes owner of the commodity. . . . With few modifications, the concepts of commodity and regulation can be used for the discussion of female sexuality in Islam." Haeri (1989) also argues that in Islam permanent marriage is a sale and temporary marriage (mainly practiced among the Shia Muslims) is a lease of female sexuality. In her analysis of marriage, Mir-Hosseini (1993: 1) in addition considers the two aspects of Islamic law: the "temporal" and the "religious." She argues that the boundaries of "sacred" and "temporal" are blurred in the case of family law, for which divine revelations are abundant: "Islamic family law is permeated with religious ideals and ethical values; it holds within itself a distinct model of family and gender relations. This model is claimed to be divinely ordained and, thus, immutable." Mernissi (1975) too argues that in Islam the male-female relationship is assumed to be highly sexual, and that female sexuality needs to be kept under control.[19] While there are very few areas of prohibition on the sexual activities of men, whether before or after marriage, sexual prohibitions abound for women and concern them in the main. Development has brought about fundamental changes in the lives of women. Female education, general improvement in women's health, and above all the increasing recognition of the value of women's economic contribution and their participation in the labor market have led to a certain freedom and power to control their own lives. These changes have restricted some of the control that men have had on women and have left them in a state of bewilderment. The consequences of such perplexity are reflected in a drastic increase in the rate of divorce, violence against women, and general social disorder, resulting in the shattering of family structure in Iran.[20] An increasing number of girls, under pressure and suffering violence from the male members of their family, choose to run away from home, and many (both boys and girls) end up in prostitution or get caught up in the trafficking of children. As Jo Boyden (2001: 177) puts it, "along with concerns about violence, crime, and subversive youth cultures, sexuality and reproduction are the spheres of youth activity and attitude that provoke the greatest moral panic and receive the greatest attention from researchers."

Policies at Odds with Themselves

Considering the genuine concern for and the amount of effort and planning put into the reproductive health of adolescents, it is ironic that it is the realities of the life of this very age group, and its reproductive experiences, which are left out of official data altogether. The unease with which the reproductive health policies approach the issue mirrors the tension between conservative and reformist forces in the society. The risks of early marriages and negative effects of early pregnancies on the physical and mental health and schooling of adolescents are well-known to health policymakers. The dilemma created by having to define their policies within an Islamic framework, and to accommodate what they themselves judge to be right, has therefore been solved through compromises, made at the cost of any acknowledgment of the sexual and reproductive health activities of the largest age group in the country; by, in other words, turning a blind eye to the actual sexual and reproductive life of young adolescents. On the one hand, any form of sexual and reproductive activity outside wedlock for young people is considered "pathological" and a real threat to the stability of society by the conservative forces. Premarital sex and reproduction by adolescents, especially girls, is socially prohibited and subject to severe punishment (Mehryar 1998: 40). On the other hand, the truth about the sexual and reproductive life of young adolescents, even their legitimate activities, seems to be too embarrassing for the modernizing policymakers to include in their data. The traditional practice of becoming sexually active at an early age under the weight of tradition and religion is deemed "pathological" by modern standards, as is promiscuous sex because of the health dangers it represents. Therefore, the compromise adopted by planners is that this age group (under fifteen years) has not yet entered sexually active life, and all it needs is education to familiarize it with its reproductive functions. Consequently, the issue of adolescent sexuality and problems associated with it are somehow ignored either by society and/or the health system. Health planners use innuendo to present the facts without being seen to put their seal of approval on them. The diffident tone of some of the health policy documents testifies to this search for acceptable ways forward. Young people, who are at the receiving end of conflicting messages, remain confused as to their identity and status in the society. Their behavior is considered pathological by both sides. Disagreements and contradictions between the two sets of values abound, and the sensitivity of the subject remains one of the major obstacles with regards to adolescent reproductive health.

There are two further obstacles in this process. First, while some information and insight into the sexual and reproductive life of young people does exist, it is incomplete. Little effort has been made to analyze what material is available or to provide quantifiable material for the policymakers to include in their data. It is often inherent in the nature of policymaking at a macro level that, unless facts can be quantified, they are of little consequence and not worth planning for. Information at a micro level is rarely treated with respect or considered relevant. The second factor is indirect resistance on the part of many of those responsible for planning or the implementation of plans, especially those who belong to the more conservative layers of society, who themselves remain unconvinced by modern policies. Many of these people, at heart, support the old values of family and fertility.

Conclusion

The preceding discussions suggest that in designing and implementing development projects, discord arises between the forces of conservatism trying to preserve the national identity, rooted in tradition, and policymakers who seek to "better" life conditions through modernization. In the case of the Population and Family Planning Program of the Islamic Republic of Iran, the usual pattern of the state versus people is further complicated by the presence of a third force, young people whose reproductive health is identified as one of the most important areas of health planning, and who are caught in the conflict between the state and its planners. The underlying factors responsible for the clash between the state and its policymakers are, above all, due to the fundamental and ideological differences between the two worldviews of society, of family structures and marriage, of age, and of gender roles within this, between conservative and modernists. The question arises as to why the same authorities, who agreed to the implementation of an enlightened and successful family planning program during its first phase, have reverted to an Islamic framework during the second phase, and are now creating restriction for policymakers. The case of Iran's population and family planning is a clear example of the interaction between politics and reproduction.

While no attempt has been made to develop a political framework for the analysis of the reproductive health policies of the Islamic Republic in this chapter, it hints at the clash between the agenda of the religious political elite and that of the modernizing bureaucrats. During the years of rapid population growth, the religious leaders, as political leaders, agreed to a population control program which they justified in the name of Islam to build up a strong, well-educated and healthy nation. To ignore population growth would in reality have meant a serious political threat to the regime and its ideology. The first phase of these population policies went ahead relatively smoothly. But, at a later stage when it became necessary to gain a real understanding of reproductive practices as lived at the grassroots, inconsistencies and conflicts between the two ideologies began to emerge. The conservative and religious leaders continued with their active support for traditional family structure and sexual and reproductive practices. In the meantime, modernity, inevitably, has disrupted these systems and alienated young people from the traditional systems of support. With the change in life conditions, young people no longer have the opportunity to learn from their parents and grandparents, and the new channels of information such as school, media, and the peer group can only provide partial information.

The authorities' (both conservative and modern) method of treating young people as children and ignorant and in need of teaching and guardianship, while they are expected to play several roles as both adults and children at the same time, has created a confusing situation for all concerned. Evidence shows that young people, of any age, play an active part in shaping their own lives, and that their behavior represents a wide range of experiences, which go beyond the "pathological" and demonstrate a profound desire to assert their existence.

Several themes emerge from the discussion: (i) attempts to devise policies for young people's sexual and reproductive life without a profound understanding of the social and cultural context in which they live are a barren exercise; (ii) a dimension often overlooked in the implementation of policies is that the attempt to teach the young the biological facts of reproduction in the hope that they will reduce their fertility does not necessarily lead to a reduction in the number children they wish to have. Decisions on sexual and reproductive activities are not easily influenced by outside factors, unless these correspond to people's own social realities and ideals; (iii) that the encounter of top-down policies with local realities tends to provoke reactions which may not be direct and active, but passive and indirect, often frustrating policies without being seen to be confrontational. In the case of Iran, active confrontation of young people against either old or modern values is on the increase in most spheres of life.

The example of Iran is by no means unique, and will be familiar to many researchers, policymakers, implementers, and to the young themselves throughout the world. The analysis of the Iranian case is used to unravel the particular model of interaction when policies meet local realities. In another context, the components may be different, but will the result differ? The question remains: will the encounter of policy with local reality ever produce the "desired" effect? Or will it continue to provoke reactions and create new and unforeseen situations, positive or negative? Perhaps the answer can be found in the following passage by David Parkin (2001: xii): "the management of reproductive life is not just a matter of formal systems of authority, control, and knowledge transmission, nor of following policy-makers' directives, nor even of integrating these with indigenous ones. It also extends to recognizing the metaphysical and cosmological understandings and practices that everywhere accompany rules, plans, and policies."

Acknowledgments

This chapter was published originally as "'And Never the Twain Shall Meet': Reproductive Health Policies in the Islamic Republic of Iran." In *Reproductive Agency, Medicine and the State: Cultural Transformations in Childbearing*, ed. Maya Unnithan-Kumar, 181–202. New York and Oxford: Berghahn Books (2004).

Notes

1. Although there is a distinct difference between *sharia* (revealed law) and *fiqh* (jurisprudence), the lines between the two are blurred. As Mir-Hosseini (1993: 5) explains, "Muslims do not normally distinguish between [the two], especially at the popular level." In Mir-Hosseini's (1993: 5) words, a distinction between the two is "central to the concept of law in Islam. . . . *Sharia* is law in the sense that it contains a divine blueprint for mankind, for both this world and the other. It is . . . the Will of God for humanity. *Fiqh*, which contains the letter of the

law, is, in Coulson's (1969: 2) words, 'the whole process of intellectual activity which ascertains and discovers the terms of divine will and transforms them into a system of legally enforceable rights and duties.'"

2. Different sources give different figures for the population growth rate, but in this chapter, I shall use the figures given by the Statistical Center of Iran, as used in the Draft Country Population Assessment Report (Mehryar 1998).
3. Homa Hoodfar has written extensively on this topic; see, for example, Hoodfar (1995). See also Makhlouf (1994).
4. See also Abbasi-Shavazi (2001).
5. See also Makhlouf (1991: 42–43) for an explanation of the history of family planning in Islam: "a clear consensus exists among all schools of Islamic law that family planning is permissible. This is based both on the absence of any prohibition against birth control in the Qur'an and on general statements in the Qur'an that God does not want to burden man but wishes to improve his life. More specifically, statements in the Hadith indicate that withdrawal (*azl*) was practiced in the Mohammad's time and that he did not discourage his followers from the practice." As Makhlouf (1991) points out, the Sunni and Shia positions on birth control are in substance the same. They derive from the work of Al-Ghazali, the most celebrated theologian of Islam, who establishes five reasons for which birth control may be allowed.
6. This view is also supported by the Draft Country Population Assessment Report (Mehryar 1998: 21).
7. The assumption cannot be made that the rise in population was happening among the poorer layers of the society only, or that the prospect of a better future had made people reduce the number of their children. Interviews with several middle-class and educated families in Tehran revealed that they had increased the number of their children. They explained this by saying, "We have just had a revolution and there is the war with Iraq. As a result, we are all out of jobs. All this will come to an end sooner or later, and we shall eventually return to work. It is a good idea to have several children now, so that by the time everything returns to normal our children will be grown up, and can help us." These quotes are from personal interviews in Tehran, conducted between 1984 and 1985.
8. Several of the United Nations agencies, especially the United Nations Population Fund, the World Health Organization, UNICEF, and the International Planned Parenthood Federation, have played an active role and closely co-operated with the Iranian authorities in their Population and Family Planning Program.
9. Iran's Family Planning Association, which is the Iranian branch of the International Planned Parenthood Federation, has been the main body writing and translating informative and teaching materials, and also carrying out research on young people.

10. Also, during an interview with officials at the Ministry of Health, it was stressed that marriages or pregnancies among the under-fifteen age group do not exist. Interviews in the summer of 2000 with marriage counselors in some of the provinces, on the other hand, confirmed that these are practiced and are not rare incidents.
11. For reference to the sensitivity of the issue elsewhere, see, for example, Mensch et al. (2001).
12. Personal interviews with counselors, August 2000.
13. *Kayhan*, London weekly newspaper, October 2001.
14. An April 2002 report issued by the Chief of Police for Greater Tehran mentions that the number of runaway children is increasing drastically, and that in the last four months alone 6,156 children have run away from home.
15. In addition, there exists a wealth of ethnographic research carried out before the 1979 Revolution, by Iranian and foreign researchers, which inter alia include ample references to the practice of early marriage. For example, see the series of monographs published by the Institute for Social Research of the Faculty of Social Sciences, University of Tehran, before the 1979 Islamic Revolution. These studies were led by H. Keshavarz for the rural areas and by Naderi Restrepo-Afshar for the tribal and pastoral nomads.
16. The main source of information is research carried out by the sociologist Jaleh Shadi Talab. Various sources, too numerous to cite here, confirm these findings. One might also point to the many articles published in Iranian journals and magazines that alert the authorities to these problems.
17. For more details on this subject, see Tremayne (2001).
18. For more information on this topic, see Moghadam (1994).
19. See also Afkhami (1994).
20. Iran is considered to have one of the highest rates of divorce in the world after the United States. One in every ten marriages ends in divorce.

References

Abbasi-Shavazi, Mohammad Jalal. 2001. "La fecondité en Iran: l'autre revolution" [Fertility in Iran: The other revolution]. *Population et Société* 373.

Afkhami, Mahnaz. 1994. "Women in Post-Revolutionary Iran: A Feminist Perspective." In *In the Eye of the Storm: Women in Post-Revolutionary Iran*, ed. Mahnaz Afkhami and Erika Friedl, 5–18. London: I.B. Tauris.

Boyden, Jo. 2001. "Scientific Conceptualisations of Childhood and Youth: Trends and Issues." In *Managing Reproductive Life: Cross-Cultural Themes in Fertility and Sexuality*, ed. Soraya Tremayne, 175–193. Oxford: Berghahn Books.

Coulson, Noel J. 1969. *Conflicts and Tensions in Islamic Jurisprudence*. Chicago: University of Chicago Press.

Country Report on Population, Reproductive Health, and Family Planning Program of the Islamic Republic of Iran. 1998. Prepared by Family Health Department, Undersecretary for Public Health, Ministry of Health and Medical Education, Islamic Republic of Iran.

Haeri, Shahla. 1989. *The Law of Desire: Temporary Marriage in Iran*. London: I.B. Tauris.

Harcourt, Wendy. 1997. "An Analysis of Reproductive Health: Myths, Resistance and New Knowledge." In *Power, Reproduction and Gender: The International Transfer of Knowledge*, ed. Wendy Harcourt, 8–34. London: Zed Books.

Hoodfar, Homa. 1995. "Population Policy and Gender Equity in Post-Revolutionary Iran." In *Family, Gender and Population in the Middle East: Policies in Context*, ed. Carla Makhlouf. Cairo: American University of Cairo Press.

Makhlouf, Carla. 1991. "Women, Islam and Population: Is the Triangle Fateful?" Working Series Paper No. 6. Harvard: Harvard School of Public Health, Harvard University.

———. 1994. "Reproductive Choice in Islam: Gender and State in Iran and Tunisia." *Studies in Family Planning* 25(1): 41–51.

Mehryar, Amir. 1998. *Country Population Assessment Report*. Plan Organization of Islamic Republic of Iran, unpublished draft with limited circulation.

Mensch, Barbara S., Wesley H. Clark, Cynthia B. Lloyd, and Annabel S. Erulkar. 2001. "Premarital Sex, Schoolgirl Pregnancy, and School Quality in Rural Kenya." *Studies in Family Planning* 32(4): 285–301.

Mernissi, Fatima. 1975. *Beyond the Veil: Male-Female Dynamics in Modern Muslim Society*. Bloomington: Indiana University Press.

Mir-Hosseini, Ziba. 1993. *Marriage on Trial: A Study of Islamic Family Law*. London: I.B. Tauris.

Moghadam, Fatemeh E. 1994. "Commoditisation of Sexuality and Female Labour Participation in Islam: Implications for Iran, 1960–90." In *In the Eye of the Storm: Women in Post-Revolutionary Iran*, ed. Mahnaz Afkhami and Erika Friedl. London: I. B. Tauris.

Parkin, David. 2001. "Foreword." In *Managing Reproductive Life: Cross-Cultural Themes in Sexuality and Fertility*, ed. Soraya Tremayne, iix–xii. Oxford: Berghahn Books.

Reproductive Health Needs Assessment of Adolescent Boys. 1998. Family Planning Association of the Islamic Republic of Iran.

Restrepo-Afshar, Naderi E. 1975. "Le Mariage dans la Tribu Bahmei (Kohgiluye-Iran)" [Marriage in the Bahmei Trible (Kohgiluye-Iran)]. Unpublished thesis. Université de Paris VII.

Sadik, Nafis. 2001. "Working Towards Gender Equality in Marriage." *Early Marriage: Child Spouses*. Innocenti Digest no. 7. UNICEF. Florence: Innocenti Research Center.

Tremayne, Soraya. 2001. "Introduction." In *Managing Reproductive Life: Cross-Cultural Themes in Fertility and Sexuality*, ed. Soraya Tremayne, 17–29. Oxford: Berghahn Books.

UNICEF. 1998. "The Situation of Children and the Young in Iran." Iranian Office of UNICEF.

———. 2001. *Early Marriage: Child Spouses*. Innocenti Digest no. 7. Florence: Innocenti Research Center.

Chapter 5

"As List E Karhayee Ke Bayad Anjame Midadam Khat Khord"

Contemporary Reproductive Body Politic in Iran

Demographic reviews of the family planning program of the Islamic Republic of Iran (1986–2006) and its outstanding success, as well as of the population policies of the pre-Revolutionary regime of the Pahlavi Dynasty, are abundant (see e.g., Hoodfar 1995, 2017). They clearly reflect the efforts made by the state to affect the nation's reproductive behavior for the purpose of nation-building. However, the long-term engagement of the state with population issues, which goes back further and dates to the late nineteenth century under the Qajar Dynasty, has not received the same exposure. In total, Iran has had five different approaches to population issues, each contradicting the previous one, but all aimed at nation-building, and remaining consistent in targeting women as the main agents responsible for ensuring the success of the policies. Today, Iran's population growth has fallen below the replacement level as many young people either have one child or none at all, a fact that has spurred the state to step in once more and adopt a pronatalist policy.

After a brief review of the past policies, this chapter uses the lens of involuntary childlessness to understand why, in a country where young generations choose voluntary childlessness, or decide to have one child only, so many women undergo hard and costly infertility treatment. By selecting two cases of infertile women, it hopes to show some of the complexities and competing demands on young people of reproductive age, the reasons for their resistance to childbearing, and the compromises they make to accommodate the pressures and expectations of family, kin, society, and the state. Young women, should they choose to have a child, justify it by saying, "*As list e karhayee ke bayad anjame midadam khat khord,*" or "I crossed it off the 'to-do' list." The chapter concludes by asking whether the new forms of resistance are a phase or are here to stay.

Introduction

On 10 October 2012, the Supreme Religious Leader of Iran, Ayatollah Ali Khamenei, did something he had rarely, if ever, done: he admitted to making a mistake. During a speech in the Khorasan province (northeast Iran), he said, "One of the mistakes we made in the nineties was population control. Government officials were wrong on this matter, and I, too, had a part. May God and history forgive us" (Karami 2012).

Following this admission, on 25 May 2014, he moved to end the two-decade-old policy of controlled population growth. He announced a fourteen-point General Population Policy decree calling on the government to take measures to ensure a higher birth rate: "On the issue of population, we should take care not to make mistakes which were made in recent years because the best situation for the enemy is a sparsely populated Iran with the elderly forming the majority of the population" (Center for Human Rights in Iran 2016).

Both the Supreme Religious Leader and then-president Mahmoud Ahmadinejad, who called the previous family planning program "ungodly" and a "Western import," were alarmed by the 2011 census showing a drastic drop in the rate of population growth, which stood at 1.3, a decline to below the replacement level (World Bank 2011). The "ungodly" "Western import" was the family planning program launched by the Islamic Republic itself in 1986, with the aim of reducing population growth, which at the time was increasing at the rate of 3.9 per annum. This program proved so successful that it brought the rate down to 2.0 in 1996, and then to 1.3. One of the leading Iranian demographers, Mohammad Jalal Abbasi-Shavazi, refers to this decline as "confounding all conventional wisdom" and explains, "the fertility rate in the Islamic Republic of Iran fell from around 7.0 births per woman in the early 1980s to 1.9 births per woman in 2006. That this, the largest and fastest fall in fertility ever recorded, should have occurred in one of the world's few Islamic republics demands explanation" (Abbasi-Shavazi, McDonald, and Hosseini-Chavoshi 2009: v).[1]

The History of Population Policies up to the Islamic Revolution

Most recorded information on population growth or decline in Iran dates to the launch of the family planning program in 1967 under the Pahlavi regime (1925–79), which aimed at reducing the population growth rate of 3.1 per annum. Iran's participation in the Third International Population Conference in Bucharest in 1974 strengthened the country's commitment to reducing the population growth further by linking the issue of population to economic development. However, this program was intended primarily for the urban middle classes and was not as successful as it might have been, due to this top-down orientation and to a distinct lack of sensitivity toward the persisting core values attached to high fertility (Hoodfar 1995; Tremayne 2004).

However, the awareness and interest of the state in achieving an ideal size of population as a component of nation-building was not new (Kashani-Sabet 2011). It dates to the nineteenth century, under the Qajar Dynasty (1785–1925). Although no substantial information exists on the demographic characteristics of the population at the time, during this period the state of the health of the population was seen as having depleted so alarmingly that by 1874 the state became actively involved in trying to improve the health of the population through promoting good hygiene. It did not formulate an explicit policy to increase population. Instead, in its pronatalist stance it focused on maternal and child health, which became the core of a hygiene movement, with health and reproduction being closely linked together. According to Firoozeh Kashani-Sabet (2011: 5), when concerns surrounding the depletion of the population were most strident, the state's pronatalist policies did not resort to formal laws regarding childbirth and its arguments were not solely based on Western concepts. Instead, the state's discourse was based on the importance of mothers' health, which appealed to Iranians because such themes could be adapted to the more familiar Islamic injunctions regarding parenting and maternity. Moreover, the awareness of women's health and infant mortality, which can be situated in the nineteenth century, brings

TABLE 5.1. Iran: Population According to Successive Censuses.

Census Year	Population	Average Annual Growth (percent)	Populations Density/km²	Proportion Urban (percent)	Household Size
1956	18,954,704	—	12	31.4	
1966	25,785,210	3.1	16	~37.5	
1976	33,708,744	2.7	20	47	5.02
1986	49,445,010	3.9	30	~54.0	5.11
1996	60,055,488	2	36	~61.0	4.84
2006	70,495,782	1.6	43	68.5	4.03
2011	75,149,669	1.3	46	71.4	3.55
2014	80,840,713	1.22	49	71.4	3

Source: United Nations (2016)

maternalism to the heart of modern Iranian thought, concepts of nationhood, and tasks of a modern government.

As the pronatalist campaign under the Qajars emphasized the importance of building up a healthy nation, so under the Pahlavi dynasty (1925–79) policies linked population to building up a prosperous nation, this time emphasizing economic development. Explicit policies did not begin until 1964 when, reversing the Qajar view, excessive population growth became a cause of concern. The state acknowledged the necessity of a family planning program as a human right and emphasized its social and economic benefits for families and society (Roudi-Fahimi 2002, 2012). Here again, women became the prime target of program efforts, with the improvement of maternal and child health reiterated as the vehicle for integrating their agency into the national interest. In the period from the late 1960s to the late 1970s, the dramatic decline in Iran's rate of population growth was initiated, as can be seen in Table 5.1.

In sum, attitudes and policies over a very long period show that in Iran the question of population and its size remained linked inextricably to politics, and that regardless of the nature of the government, influencing population size remained a political objective. While on one side, arguments in favor of reducing the number of children maintained that an over-populated country remained weak, poor, and dependent (on the West), the same threat was used when encouraging people to have more children, so that the country did not become weak, dependent, and subject to attacks by foreign powers. Two common points emerge, regardless of whether governments were pro- or anti-natalist. First, at no point did these campaigns resort to coercive measures—unlike, for example, the pronatalist policies of Ceausescu in Romania, or the anti-natalist one-child policy in China. Arguments used in Iran have been based on advocacy, emphasizing reproduction as a core cultural value. The ideals of helping build a strong nation are presented, to varying degrees, as the responsibility of each individual. The second common point, more particularly, is that the key individuals to which policies have been addressed were women, who were seen directly or indirectly as the main agents responsible for policy success or failure.

The pronatalist policies of the early years of the Islamic Republic of Iran continued these themes, at first reversing previous pronatalism, before then returning to it, and later again embracing pronatalism. Initially, there was not a coherent policy. The new Islamic Republic simply dismantled the family planning centers, while Ayatollah Khomeini encouraged people to have more children so that Iran could have "an army of 20 million" (a reference to the necessity of having a large army during the Iran–Iraq War of 1980–88). A second, anti-natalist phase, from 1986, while installing some disincentives to childbearing, did not make it compulsory for people to reduce the number of children they wanted. It argued that, by having fewer children, the country could remain independent, not poor and subject to the colonial powers. Finally, the current return to pronatalist policies has also been based on the ideals of nationhood and citizenship. Interestingly, unlike the previous campaign, the authorities now seem to resort less to religious arguments to promote growth, as the previous campaign had already exhausted them in arguing in favor of reducing population growth. We now look in turn at each recurring *volte face*.

The Islamic Revolution (1979 to Date)

The period since the Islamic Revolution has witnessed the radical fall of fertility from over six births per woman, to less than two. The remarkable character of this decline, when compared to fertility change in other regions, is evident in Figure 5.1. Yet the progression of population policies over the same period did not follow the same seemingly smooth trend of the decline. Under the Republic, family planning programs have undergone three contradictory phases.

Phase 1 (1979–1986)

In the early days of the Islamic Revolution, Ayatollah Khomeini ordered family planning programs to be closed, explicitly encouraging larger families and reminding women that their role, above all, was that of being a good mother and of producing and bringing up children. The Republic lowered the age of marriage to nine for girls and to fifteen for boys, in keeping with Islamic law (*sharia*). It also offered maternity benefits, provided incentives for families to have more children, and outlawed sterilization and abortion, which are not allowed unconditionally under Iranian law. Among other propaganda, the walls of the cities were covered with the slogan, "Paradise is at mothers' feet." This phrase has been interpreted in different ways by Muslim scholars from different countries. In its Iranian context, it is understood to convey the message that bringing up children fit to go to paradise is in the mothers' gift: responsibility for shaping the nation's children rests with women.

Phase 2 (1986–2006)

This phase substantially reversed Phase 1, aiming to control population growth. Health planners and policymakers responsible for the implementation of the family planning program now collaborated with leading Islamic jurists to justify the aims of the program. The jurists, in their deliberations on the permissibility of family planning, relied on scholarly Islamic sources, concluding that the faith does not necessarily advocate large families, but encourages better quality of life and health for mothers and their children. They insisted that this is best achieved by having fewer children (Makhlouf-Obermeyer 1991; Hoodfar 1995). The program, again recognizing that to succeed required the inclusion and cooperation of women, placed great importance on addressing women directly and making them responsible. Interestingly, trying to persuade women to have fewer children proved to be an easier ask than anticipated—as long as women could justify family planning to their husbands, a considerable number of whom were not happy with the motto of the campaign, which was "Two children only." However, the endorsement of the religious authorities at the highest level gave the women the license they needed to stand up to their men and tell them that "*agha*" (meaning "Sir," referring to Ayatollah Khomeini) had himself said that women should not have more than two children.

The author's research over the past three decades shows that almost none of the tens of women interviewed wanted many children, but they had no real way of standing up to their husbands if they insisted on larger families. This tendency varied substantially by social class, level of education, and degree of conservatism. The educated, secular, middle classes had started reducing the number of their children before the campaign of 1986 (Ladier-Fouladi 1997; Abbasi-Shavazi 2001; Tremayne 2004). Even eight years into the family planning program, the author came across such women, who were subjected to violence and having their contraceptive pills taken away by their husbands. Often these women conspired with the health workers, who gave them pills, which they then hid from their husbands. A more nuanced discussion of why some women nonetheless submitted to their husbands' demands for more children can be found elsewhere (Tremayne 2006).[2]

The educational strand of the campaign also played a crucial role in anchoring the value of having smaller families. A noticeable outcome has been the emergence of greater uniformity in the childbearing values among the young generation of reproductive age, regardless of their social and educational background. This was reflected in the census of 2011 and, indeed, the 2016 census: by that time, rates of growth had moved substantially below replacement level, being even lower in rural areas (at 0.73) than urban (at 1.2); the rate of total growth (at 1.2) had, however, risen slightly higher than in 2011 (Statistical Center of Iran 2016). These results were also confirmed, for example, by the findings of a survey carried out by the Iranian Center for Research on Asian and Oceanic Population:

> Those couples who have just married and those who have been married for up to three years show no inclination to have any children at all, or perhaps just one. This tendency over the past decade illustrates that for women of urban and rural backgrounds, from different social classes, the poor and the rich, illiterate and literate, all have a similar attitude to giving birth these days, leading to the rapid downward trend in the Iranian TFR [total fertility rate]. (Tabnak 2013)

To illustrate the impact of education on children, in 1997 (over a decade after the start of the 1986 campaign), when the author was on a mission working with the Iranian Bureau of Women's Affairs, several female employees of the Bureau, most of whom were of conservative, if not fundamentalist, upbringing, related that their children now come back from school to tell them, "Please don't have more than two children. We are ashamed to go to school and tell our friends that there are more than two children in our family."

Or, teenage children would tell their mothers, "You are not a battery hen, why are you having more than two children?" When the Supreme Religious Leader, Ayatollah Khamenei, subsequently reversed the two-decade-old policy of controlled population growth, announcing publicly that it must end, he was thus challenging what had become deep-seated values in the younger generation, who had grown up believing in the advantages of fewer children. The Supreme Leader was emphatic that Iran's goal should be to reach a population increase from the current 80 million to 150 million by 2050 (Karami 2012).

Phase 3 (2011 to Date)

This latest phase of state population policy, in reverting to policies of the early days of the Revolution, is a direct response to the sharp drop in childbearing among the young married couples tracked in Figure 5.1. As discussed in "Phase 2 (1986–2006)," the one- or no-child trend applies to both the rural and urban populations. In fact, the urban population of Iran stands at 74 percent, and those living in rural areas are predominantly the elderly and the very young (which doubtless contributes to the higher figures shown for the decline in rural areas). As Heidar Ali Abedi, a member of the Parliament's Health and Treatment Commission, has remarked, "the total fertility rate (TFR) for the average number of children born to a woman in her lifetime is now 1.8 in Iran, which is the

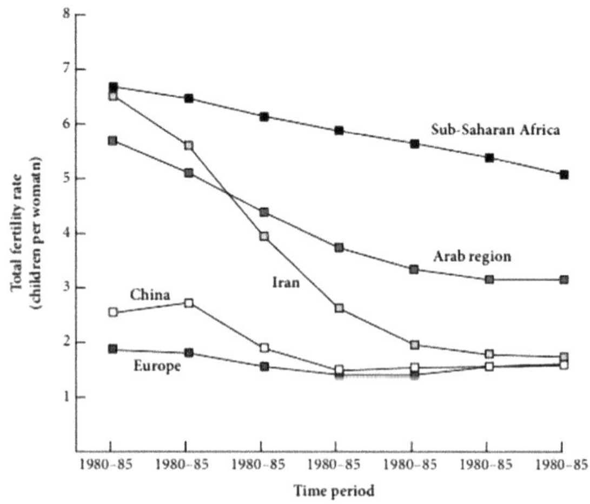

FIGURE 5.1. Iran and Selected International Fertility Trends.
Source: United Nations Department of Economic and Social Affairs (2017)

lowest among Islamic countries, and even below the world average of 2.1 births per woman" (Iran Project 2016b). To promote the culture of a multi-child family, he suggests increasing maternity leave, providing more nurseries near workplaces, free medical checks in pregnancy and care services, coverage of all medical and social care costs of children under eighteen, and financial support for infertile couples, whose number he estimated at around 3 million. As is clear from these suggestions, women remain the focus. There are, of course, some measures, such as the ban on vasectomy, which apply to men, but by and large men are less visible in the policy statements. The main responsibility for reproducing the nation continues to fall on women.

Prior to the Supreme Religious Leader's fourteen-point decree, in 2010 President Ahmadinejad had already raised the alarm, drawing attention to the fertility decline and proposing new measures to encourage population growth. His government promised to open a bank account for every newly born child and to continue paying into it until the child reached age eighteen. The authorities also started increasing pressure on women by asking them to take part-time jobs, or to cease work altogether so that they could be free to have more children (thereby also providing more jobs for men). These pleas evidently fell on deaf ears, as the evidence of Figure 5.1 shows: young people of reproductive age did not produce more children in that, or subsequent, periods.

Moreover, many went further in their resistance to the government's wishes, giving up the very idea of marriage, instead cohabiting with their partners, a practice which is referred to as "white marriage" (*ezdevaj-e sefid*).[3] This increasing trend among young Iranians is a bold one, considering that under the Islamic theocracy any sexual relationship between men and women outside wedlock is considered adultery, which is punishable by death. Any children born out of such a relationship are considered illegitimate. There can be little doubt, however, of the major importance of this development. The demographic situation was recently summarized by the Head of the Information Statistics Department of the National Organization for Civil Registration, Ali Akbar Mahzoon, in an interview with Faranak Bakhtiari (2019). There are more than 11 million unmarried youths in Iran in the customary range of ages for marriage. This is between twenty and thirty-four for men and fifteen and twenty-nine for women. In this group, 46 percent of men and 48 percent of women remain unmarried, and marriage rates had declined in the previous 3.5 years—down by 1.9

percent in 2012, by 5.1 percent in 2013, by 6.7 percent in 2014, and by 7.2 percent in the first months of 2015.

The reasons for such a decline are many, most commentators emphasizing the rise in female education and economic hardship. But these reasons, while true, are an over-simplification of a more complex set of factors. Here, we turn to the central focus of this chapter, on the emerging ways that young people respond to societal pressures by often deviating from existing cultural norms and practices, and on the implications of these newfound solutions for women. First, growing recognition of the issue will be traced briefly in the academic literature, and in the response of the Islamic government. Second, we focus on one of the most striking changes, given the sharp disapproval of white marriage: the increasing recognition of infertility as both a woman's predicament and as a medical concern. Having outlined this context, two detailed case studies are then presented to illustrate the complexity of women's handling of the pressures on them in relation to childbearing.

Recent Discussion of White Marriage in the Public Sphere

Reasons often cited for the rise of white marriage often point to practical conflicts that would plausibly lead young people to prefer cohabitation over marriage. These include, for example: the high expectation of marriage and the financial costs involved; the high rate of divorce, which is often a heavy financial and legal burden on both men and women; and concerns over long-term commitment to a partner one does not know. In addition, a considerable shift in the status of women is remarked, which has led women to realize increasingly that their identity and personhood do not depend solely on, and are not limited to, motherhood. They now have many other choices open to them to express their identity. Thus, according to Abbasi-Shavazi, McDonald, and Hosseini-Chavoshi (2009: 187), "The higher status of women in Iran will also tend to have a negative effect on fertility in the future. This is in line with the 'gender equity' argument made by McDonald (2000) and supports Dyson's (2002) hypothesis that one of the main factors of the fall of fertility in developing countries is that 'women become more like men.'" More generally, the shift in marriage practice is recognized as a historical fact relating to a particular conjuncture in Iran's development. According to Said Peyvandi, a professor of social sciences:

> The youths' reduced interest in marriage stems in part from the "living condition of Iranian youths born in the 1980s and 1990s.

> Economic and cultural middle classes of society have experienced astronomical growth in technology and freedom in social relationships. Therefore, the youth have more opportunities to engage in romantic and sexual relationships while they are single. They are not willing to lose these opportunities by committing themselves to marriage." (*Al-Monitor* 2015)

Finally, as the Iranian sociologist Shadi-Talab (2001) notes, the changes reflect more pervasive normative changes in the family and its power structures as women negotiate wider movement in society: "Iranian girls gradually practice democracy within the family, and patriarchal power is slowly diminishing. Although, attitude change is a very slow process, the interaction between education and changes in norms and value systems is observable in the share of girls' participation at universities from the most deprived provinces and far from their home town." Hence, as the Iranian sociologist Mehrdad Darvishpour remarked to the BBC, "The government might try to use force to stop this [white marriage], just as they tried to impose stricter adherence to the rules on wearing a hijab [headscarf] on young women, but young people will continue to move forward. Modernity can't be stopped" (Rahimpour 2014). The response of politico-religious leaders to cohabitation, in contrast, has been one of outright condemnation. Ayatollah Khamenei has called white marriage "shameful" and has issued a warning to the public, calling on the police and the judiciary to "show no mercy" to cohabiting couples. He added, "It won't take long for people who have chosen this lifestyle to have wiped out a legitimate generation with an illegitimate one" (*The Week* 2014). The irony of this statement lies in the fact that cohabitation is not necessarily about having or not having children, but about living free of the many complicating bonds of marriage. Having a child out of wedlock, of course, is bound to alert the authorities to the existence of a white relationship. The effect is to further discourage childbearing at the very time the government is trying to promote higher fertility.[4]

Beyond the backlash of the religious leaders and the reactions of officials, the attitudes of young women's parents also seem to point to a widening gap in values and outlook to life between generations. Parents, after all, still feel responsible for their children's well-being. For men, cohabiting with a woman carries no major stigma, even though it is illegal, nor does it carry serious negative social consequences if the relationship breaks down. However, the situation differs greatly for women. This is especially true for those women who are from conservative or religious backgrounds who are coming to larger cities, now living a relatively anonymous life. These young women keep their white marriages secret from their parents, who would vehemently disapprove. By cohabiting, in addition to breaking the law, they run the risk of damaging their reputation and possible later chances of marriage, additionally jeopardizing relationships with their wider kin group, who would reject them as prostitutes. There is always a possibility that some more conservative parents may resort to honor killing, which still happens in some highly conservative families. However, it is noteworthy that some parents from secular and educated groups in society do support their children in the choice of white marriage. Although there is no accurate information of the extent of this approval, interviews with young people themselves indicate that supportive parents form a very small group at present (personal interviews with young couples in a white marriage arrangement, with unmarried young women, and with married couples in Tehran and in Iranian diaspora).

The Emergence of Infertility as an Issue

Beyond the question of cohabitation, the state's response to the decline in fertility must be regarded as a set of drastic measures, which none of the previous campaigns had adopted. Among these are: the dismantling of the family planning program, the reversal of previous progressive laws on family planning, outlawing voluntary sterilization, and restricting access to contraceptives. Iran stopped subsidizing vasectomies, free condoms, and affordable contraceptives, as well as countrywide education on sexual health and family planning and rerouted funds allocated to the previous family planning campaign to promote pronatalist policies. The Iranian parliament is now considering two separate bills aimed at boosting population. Amnesty International has warned that these proposals, if approved, would "entrench discriminatory practices" and expose women to health risks (Dehghan 2015). As part of its effort to boost population growth, the state is considering granting citizenship to potentially millions of migrants and refugees (see Ladier-Fouladi 2017).

Recent historical and anthropological demography has shown that, in a great many contexts, infertility is a key and neglected constituent of modern population dynamics, particularly in relation to fertility declines.[5] Iran has not been an exception, even though in the past only a passing reference was made to infertility in its 1986 campaign, and little action was actually taken toward its treatment. At the time, the extent of infertility was unknown, although Ayatollah Khamenei issued a fatwa in 1999 sympathetic to the introduction of new reproductive technologies (Tremayne and Akhondi 2016). However, the treatment of infertility was left to the private sector and remained so until the "crisis" of the decline in fertility growth became apparent.

At the same time that the census of 2011 raised the alarm on the fall in population growth, a survey of 17,000 households was carried out by Avicenna Research Institute (Akhondi et al. 2013). Following a conventional demographic definition of infertility as couples experiencing a year of sex without conception and without using contraception, the estimated prevalence of infertility among married couples in the general population of Iran was shown to be around 20 percent (19.9 percent in urban areas and 22 percent in rural areas).[6] These figures are considerably higher than those estimated for infertility between reproductive-age couples worldwide, which is between 8 and 12 percent (Ombelet et al. 2008).

With the publication of the results of the 2011 census and as part of the new pronatalist policies, the authorities started to take infertility more seriously. A plan called *Barekat-e Khanevadeh* (Family blessing) was put in place in 2015, targeting the country's underprivileged areas in ten provinces; infertile couples between twenty and twenty-four years of age would now be treated free of charge. The government has also encouraged insurance companies to cover some of the costs involved in infertility treatment, which had previously been listed as cosmetic rather than a disability, and therefore not eligible for claims (Tremayne and Akhondi 2016). Likewise, the government is also actively engaged in increasing the number of infertility clinics within the public hospitals in the poorer regions in the country (Iran Project 2016a).

White Marriage in the Lens of Infertility

The preceding review of policy and opinion on population decline and voluntary childlessness sets the stage to explore the cases of two infertile women, who had initially opted for white marriage and childlessness, but subsequently sought infertility treatment. This might appear an abrupt departure from the problems surrounding white marriage, but infertility is not merely a matter for those few women in a population who are unable to conceive naturally. As the cases show, infertility is intimately bound up with the emergence of cohabitation and the effects of government policies which heavily restrict women's options. Put schematically: cohabitation can lead readily to pregnancies that cannot be made public and which, in turn, lead to abortion and medical complications. Infertility is a major case in point and is, so to speak, a lens which clarifies a very different picture to the black-and-white image prevailing in official discourse. That is, in spite of the increasing number of young people who choose cohabitation over legal relationships, and the real and sometimes unhappy consequences of such relationships, it becomes clear that core values attached to reproduction persist. Even though attitudes to childbearing may have changed their form, and regardless of the number of children a person may have, reproduction per se remains the cornerstone of social relations fundamental to kinship, family, and society. The two case studies are drawn from the longitudinal study carried out by the author since 2004 on infertile couples, both in infertility clinics and through qualitative methods in other settings. The second case is selected from among a number of cases of Iranian women refugees in the United Kingdom, for whom the author has acted as expert witness in courts.

As mentioned in the sections "The Islamic Revolution (1979 to Date)" and "White Marriage in the Lens of Infertility," in referring to white marriages, a conservative academic has predicted that women practicing them, once old and no longer beautiful, would end up as sex workers. That sex outside marriage leads women to prostitution is an old trope in many parts of the world, and Iran is no exception. However, the two case studies presented here are the stories of two such women and show a very different picture of the twists and turns their lives have taken. Prostitution has not been a consideration at any point for them, once their cohabitation phase has been over. The cases presented here are, of course, not a random sample, and hence cannot be taken as representative of the majority of infertile women who come to clinics seeking treatment. Quite the opposite: they are chosen because their stories lift the veil on the "free" lifestyle chosen by a growing number of young women, against the backdrop of over a century of being treated as reproductive machines of state. As noted, the repeated reversal of state reproductive policies, presupposing that childbearing can be switched on and off at the state's whim, has been an affront which has led to resistance against the state's dictates. In contrast, the case studies reveal how cultural, societal, and legal constraints continue to determine women's life courses. When we look beneath the publicly authorized condemnation of white marriage, there is at least a hint of possibility that this development may just be a phase and rebellion, rather than a real choice—as long as women have to live under an Islamic theocratic regime.

The author met Afsaneh in 2012. She was staying with the author's cousin in Tehran, who had told her about the author's study of infertility and the use of assisted reproductive technologies. Afsaneh showed an interest in this study and, after some time, indicated that she was undergoing treatment for infertility herself. She and the author arranged to meet again and, after a few meetings, when the author felt that a few personal questions could be asked, it was enquired what kind of treatment she was seeking at the clinic. She said that she hopes to be able to conceive through IVF (in vitro fertilization). She then volunteered the full story leading to her infertility, which was diagnosed as blocked fallopian tubes. The doctor had told her that he was not sure that the treatment would be successful and that she will conceive. She continued, "I think that those backstreet abortionists did something wrong, which caused this problem." "Why did you go to backstreet abortionists?" the author asked. "I could not ask a normal doctor to do it. As you know, abortion is illegal in Iran and doctors normally refuse to do it." Further: "I could not go to normal doctors, even though some of them carry out abortions for married women. I was not married at the time. After one of the abortions, I suffered from pain and infections, which may be the cause of my infertility."

Afsaneh comes from Mashhad, northeast Iran. Her father is an engineer working for a construction company and her mother is a nurse working in a public hospital. She has a younger brother, too. The parents are religious and fairly conservative. After her secondary education, Afsaneh came to Tehran to study at one of the universities and rented a flat with some of the other girls in her class. She met her first boyfriend at the university and had a brief relationship with him. By the time she completed her studies, she had had three boyfriends and had lived with the last two for several months each time. During these years, she had become pregnant twice and had resorted to backstreet abortionists. While her first abortion was with the agreement of her boyfriend, the second one ended acrimoniously, as the boyfriend became aggressive and turned violent when she told him that she was pregnant, did not want another abortion, and suggested that they get officially married. He had no intention of marrying her and left her with no choice but to resort to abortion. Her parents had no knowledge of her lifestyle, otherwise she would have been in deep trouble. After her studies were completed, she could not get a job in Tehran and had no money, so had to return to Mashhad. Once back home, her family members started looking around for a suitable husband for her. Here is Afsaneh's full story:

> Almost every day my mother would talk about our neighbor's son, who had completed his education and had returned to Mashhad, as a possible husband for me. My maternal aunt would come round and mention that time had come for me to get married. She had a few candidates of her own. My father too gave me sideways glances in a disapproving way, implying that, now that I had finished my studies, "I must think of more important things in life," meaning getting married and having a family. At almost every female gathering the talk was about the potential suitors for me and, sometimes, I was not even included in the conversation, in spite of trying hard to tell them this was my life and I am the one who should make the decision. Nobody took what I said seriously, and they went on oblivious to my protests, interpreting my reluctance as shyness. Finally, having met some of the potential husbands, I saw that getting married for me was a way out of this relentless pressure. These men came from relatively conservative families and neither they nor their families would accept a wife who has had boyfriends and was not a virgin. The next step to freedom for me, therefore, was to resort to repair of the hymen. A trip back to Tehran "to visit my friends" allowed me to restore my virginity and I was finally ready to get married.
>
> My husband was a kind man, content with working and coming home, having a meal, watching TV, and going to bed. Our social life was solely with both our families with little excitement or interest for me. A rather dull life! I tried hard to find a job, but, having studied social sciences at the university, it was difficult to find anything suitable or relevant to my interests. Besides, my husband was not too keen for me to work. A few months into the marriage, queries started from all around on when I was going to have a child. The growing chorus of mother, aunt, and this time mother-in-law, all in a kind and gentle way querying constantly whether there was something wrong, was I not happy with him (referring to my husband), and so on. The reality was that I did not want a child and my husband was content to wait for a while, but he too wanted to have children before long. Finally, I decided to end the torture of the increased pressure and try to have a child. The idea was to use the child to liberate myself and be able to get away from the expectations that I have to be

a mother. However, after trying for nearly eighteen months, nothing happened, and I decided to come to one of the infertility clinics in Tehran to find out the reason for my inability to conceive. I chose to do this outside Mashhad, as there is no privacy there, although good infertility clinics exist. The news would have spread one way or another to everybody in my social network. Having seen the doctors in Tehran, I was told that the fallopian tubes are blocked, and all I can think of is those abortions, which must have caused it. The doctors did not promise that IVF will work, but "we are going to try."

The author has lost touch with Afsaneh and does not know whether the treatment worked and she has conceived.

The second case study is that of Parvin, an Iranian refugee woman, who had come to the United Kingdom seeking asylum, having run away from Iranian courts, which had summoned her. She was accused of having abducted her own child. The author acted for Parvin as expert witness in the United Kingdom. Her story is different from that of Afsaneh in some ways, but also similar in others. Both women have ended up in unwanted, even precarious situations, which is the price they have had to pay for their desire to live a life of their choice.

Parvin is from Rasht, the capital of Guilan province, north Iran. She was forced by her parents to marry a man much older than herself when she was fifteen years old, but the marriage did not last, as she did not have a child. She then trained as an accountant and moved to Tehran and started working and earning enough to have a comfortable life. She also worked as a karate teacher, where she met her future lover and started a long-lasting affair with him. He was a married man with grown-up children. When his wife found out that he was having an affair with Parvin, she sent her son to threaten her and tell her to give up the affair. Parvin's lover's visits became less frequent and in order to keep the relationship going, Parvin thought of having a child. But, having failed to conceive in the past, she needed to seek infertility treatment and persuaded her lover to enter into temporary marriage[7] with her, as she could not seek treatment as a single woman, conception outside wedlock being illegal under the Islamic law. He agreed reluctantly, in the belief that she would not be able to conceive. When the IVF proved successful and she became pregnant, he was unhappy and turned violent. It became clear that all he wanted was a relationship, and not another family. He almost stopped visiting her. When she found out where he lived and went to see him, she was beaten and thrown down the stairs by his first wife and son. The story of what went on between the lover's main family and Parvin is too long, but it ended with him taking the child away, which, as the father, and therefore the owner, of the child, he was entitled to do. He then tricked her into giving him her share of the house, which they owned jointly, in exchange for the child, to which she agreed. As soon as she transferred the deeds, he called the police on the grounds that she was harassing him. The fight to regain custody of her child became fierce and everything Parvin did made her situation worse. Eventually, she abducted the child. This gave her lover the perfect excuse to threaten her that he would tell the judges that she had been living with him without being married to him. This would have meant facing the Revolutionary Courts and the prospect of being stoned for adultery. Knowing that he was a conservative man and had access to some of the senior judges, she believed his threats, and when she received a summons from the courts, she knew that she did not stand a chance of winning her child back, even if she was lucky enough not to be sentenced only to imprisonment. Finally, having been subject to the violence of her lover's family, she arranged to be smuggled out of Iran and came to the United Kingdom, where she sought asylum.

Conclusion

This chapter has traced the long history in which women have been the main target of various population control strategies or policies of the Iranian state, starting in the nineteenth century. All of these policies, regardless of their ultimate purpose to increase or decrease population, have treated women as the main agents responsible for producing citizens needed for the nation-building aims of the state. Currently, population growth has fallen to below replacement level, yet no amount of effort on the part of government planners has succeeded in persuading young people of reproductive age to have larger families. On the contrary, many young, married couples opt for one child or none at all, and an increasing number now co-habit without formalizing their relationship, despite white marriage being viewed legally as adultery and subject to heavy punishment.[8] In the face of such sanctions, there can be little surprise that these young people choose to remain childless, as their children will be treated as illegitimate.

Documentation of the extent of white marriage, however, is scant, and based largely on reports in the media. Even if cohabitation is widespread, it can only be one of a number of factors behind the drop in population growth. This has not kept it from being used to justify stigmatization. What is clear is that white marriage tends to become a vicious circle, in which women end up where they started, i.e., conforming to norms by getting married and willingly or unwillingly having a child to "tick the box" and regain not only their respectability, but freedom from the scrutiny of family, kin, and society. The alternatives for these "white brides" are not always promising.

Contemporary Iranian demography indicates that the majority of women seem to be reducing their reproduction to a minimum, yet still managing in most cases to have one child. The dictates of the state to have more than one child—which, as we have seen, are powerfully promoted and legally reinforced—are evidently being subverted. Meanwhile, the (often unrelenting) pressures of family, kin, and social norms likewise enjoin higher fertility, but seemingly to no avail. When we talk to young women at the center of this issue, however, their adoption of white marriage and a de facto no-child policy turn out not to be a simple rejection of prevailing childbearing norms. Their objection is to the social and economic disenfranchisement that accompanies such norms, particularly as they relate to marriage. The unhappy consequences of their attempts to obtain real agency over their life course, and yet also to have at least one child, are a heavy price for them to pay. This is the real outcome of the present impasse. While very low fertility and childlessness remain central to the demography of this impasse, they do not appear to reflect a fundamental shift in reproductive values, but are a consequence of the legal and social barriers young women face. That said, the changes in attitudes that have led to new marriage practices are fundamental, and whether they continue to discourage reproduction will require a very different official response.

Acknowledgments

This chapter was published originally as "'*As List E Karhayee Ke Bayad Anjame Midadam Khat Khord*': Contemporary Reproductive Body Politic in Iran." In *The Anthropological Demography of Health*, ed. Véronique Petit, Kaveri Qureshi, Yves Charbit, and Philip Kreager, 183–203. Oxford: Oxford University Press (2020).

Notes

1. However, earlier on, Abbasi-Shavazi (2001) had noted that this decline cannot be linked only to the population policies, and that the decline had started among the urban middle classes before the campaign. This has also been confirmed by Ladier-Fouladi (1997). Since this chapter was first presented in March 2017, Abbasi-Shavazi, in an interview given in December 2017, mentioned that, according to in-depth research, the fertility rate has more recently shown a growing trend, and that replacement-level fertility has almost returned. He continued: "Looking into the figures and numbers pertaining to fertility rate before the (13)90s (i.e. in the Iranian calendar, or around 2011), the rates have gone up over the past six years. From 2014 to 2016 the rate has grown to 2.08 while in a five-year period the rate has reached 2.01" (*Tehran Times* 2017).
2. Given the long politicization of contraception in Iran, the extent to which representative data on usage may actually be collected is, at best, uncertain. Local studies, which may perhaps be more reliable, reveal high levels of usage (at over 80 percent in both urban and rural samples) involving not only modern, but also considerable recourse to "traditional" methods, such as withdrawal (Sarvestani et al. 2017). However, the decline in population growth was not solely due to the use of contraception, but to a combination of methods and outstanding coordination between various sectors. This included an effective health network, widespread education, and making various methods of contraception available to married couples free of charge (see Hoodfar 1995 and Tremayne 2004).
3. This choice of the word "white" does not have a symbolic significance in Islam but stems from the fact that marriages are registered in individuals' birth certificate booklets. Since "white marriage" is not officially registered, the page pertaining to the civil status is blank, as is the marriage certificate.
4. The visibility of out-of-wedlock births also influences reportage of Iranian demographic data. As Ladier-Fouladi (1997: 198) remarks, "fertility outside marriage is non-existent in Iran." In other words, Islamic law forbids it, leading to abortions.
5. See e.g., Kreager and Schroder-Butterfill (2004) and Szreter (2019).
6. These percentages refer to "primary infertility," which Akhondi et al. (2013: 1398) define as "a condition in which a couple have not been able to conceive a child after one year of unprotected intercourse." The measure is thus not a statement about natural infecundity (i.e., a biological inability to conceive), nor about the percentage of women who remain, or are likely to remain, childless at age forty-five. Demographers consider natural infecundity constant at about 3–4 percent of couples, rising gradually with a woman's age, whereas childlessness at

age forty-five may reflect many social factors (Kreager 2004). Primary infertility is also sometimes defined as a period of difficulty conceiving at any point over the life course, so comparison of figures from different sources can contain many potential sources of ambiguity. One such ambiguity, of course, is couples disguising the fact that they are using contraception—which is, after all, a greater factor in very low fertility than infertility (Hoodfar 2017). What is clear is that measures of primary infertility give results likely to exaggerate actual lifetime reproductive experience in a population, although in so doing the authors give support to the government's concerns.

7. Temporary marriage or *sigheh* in Persian is unique to the Shia school of Islam and is recognized as legal. It is a form of marriage whereby a man and a woman agree to enter into marriage with a time limit on it, anything between one hour and ninety-nine years. Once the time agreed comes to an end, the marriage becomes null automatically. Although, legally, this form of marriage should protect women and entitle them to some form of payment, in reality men in many cases decline payment and women are left with no protection. Children resulting from temporary marriage are recognized as legitimate and the responsibility of the father. For more information, see Haeri (1989).
8. People who are cohabiting could give their cohabitation a legal appearance by entering into temporary marriage, but rarely do so. However, sometimes, when confronted by the police, they may claim to be temporarily married to avert the consequences.

References

Abbasi-Shavazi, Mohammad Jalal. 2001. "Fertility Revolution in Iran." *Population et Société* 373: 1–4.

Abbasi-Shavazi, Mohammad Jalal, Peter McDonald, and Meimanat Hosseini-Chavoshi. 2009. *The Fertility Transition in Iran: Revolution and Reproduction*. Dordrecht: Springer.

Al-Monitor. 2015. "Why Are Young Iranians Losing Interest in Marriage?" 2 June. Retrieved 19 September 2021 from https://www.al-monitor.com/originals/2015/06/iran-birth-rate-marriage-decline-divorce.html.

Akhondi, Mohammad Mehdi, Koorosh Kamali, Fahimeh Ranjbar, Mahdi Shirzad, Shiva Shafeghati, Zohreh Behjati Ardakani, Abolfazl Goodjani, Mahboubeh Parsaeian, and Kazem Mohammad. 2013. "Prevalence of Primary Infertility in Iran in 2010." *Journal of Public Health* 42(12): 1398–1404.

Bakhtiari, Faranak. 2019. "Iran Facing Population Decline; Is it Possible to Reverse the Trend?" *Mehr News Agency*, May. Retrieved 19 September 2021 from https://en.mehrnews.com/news/145496/Iran-facing-population-decline-is-it-possible-to-reverse-the.

Center for Human Rights in Iran. 2016. "Officials Seek to Confront Iran's Increasingly Popular 'White Marriages.'" 6 June. Retrieved 19 September 2021 from https://www.iranhumanrights.org/2016/06/white-marriage-2/.

Dehghan, Saeed Kamali. 2015. "Iran Aims to Ban Vasectomies and Cut Access to Contraceptives to Boost Births." *The Guardian*, 11 March. Retrieved 19 September 2021 from https://www.theguardian.com/world/2015/mar/11/iran-ban-voluntary-sterilisation-contraceptive-access-block-boost-population.

Dyson, T. 2002. "On the Future of Human Fertility in India." Paper prepared for the Expert Group Meeting on Continuing the Fertility Transitions, Population Division of the United Nations, New York, 11–14 March.

Haeri, Shahla. 1989. *The Law of Desire: Temporary Marriage in Shi'i Iran*. Syracuse, NY: Syracuse University Press.

Hoodfar, Homa. 1995. "Population Policy and Gender Equity in Post-Revolutionary Iran.' In *Family, Gender and Population in the Middle East: Policies in Context*, ed. Carla Makhlouf, 105–135. Cairo: American University of Cairo Press.

———. 2017. "Turning Back the Clock: Population Policy and Human Rights in Iran." In *Routledge Handbook on Human Rights and the Middle East and North Africa*, ed. Anthony Tirado Chase, 230–242. London: Routledge and Taylor & Francis Group.

Iran Project. 2016a. "Free Infertility Treatment Brings Hope to Many Families." Retrieved 19 September 2021 from http://theiranproject.com/blog/2016/06/22/free-infertility-treatment-brings-hope-many-families.

———. 2016b. "Single Child Families Challenge Iran's Population Growth." Retrieved 19 September 2021 from http://theiranproject.com/blog/2016/08/14/single-child-families-challenge-iran-population-growth-rate/.

Karami, Arash. 2012. "Khamenei on Population Control: 'May God and History Forgive Us.'" *Al-Monitor*, 17 October. Retrieved 19 September 2021 from https://www.al-monitor.com/pulse/fr/contents/articles/originals/2012/al-monitor/iran-population-control.html.

Kashani-Sabet, Firoozeh. 2011. *Conceiving Citizen: Women and the Politics of Motherhood in Iran*. Oxford: Oxford University Press.

Kreager, Philip. 2004. "Where Are the Children?" In *Ageing without Children: European and Asian Perspectives*, ed. Philip Kreager and Elisabeth Schröder-Butterfill, 1–48. Oxford: Berghahn Books.

Kreager, Philip, and Elisabeth Schröder-Butterfill, eds. 2004. *Ageing without Children: European and Asian Perspectives*. Oxford: Berghahn Books.

Ladier-Fouladi, Marie. 1997. "The Fertility Transition in Iran." *Population. An English Selection* 9: 191–214.

———. 2017. "La Nouvelle Politique de Population de la Republique Islamique: Enjeux et Defies" [The new population policy of the Islamic Republic: issues and challenges]. *Bulletin de l'Association de Géographies Français* 94: 4.

Makhlouf-Obermeyer, Carla. 1991. "Women, Islam and Population: Is the Triangle Fateful?" Working Series Paper No. 6. Harvard: Harvard School of Public Health, Harvard University.

McDonald, Peter. 2000. "Gender Equity in Theories of Demographic Transition." *Population and Development Review* 26(3): 427–439.

Ombelet, Willem, Ian Cooke, Silke Dyer, Gamal Serour, and Paul Devroey. 2008. "Infertility and the Provision of Infertility Medical Services in Developing Countries." *Human Reproductive Update* 14(6): 605–621.

Rahimpour, Rana. 2014. "Can Iran 'Control' its Cohabiting Couples?" BBC, 10 December. Retrieved 19 September 2021 from http://www.bbc.co.uk/news/world-middle-east-30391593.

Roudi-Fahimi, Farzaneh. 2002. "Iran's Family Planning Program: Responding to a Nation's Needs." *Population Reference Bureau* 31: 1–8.

———. 2012. "Iran is Reversing its Population Policies." *Viewpoints* 7, 28 August, Woodrow Wilson International Center for Scholars.

Sarvestani, Khadijeh Asadi, Suet Leng Khoo, Noor Malina Malek, Suziana Mat Yasin, and Aliyar Ahmadi. 2017. "Determinants of Contraceptive Usage among Married Women in Shiraz, Iran." *Journal of Midwifery and Reproductive Health* 5(4): 1041–1052.

Shadi-Talab, Jaleh. 2001. "Iranian Women: Rising Expectations." Paper Presented at Middle East Studies Association Annual Meeting, 27–28 November, Florida.

Statistical Center of Iran. 2016. *Iran Statistical Yearbook 2015–2016*. Tehran: Statistical Center of Iran.

Szreter, Simon, ed. 2019. *The Hidden Affliction: Sexually Transmitted Infections and Infertility in History*. Rochester: University of Rochester Press.

Tabnak. 2013. "Iran's Population Crisis Awaits the Iranian People." In Persian. 24 September. Retrieved 19 September 2021 from http://www.tabnak.ir/fa/news/346841.

Tehran Times. 2017. "Iran's Fertility Rate Reaches Normal Levels." 29 December. Retrieved 19 September 2021 from http://www.tehrantimes.com/news/419793/Iran-s-fertility-rate-reaches-normal-levels-expert.

The Week. 2014. "White Marriages: Iran's Cohabiting Couples Defy Sharia Law." 10 December. Retrieved 19 September 2021 from http://www.theweek.co.uk/middle-east/61738/white-marriages-irans-cohabiting-couples-defy-sharia-law.

Tremayne, Soraya. 2004. "'And Never the Twain Shall Meet': Reproductive Health Policies in the Islamic Republic of Iran." In *Reproductive Agency, Medicine and the State: Cultural Transformations in Childbearing*, ed. Maya Unnithan-Kumar, 181–202. Oxford: Berghahn Books.

———. 2006. "Modernity and Early Marriage: A View from Within." *Journal of the Middle East Women's Studies* 2(1): 65–94.

Tremayne, Soraya, and Mohammad Mehdi Akhondi. 2016. "Conceiving IVF in Iran." *Journal of Reproductive Biomedicine and Society Online* 2: 62–70.

United Nations. 2016. *Demographic Yearbook*: "Demographics of Iran." Retrieved 19 September 2021 from http://www.worldometers.info/world-population/iran-population/.

United Nations Department of Economic and Social Affairs. 2017. "World Population Prospects: Key Findings and Advance Tables." Retrieved 11 October 2021 from https://population.un.org/wpp/Publications/Files/WPP2017_KeyFindings.pdf.

World Bank. 2011. "Population Growth (Annual Percent)—Iran, Islamic Republic." Retrieved 19 September 2021 from https://data.worldbank.org/indicator/SP.POP.GROW?locations=IR.

Chapter 6

"The Only Thing [the State Is] Good at Is Intruding in People's Beds"

Citizens as Tools of Reproduction

Introduction

In 2011, Iran made an abrupt policy shift; after two decades of encouraging families to limit reproduction, it suddenly moved to emphasize procreation as a national imperative. Through the lens of infertility, this chapter examines the Iranian state's increasingly coercive efforts to control the reproductive lives of its citizens to meet its overall political agenda.

In November 2021, just three months after his election in August 2021, hardliner president Ebrahim Raisi submitted a bill to parliament called "The Rejuvenation of the Population and the Protection of Family." The media reported this legislation as: "Approved in accordance with Article 53 of the Constitution by the Joint Commission without being discussed during an open parliamentary session, the plan offers some financial and employment benefits to those who have children, while imposing stricter restrictions on contraception and abortion" (*Middle East Eye* 2021).

Compared to its preceding pronatalist policies, discussed in this chapter, Iran's new draconian law is ringing alarm bells across the country. Health officials warn of its potential dangers, including risks to the health of young people of reproductive age and lasting damage to the health of future generations. Human rights activists consider the new law a violation of reproductive rights and point out that, while the law affects both men and women,

women remain its ultimate casualty. According to United Nations experts, "The consequences of this law will be crippling for women and girls' right to health and [represent] an alarming and regressive U-turn by a government that had been praised for progress on the right to health" (OHCHR 2021). Moreover, "It is shocking to see the extent to which the authorities have applied criminal law to restrict women's fundamental rights" (OHCHR 2021).[1] However, the state's message is clear: citizens must produce their due share of children to save the nation from extinction.

The Population and the State

As discussed in Chapter 5, throughout history, the Iranian state's approach to population has been driven by the ideals of nation-building. Since the late nineteenth century, this interest has fluctuated between being indirect and uncoordinated at times and cohesive and assertive at others. Regardless of its approach, Iran has reversed its positions and policies five times, adopting anti- or pronatalist stances alternately over the past century. The state's body politic started in the late nineteenth and early twentieth century, under the rule of the Qajar Dynasty (1785–1925), when the state became aware of a serious decline in population. At this time, Iran adopted a pronatalist approach and took various measures to improve the health of the nation. As US-based Iranian historian Firoozeh Kashani-Sabet (2011: 4) explains in her analysis of the state's attitudes toward the improvement of the nation's health, "embedded in this analysis is a general consideration about the political and professional visibility of women and the rise of ideologies that appropriated motherhood for political purposes." She further argues that maternalism became an ideology that promoted motherhood and maternal well-being not only within the framework of the family but also in nationalist contexts: "the awareness of women's health and infant mortality, which can be situated in the nineteenth century, brings maternalism to the heart of modern Iranian thought, concepts of nationhood, and tasks of a modern government" (Kashani-Sabet 2011: 4).

The Qajar Dynasty was followed by the Pahlavi Dynasty (1925–79), which initially continued to focus on maternal and child health and, to this end, set up the first family planning clinics in 1958 (Abbasi-Shavazi et al. 2009; Hoodfar and Assadipour 2000). During the latter part of the Pahlavi era, Iran underwent a process of reform aimed at modernizing Iranian society. In 1966, government statistics indicated that the population was growing at the rate of around 3.1 percent per annum. As a result, Iran introduced a family planning program to slow population growth. With the establishment of the Islamic Republic in 1979, the previous family planning programs were dismantled and, as Abbasi-Shavazi et al. (2009: 24) explain, "although the new government did not develop a specific pronatalist policy, several socio-cultural and economic changes were made that were effectively pronatalist in nature." As a result, by 1986 the census showed the rate of population growth to have reached 3.9 percent per annum. Such a rapid increase led to the launch of a massive anti-natalist campaign in 1989, which succeeded in bringing the rate of growth down to 2.1 within ten years of its implementation.[2] This decline continued until the 2011 census showed a drop in the total fertility rate to 1.5, below the replacement level. The decline was due, inter alia, to the educational strand of the population policies, which had highlighted the advantages of having smaller families. This advocacy proved highly effective in transforming the reproductive behavior of the current generation of reproductive age. However, the 2011 census data led the state to again reverse its pronatalist policies.[3]

While espousing different goals, these policies shared some common features. First, their adoption indicates that Iran remains concerned fundamentally with nation-building rather than with the well-being of its citizens. With each population policy articulation, the Islamic Republic has aimed to persuade citizens to adjust or even reverse their reproductive norms and practices to suit the state's ideals by emphasizing "the need for building a strong and independent nation" and by pointing to the responsibility of the citizens to cooperate with the state for the "common good" (Hoodfar 1995). Second, none of the population policies considered infertility to be a constituent of modern population dynamics. While the 1986 campaign made a passing reference to infertility, it failed to take any effective steps toward its treatment. One underlying reason for this inaction stems from the deeply rooted cultural belief that infertility is a divine damnation and a matter of private—not public—concern. Although the shame and stigma of infertility may be widespread throughout the world (Inhorn and Van Ballen 2002), in the Middle East, traditionally, biological relatedness has been the only acceptable form of reproduction. Having one's own children has been imperative, and voluntary childlessness has not been an option. While the stigma of infertility and childlessness persists in

Iran, with many infertile couples desperate to conceive, a new phenomenon has also emerged in the past few decades in the form of voluntary childlessness. Couples choosing to remain childless do not carry the same stigma, and women often use childlessness as a badge of honor conveying the message that their status and identity no longer depend on, or are limited to, their reproductive abilities. Deliberate childlessness also sends a warning to the authorities to keep out of the couples' most intimate sphere of life. However, in the long run and a few years into their relationships, these couples usually end up having at least one child.

Despite considerable changes in reproductive norms and practices in Iran, family values remain firmly rooted in tradition, which continues to prioritize family and kinship based on biological relatedness. A child who is not biologically related to the family is rarely considered a "real" family member by the kin group and by society. Iran's law of inheritance further illustrates this emphasis on biological relatedness. Someone who is not related by blood to the rest of the kin group has no legal claim to inheritance. In light of the paramount importance of biological relatedness in Iranian culture and in the absence of significant state assistance with infertility treatment, the private sector's introduction of in vitro fertilization (IVF) to Iran in the late 1980s was met with great anticipation.

Infertility and Reproductive Technologies

In 1978, a new method of conception was offered to infertile couples in the United Kingdom: in vitro fertilization (IVF), which is now a routine medical treatment, was a revolutionary technology at that time. Its introduction to Iran in 1989 coincided with Iran's anti-natalist population policies. The pioneering medical practitioners who introduced IVF to Iran were mindful of the pronatalist Islamic beliefs on reproduction and sought the opinion of Iran's Islamic jurists on the permissibility of its use. Unlike most secular countries, where the responsibility for legitimizing innovative biotechnologies falls on a committee of experts and the parliament, in Iran, their legitimization often falls under the jurisdiction of Muslim jurists (*foqaha*), who are recognized by their peers as the sources of emulation (*maraje-e taqlid*, singular: *marja*). By resorting to independent interpretation of Islamic sources (i.e., the practice of *ijtihad*), these jurists issue religious edicts (*fatwas*) on a wide range of issues.

Many of these sources approved of IVF on the condition that its practice remained limited to heterosexual married couples, as conception outside marriage in Islam is equivalent to adultery and the resulting child is considered illegitimate or a bastard (*valad-e zena*). At this juncture, judicial debates on IVF were not particularly controversial and its practice did not attract the attention of the world outside the medical practice. But the introduction of third-party gamete donation led to a more profound exploration of the permissibility of these state-of-the-art technologies and their implications for the entrenched cultural and religious beliefs surrounding reproduction. Because the inclusion of a third party's gamete in reproduction was viewed as problematic, the jurists needed to find valid arguments to justify the procedure, which allowed procreation and the continuity of the family line while threatening the purity of lineage. However, although some jurists found ways to legitimize third-party donation, they did not reach a unanimous verdict and, to date, opinions on this topic remain divided.[4] Paradoxically, those jurists who justified the practice in the name of creating happy families, thus conforming to the Islamic ideology, effectively deviated from the very Islamic imperatives of the sanctity of the family and purity of blood they were trying to protect.

While the permissive *fatwas* paved the way for the use of all kinds of assisted reproductive technologies, a law was needed to legalize embryo donation as no amount of *ijtihad* could justify its practice. In 2003, embryo donation was legalized through an act of the parliament, which is also, in theory, supposed to apply to all the other forms of third-party donation, previously approved through *fatwas*. However, in practice, the enforcement of the law has proved ineffective due to the differences of views between various sources of emulation, whose contradictory opinions are equally valid; the freedom of the followers to choose the source of emulation; and a lack of clarity on who the donors and recipients can be, all offering unlimited choices to all parties involved. Thus, the practice of third-party gamete donation remains in flux.[5]

The jurists who approved of third-party donation were unanimous in their belief that a child conceived through third-party donation belongs to his biological parent, meaning the gamete donor, not the gamete recipient. They also allowed all forms of IVF on the condition that fertilization of the gamete take place outside the body and that no touch or gaze transpire between the parties involved.[6] The emphasis on "outside the body" initially led to the classification of infertility treatment as cosmetic surgery and made it ineligible for financial contribution by the health insurance providers. At this stage, the state's contribution to infertility treatment remained limited to allowing some public hospitals to set up infertility clinics, which covered only costs of the medication but not the treatment itself.[7] As infertility treatment had remained predominately within the private sector, costs remained high and unreachable for most infertile couples. As a result, these couples had to turn to their kin group for financial assistance, an act that justified involving relatives in the treatment and added to the confusion and increasing legal and ethical complications for all the parties involved. Considering the close-knit structure of kinship in Iran, a couple's infertility is often considered a problem for the kin group, too, which feels that it must support its infertile relative to ensure the continuity and purity of lineage.[8] In cases of financially pinched infertile couples, relatives frequently feel obliged to provide financial help, even at the cost of selling their own cars or houses, acts that are seen as justifying their involvement. The lack of an enforceable law and the ambiguity of *fatwas* on gamete donors and recipient practices comprise a small fraction of the myriad legal, ethical, religious, psychological, and other issues that arise regularly in the course of infertility treatment. These complications pose problems that often fall beyond the control or power of the clinics to resolve due to the absence of authoritative and uniform legislation.[9]

Iran's Reproduction Reversal

Amid this climate of uncertainty, the results of the 2011 census were published, introducing a turning point in Iran's approach to population growth and infertility treatment. The census showed a sharp decline in population growth to 1.5 percent per annum, below replacement level. Several studies confirmed the uniformity of this decline among the generation of reproductive age, across the country. For example, according to the following report by the Iranian Center for Research on Asian and Oceanic Population:

> Those couples who have just married and those who have been married for up to three years show no inclination to have any children at all, or perhaps just one. This tendency over the past decade illustrates that for women of urban and rural backgrounds, from different social

> classes, the poor and the rich, illiterate and literate, all have similar attitudes to giving birth these days, leading to the rapid downward trend in the Iranian total fertility rate (TFR). (Tabnak 2013)

The decline in population growth proved alarming and led Supreme Religious Leader Ayatollah Khamenei to announce publicly that "it was wrong to continue with the family planning program and that the two-decade old policy of controlled population growth must end" (Tabnak 2013). The Supreme Leader admitted that "one of the mistakes [Iran] made in the nineties was population control" (Tabnak 2013). He also stressed the necessity of building a strong nation and articulated Iran's goal to increase its population from 85 million to 150 million by 2050 (Tabnak 2013). In reversing the family planning program of the 1980s, the Supreme Leader was challenging values that had, by now, become deep-seated in the generation that had grown up believing in the advantages of having fewer children. The conservative Iranian president Mahmoud Ahmadinejad announced a new pronatalist approach, calling the anti-natalist policies ungodly and a Western import.[10] The previous family planning programs were dismantled, and their funding was rerouted to promote the new policies. Earlier measures included the introduction of two bills to the parliament aimed at limiting couples' access to voluntary contraceptive measures, such as sterilization. Bill 446, aiming to increase fertility rates and prevent population decline, and Bill 315, aiming predominantly to curtail women's access to family planning and limit their employment opportunities outside the home, passed with an overwhelming majority in August 2014 and 2015, respectively. Iran's new policies also included incentives to encourage couples to procreate. The government offered to give newborn babies gold coins, grant them financial loans, and open bank accounts for them until they reach the age of eighteen. However, these measures did not yield significant results, and population growth continued to decline. In June 2021, the head of the Center for Strategic Research on Population expressed his concern in an interview:

> Saleh Ghasemi, head of the Center for Strategic Research on Population, told a local news agency that the current birth rate is 1.6 for each woman at the age of fertility. He added that in [the] mid-1980s Iran had a 6.5 birth rate, one [of] the highest in the world, but it has been declining since. . . . He added that the population growth rate is currently 0.6 percent but is expected to decline to zero in the next 10–15 years. . . . He went on to say that women born in the 1980s

> are dropping out of the child-bearing age. This, coupled with change in people's preferences and lifestyle, will continue to reduce births. (*Iran International* 2021)

Realizing the failure of these pronatalist policies, President Ebrahim Raisi submitted a bill introducing further measures to boost population growth. The new law passed in November 2021, while offering financial help and providing facilities for couples to have more children, is extremely coercive, essentially granting the state control over the reproductive lives and rights of couples. The law prevents families' access to any form of contraception and limits women's access to sexual and reproductive health care. One of the harmful outcomes of the ban, among many others, is unwanted pregnancies leading to illegal abortions. Under the new law, a panel comprised of a judge and two medical professionals will determine the legality of all abortion cases. Any use of contraceptives is limited and subject to the judgment of a committee of experts; necessity is based on medical, not contraceptive, purposes. The law further bans women's access to prenatal genetic testing, increasing the number of children being born with genetic defects.[11] Health experts point to further risks involved in banning contraceptives, such as the wide spread of sexually transmitted diseases, including AIDS (Radio Free Europe 2021). These new policies also instruct the laboratories that process blood tests to record and share information about patients, particularly pregnant women, with the government, a move interpreted as the state trying to keep tabs on pregnant women in order to discourage or prevent abortions. As Simin Kazemi, an Iranian demographer and health sociologist, pointed out, "women remain the main target of pronatalist policies," and "they are seen as tools for reproduction at the service of government" (Esfandiari and Ravanshad 2021). Clerics are also preaching from the pulpit on these issues, encouraging young couples, for example, to reproduce, hold prayer sessions, and choose auspicious religious dates for mating to increase the chance of conception. The state is also providing five-year loans for young unmarried couples, between men younger than twenty-five and women younger than twenty-two.[12]

Iran's draconian pronatalist policies recall those of Ceausescu's Romania. According to Gail Kligman (1998), between 1965 and 1989, dictator Nicolae Ceausescu enacted some of the most repressive pronatalist policies in history to force population growth in the country. For example, Ceausescu required each family to produce at least four or five children and prohibited abortion (Kligman 1998:

1). His draconian policies failed to increase population growth and came at a high cost to the health of women and families. Romania had the highest maternal mortality rate in the world at that time as women resorted to every means available to abort their unwanted fetuses. In Iran, the state's drive to force population growth has so far fallen on deaf ears, with the younger generation of reproductive age remaining defiant and ignoring the state's actions by finding ways to bypass them. As one young woman, representative of her generation, commented, "We are used to restrictions in this country, and we always find ways to get around them." Another young woman, who has been married for eight years said, "They have put their knees on people's necks and told them to have children," and added, "The only thing they are good at is intruding in people's beds" (*Middle East Eye* 2021). However, it is too early to assess the effectiveness of these policies.

Iranian authorities attribute the delay in the age of marriage, decline in fertility growth, and considerable increase in voluntary childlessness to economic hardship. However, this is a reductionist interpretation of a more complex situation. Instead, these trends are rooted in a multitude of factors, including: the resistance of young people to reverse their reproductive behaviors to meet the state's nation-building goals, due largely to the impact of the family planning programs of the 1980s and 1990s; a successful literacy campaign, especially a rise in female literacy and education, during this time; an increase in female participation in the labor market; a high rate of urbanization, depriving young couples of the support of their traditional networks, including the help of the older generation with childcare; and a major shift in the status of women in the family and society at large.[13] Even if couples, including those who have opted for voluntary childlessness, respond to the state's plea and have one or two children, their contribution will not be enough to help the state meet its population goals. Population growth can be achieved only if every couple has more than two children. Furthermore, there exists another relatively small group, that of cohabiting couples who would like to have children but cannot because conceiving outside of wedlock is equivalent to adultery and carries severe punishment. Among this group, most pregnancies end up being aborted illegally. Some of these couples, who wanted to have children, have been forced to leave the country for places that permit bearing children out of wedlock (Nazari 2021).

Iran's new pronatalist policies have altered the state's approach to infertility and its treatment. The state's initial search for solutions to boost population growth in 2013 coincided with the publication of a large survey on infertility carried out by Avicenna Research Center, a leading center for infertility treatment. The survey of 17,000 households showed the prevalence of infertility among married couples to be 19 percent in urban and 22 percent in rural areas (Akhondi et al. 2013), which was considerably higher than the average 15 percent global figures given by the World Health Organization. Further figures released by health officials also put the number of infertile couples at around 2 million (Nazari 2021). The state saw in these high infertility rates an opportunity to further implement its pronatalist policies. It considered infertility to be a matter of public health and incorporated its treatment into the nationwide programming. The Ministry of Health set up an infertility treatment plan called *Barekat-e Khanevadeh* (Family blessing) in 2015, aiming to provide treatment for all infertile couples between the ages of twenty and forty, free of charge, in underprivileged areas in ten provinces. The foundation that implemented this plan was affiliated with Setad, a special office for executing the decrees of Imam Khomeini that seek to help the underprivileged. According to the head of the Infertility and Reproductive Health Research Center at Tehran's Shahid Beheshti University, "The infertility treatment program conducted jointly by the Health Ministry and the Barekat Foundation . . . is in line with the general population policies to enhance population growth set by the Leader, Ayatollah Seyyed Ali Khamenei in June 2014" (*Financial Tribune* 2016). Health officials also released further information on the status of infertility in the country. For example, according to one official, "Based on the latest surveys conducted, it is estimated that there are 450,000 infertile couples in the rural areas and some of them cannot afford to pay for the costly infertility treatments." Furthermore, the deputy Health Minister was quoted as saying: "As of today, all infertile Iranian couples, who number about two million couples, can enjoy the coverage of their expenses and state insurance will cover 85 percent of the costs, the first time infertility treatments have been covered—and the government has allocated around $30 million (27 million euros) for the project."[14] Until 2016, infertility treatment, by and large, was in the hands of private practitioners and a total of sixty-one infertility clinics in the country, twenty-four of which were public and thirty-seven private. Since 2013, the state has continued to invest in public clinics, which now number approximately 100, and fully covers the costs of up to three cycles of treatment for those who cannot afford them.

Although this sudden turnaround by the state diminished the private sector's involvement in infertility treatment, the move was welcomed by health practitioners, who hoped that this new government oversight would introduce standards of uniformity and help clarify some of the nebulous areas that had emerged over the past three decades of practice. However, with the state determined to increase population growth at all costs, a new form of chaos has emerged regarding infertility treatment. Confidential interviews carried out with leading physicians reveal that the state has instructed infertility clinics to increase the success rate in treating infertile couples. According to one leading clinician, "Following the state's policies on increasing population growth, at present anything goes in infertility clinics, which are instructed not to scrutinize too closely the medical and ethical standards concerning third-party gamete donation and some of the less scrupulous clinics are only too happy to oblige. The priority is now to appease the state's urge for producing more children at any cost." At present no data is available on whether infertility treatment financed by the state is yielding the expected results, and several questions remain unanswered. For example: considering that the chance of successful treatment is around 25 to 30 percent, will the number of children born as a result of IVF treatment contribute significantly to Iran's population growth? Furthermore, in the event of an unsuccessful first round of treatment, would the couple want to undergo a second? Would they succeed? If so, at what cost to the state? And, considering the absence of any enforcement, what is the likelihood that more ethical and legal problems will emerge and lead to long-term complications? In the meantime, concerns on following the Islamic rules of conception through biological relatedness and purity of lineage seem to have taken a backseat.

Reflections on Reproduction and the State's Population Policies

The journey of infertility treatment in Iran from the private sector to the public domain traces the state's extensive use of reproduction to achieve its body politic. This chapter yields two main findings. First, when Iran's population policies aligned with people's aspirations and respected their reproductive norms and values, they succeeded. For example, Iran's anti-natalist approach of the 1990s, which won Iran a United Nations award for their outstanding success, did not lead the state to resort to force; instead, they persuaded people to reduce the size of their families through advocacy and other methods (see Chapter 4). Ultimately, they were successful because they aligned with the needs and priorities of women and families. The latest pronatalist policies, on the other hand, which initially led the state to adopt a combination of incentives and coercive approaches, expected citizens of reproductive age to reverse the very values advocated by the state two decades earlier. Thus, they were ignored, forcing the state to resort to draconian measures of coercion, thus far unsuccessful.

Second, the Iranian regime's legitimization of third-party gamete donation—in other words, its permission for couples to conceive through the assistance of strangers—further illustrates the extent of its pronatalist commitment. While it permits these controversial procedures with the intention of conforming to the Islamic rules of creating happy and stable families, it simultaneously transgresses the very lineage principles it means to protect. In its anxiety to conform, not only does its justification of gamete donation by strangers disrupt the purity of biological lineage, it introduces legal and ethical quandaries. For example, it complicates definitions of "confidentiality" and "anonymity" concerning gamete donors and recipients. This ambiguity has had major implications on the considerable number of actors involved in the process of procreation, as well as on institutions of family and kinship. Finally, the endorsement of independent Islamist jurists of third-party donation has emerged as a useful tool in the hands of the theocratic state in its drive to increase population growth. However, this also presents a conundrum for religio-political authorities, such as the members of the Guardian Council, which consists of a majority of ultra conservative members, who, while equally anxious to increase population growth, also object to the intrusion of a third party into what they see as the sanctity of the family.[15]

Conclusion

Through a brief comparison of the body politic of various Iranian states, from the late nineteenth century to the present, this chapter shows the issue of population to be inextricably linked to the ideals of nation-building. Overall, policy approaches toward population size, under two monarchies and the Islamic Republic, cover five episodes, each contradicting the previous one and all expecting citizens to reverse their reproductive behaviors to meet the goals of the state. Throughout, attention to the reproductive well-being and rights of the citizen has either gone unacknowledged or has been exploited for political purposes. This is particularly true in the case of women, who, according to Hoodfar (2017: 230), "are being essentially directed through these policies to increase their fertility as a national and religious duty in order to achieve the political goals of the state." Although any state's body politic is political by nature, Iran's case is unique. The Iranian state, which had initially relied on advocacy to gain the collaboration of the nation, is now becoming increasingly ruthless in using its citizens as tools of reproduction for political purposes. The recognition of the reproductive rights of the citizens has vanished in the face of the state's drive to increase the population. This study provides a clear example of how a state that is desperate to preserve power at all costs believes, wrongly, that it can manipulate and coerce the nation to change its reproduction values every few decades to align with its own political agenda.

However, while there is no denial that many people of reproductive age, especially women, are increasingly harmed by the state's pronatalist policies, members of this age group have taken control of their own reproductive lives by ignoring the demands of the state and refusing to have more children than they want. In the process, these young people have confirmed an age-old Iranian belief that one's rights are not given and have to be taken (*Haq guereftani ast na dadani*). Although from the perspective of human and reproductive rights these pronatalist policies may be a breach of individual liberties, Iranians of reproductive age have chosen the path that best fits their vision of reproduction, which means overriding or bypassing state dictates. In managing its own reproductive life, this generation is sending a message to policymakers that, in David Parkin's (2001: xii) words, "the management of reproductive life is not just a matter of formal systems of authority, control and knowledge transmission, nor of following policymakers' directives, nor even of integrating these with indigenous ones. It also extends to recognizing the metaphysical and cosmological understandings and practices that everywhere accompany rules, plans, and policies."

Notes

1. For more information, see Esfandiari and Ravanshad (2021).
2. Some scholars, such as Abbasi-Shavazi (2001), Ladier-Fouladi (2003), and Hoodfar and Assadipour (2000), have argued that, although the population policies are viewed as responsible for a sharp drop in population growth, in reality this decline had started around 1984, before the implementation of the policies, especially in urban areas, due to a number of sociocultural and economic factors.
3. As mentioned above, in addition to the state's educational program, other socioeconomic factors played a significant role in the reduction in the size of the family.
4. For more information on various solutions suggested by the jurists to legitimize third-party gamete donation, see Inhorn and Tremayne (2012).
5. Interestingly, during my fieldwork, I came across a couple whose *marja* was against third-party gamete donation, but who recommended another *marja* from whom the couple could seek permission. Tappan (2012) also recounts such incidents. Finally, the director of one of the leading clinics also confirmed that they frequently observe this practice among their patients.
6. Some *marjas* put forth other solutions to legitimize gamete donation, for example the use of temporary marriage to the donor of the gamete. See Tremayne (2009: 144–164).
7. The majority of public clinics were housed within public hospitals and operated under the supervision of university medical departments.
8. Personal observation during the fieldwork in the clinics.
9. Najmabadi (2013) explains a similar situation in cases of transgender surgery in Iran, whereby regulation gaps allow room for maneuver by homosexuals to use the situation to their own benefit.
10. From a speech made by Ahmadinejad during a trip to Alborz Province on 6 January 2011, reported by London weekly *Kayhan*.
11. https://www.bbc.com/persian/iran-59331496.
12. For more details on Iran's coercive anti-contraception measures, see Esfandiari and Ravanshad (2021), Human Rights Watch (2021), Motamedi (2021), and Radio Free Europe (2021).
13. For a fuller explanation of the change in women's status, see Shadi-Talab (2005).
14. https://www.al-monitor.com/pulse/contents/afp/2016/08/iran-health care-infertility-politics.print.html.
15. See Inhorn and Tremayne (2012) and Tremayne (2015); for more details, also see Tremayne and Akhondi (2016).

References

Abbasi-Shavazi, Mohammad Jalal. 2001. "La Fécondité en Iran: L'autre Revolution" [Fertility in Iran: The other revolution]. *Population et Societé* 373.

Abbasi-Shavazi, Mohammad Jalal, Peter McDonald, and Meimanat Hosseini-Chavoshi. 2009. *The Fertility Transition in Iran: Revolution and Reproduction*. Dordrecht: Springer.

Akhondi, Mohammad Mehdi, Koorosh Kamali, Fahimeh Ranjbar, Mahdi Shirzad, Shiva Shafeghati, Zohreh Behjati Ardakani, Abolfazl Goodjani, Mahboubeh Parsaeian, and Kazem Mohammad. 2013. "Prevalence of Primary Infertility in Iran in 2010." *Journal of Public Health* 42(12): 1398–1404.

Esfandiari, Golnaz, and Elahe Ravanshad. 2021. "'It's My Decision': Iran's New Population Law Blasted for Restricting Access to Contraceptives, Abortions." Radio Free Europe, 18 November. Retrieved 20 January 2022 from https://www.rferl.org/a/iran-abortions-sterilizations-contraceptives/31568161.html.

Financial Tribune. 2016. "Advanced Treatment for Infertility Available in Iran." 28 September. Retrieved 27 April 2022 from https://financialtribune.com/articles/people/50678/advanced-treatment-for-infertility-available-in-iran.

Hoodfar, Homa. 1995. "Population Policy and Gender Equity in Post-Revolutionary Iran." In *Family, Gender and Population in the Middle East: Policies in Context*, ed. Carla Makhlouf, 105–135. Cairo: American University of Cairo Press.

———. 2017. "Turning Back the Clock: Population Policy and Human Rights in Iran." In *Routledge Handbook on Human Rights and the Middle East and North Africa*, ed. Anthony Tirado Chase, 230–242. New York: Routledge.

Hoodfar, Homa, and Samad Assadipour. 2000. "The Politics of Population Policy in the Islamic Republic of Iran." *Studies in Family Planning* 31(1): 19–34.

Human Rights Watch. 2021. "Iran: Population Law Violates Women's Rights: Denies Access to Essential Reproductive Health Care, Information." 10 November. Retrieved 20 January 2022 from https://www.hrw.org/news/2021/11/10/iran-population-law-violates-womens-rights.

Inhorn, Marcia C., and Frank Van Ballen, eds. 2002. *Infertility Around the Globe: New Thinking on Childlessness, Gender, and Reproductive Technologies*. Berkeley: University of California Press.

Inhorn, Marcia C., and Soraya Tremayne. 2012. *Islam and Assisted Reproductive Technologies: Sunni and Shia Perspectives*. New York: Berghahn Books.

Iran International. 2021. "Official Warns Population Growth Rate Fast Declining in Iran." 25 October. Retrieved 20 January 2022 from https://www.iranintl.com/en/20211025107012.

Kashani-Sabet, Firoozeh. 2011. *Conceiving Citizens: Women and the Politics of Motherhood in Iran*. Oxford: Oxford University Press.

Khamenei, Ali. 1999. *Ojoubeh Al-Esteftaat*. Questions 1271 to 1277. Amir Kabir.

Khomeini, Ruhollah. 2001. *Tahrir-Al-Vasilah*. Qom: Islamic Publishing.

Kligman, Gail. 1998. *The Politics of Duplicity: Controlling Reproduction in Ceausescu's Romania*. Berkeley; Los Angeles: University of California Press.

Ladier-Fouladi, Marie. 2003. "Population et Politique en Iran: De la Monarchie a la République islamique" [Population and politics in Iran: From the monarchy to the Islamic republic]. *Les Cahiers de L'INED* (Institut National des Etudes Demographiques) 150(2).

Madani Tabrizi, Yousef. 2009. *Al-Massael-al-Mostahadasseh* 3. Tehran: Ayatollah Madani Tabrizi's Office, 212–228.

Middle East Eye. 2021. "Iran Pushes for Baby Boom by Curtailing Access to Contraceptives and Abortions." 5 December. Retrieved 20 January 2022 from https://www.middleeasteye.net/news/iran-contraceptive-abortion-access-curtailed-push-baby-boom.

Motamedi, Maziar. 2021. "UN Experts Call on Iran to Repeal 'Anti-Abortion' Population Law." *Al Jazeera*, 16 November. Retrieved 20 January 2022 from https://www.aljazeera.com/news/2021/11/16/un-experts-call-on-iran-to-repeal-anti-abortion-population-law.

Najmabadi, Afsaneh. 2013. *Professing Selves: Transsexuality and Same-Sex Desire in Contemporary Iran*. Durham, NC: Duke University Press.

Nazari, Sarbas. 2021. "Iran: The Painful Choices of Being Pregnant and Unmarried." BBC News, 24 October. Retrieved 20 January 2022 from https://www.bbc.com/news/world-middle-east-58957045.

OHCHR (United Nations Office of the High Commissioner on Human Rights). 2021. "Iran: Repeal 'Crippling' New Anti-Abortion Law – UN Experts." 16 November. Retrieved 19 January 2022 from https://www.ohchr.org/EN/NewsEvents/Pages/DisplayNews.aspx?NewsID=27817&LangID=E.

Parkin, David. 2001. "Foreword." In *Managing Reproductive Life: Cross-Cultural Themes in Fertility and Sexuality*, ed. Soraya Tremayne, iix–xii. New York: Berghahn Books.

Radio Free Europe. 2021. "Iran Condom Ban Sparks Fears of Disease, Unwanted Pregnancies, and a Black Market." 21 December. Retrieved 20 January 2022 from https://www.rferl.org/a/iran-condom-ban-sparks-fears-of-disease-unwanted-pregnancies-and-a-black-market/31621377.html.

Shadi-Talab, Jaleh. 2005. "Iranian Women: Rising Expectations." *Critique Critical Middle Eastern Studies* 14(1): 35–55.

Tabnak. 2013. "Iran's Population Crisis Awaits the Iranian People." In Persian. 24 September. Retrieved 26 September 2021 from www.tabnak.ir/fa/news/346841.

Tappan, Robert. 2012. "Ethical Decision-Making in Iranian Fertility

Clinics." In *Islam and Assisted Reproductive Technologies: Sunni and Shia Perspectives*, ed. Marcia C. Inhorn and Soraya Tremayne, 103–129. New York: Berghahn Books.

Tremayne, Soraya. 2004. "'And Never the Twain Shall Meet': Reproductive Health Policies in the Islamic State of Iran." In *Reproductive Agency, Medicine and the State: Cultural Transformations in Childbearing*, ed. Maya Unnithan-Kumar, 181–202. New York: Berghahn Books.

———. 2009. "Law, Ethics and Donor Technologies in Shia Iran." In *Assisting Reproduction, Testing Genes: Global Encounters with New Biotechnologies*, ed. Daphna Birenbaum-Carmeli and Marcia C. Inhorn, 144–163. New York: Berghahn Books.

———. 2015. "Whither Kinship? Assisted Reproductive Technologies and Relatedness in the Islamic Republic of Iran." In *Assisted Reproductive Technologies in the Third Phase*, ed. Kate Hampshire and Bob Simpson. New York: Berghahn Books.

Tremayne, Soraya, and Mohammad Mehdi Akhondi. 2016. "Conceiving IVF in Iran." *Reproductive Biomedicine & Society Online* 2: 62–70.

United Nations. 2016. *Demographic Yearbook*: "Demographics of Iran." Retrieved 19 September 2021 from http://www.worldometers.info/world-population/iran-population/.

Yazdi, Mohammad. 1996. "Infertility Treatment and its Jurisprudential Approach." *Figh-e-Ahl-e-Beit* 5: 5–6.

Part III

Kinship, Family, Gender

Chapter 7

THE "DOWN SIDE" OF GAMETE DONATION

CHALLENGING "HAPPY FAMILY" RHETORIC IN IRAN

Introduction

The use of assisted reproductive technologies (ARTs) for infertility treatment has been made possible in the Muslim countries of the Middle East by the endorsement and strong support of the religious leaders, as observed by Inhorn (2003: 1), who also notes that "nowhere is this globalization process more evident than in the nearly twenty nations of the Muslim Middle East." These technologies, however, have remained limited in their application in most Muslim countries to in vitro fertilization (IVF) treatment for married couples only, and no third-party donation is allowed among Sunni Muslims (Inhorn 2005a; Clarke 2006a). Iran, which is a Shia theocracy, on the other hand, has adopted these technologies with open arms and has legitimized almost all forms of third-party donation including that of sperm and egg donation, embryo donation, and surrogacy, and more recently stem cell research and sex selection. ARTs have been practiced in Iran for over twenty years, and demand for them continues to grow. As Inhorn (2005b) notes, "Iran is definitely in the lead among the Muslim countries in the Middle East in the application of these technologies."[1] The reasons for and the process of legitimizing ARTs in the Muslim Middle East have been documented extensively elsewhere (Inhorn 2003, 2005a, 2006a, 2006b; Clarke 2006a, 2006b, 2009; Serour 1993; Tremayne 2005, 2006a, 2006b, 2009 among others). A brief explanation of the difference between Shia Iran and the rest of the Muslim world is that the majority of Sunni Muslims, in considering such practices, have concluded that the practice of third-party gamete donation would lead to confusion in the lineage (*nasab*), which forms the foundation of the Muslim family, and would be equal to incest or adultery and, therefore, a threat to the stability of social relations (Inhorn 2005a; Clarke 2009; Tremayne 2009).

The Shia religious leaders in Iran, on the other hand, have been able to find solutions to legitimize third-party donation without breaking any of the Islamic rules concerning adultery and incest. In doing so, they have focused on an in-depth examination of what constitutes *nasab*,[2] and whether the practice of ARTs with all its ramifications would confuse the line of lineage. To do so, the senior Shia clerics resorted to *ijtihad*, and concluded that certain forms of third-party donation could be allowed without breaching any divine rules (Tremayne 2009). ARTs are therefore currently practiced in Iran with the full approval of the ruling religious leaders, although the use of donor sperm remains a more contentious issue, as will be discussed further down, and its practice is limited. However, not all religious leaders in Iran are in agreement with the interpretations that have led to legitimizing third-party donation. Similar to the Sunni religious leaders, the opponents of such practices in Iran remain uncompromising in their interpretations of the Qur'an and forbid the use of third-party donation. Iran being a theocracy, a distinction has to be made between the views of those leading clerics who are also the political rulers and law makers and represent the "official" position on religious and juristic matters, and those who are equally, if not more, qualified in *fiqh* and are sources of emulation with a large following, but are not in a position to enforce their views.[3] It is therefore the ruling of the religio-political rulers, with support from some of the more progressive apolitical clerics, that has opened the door for the use of ARTs.

The official endorsement of third-party donation of gametes, issued by the supreme religious leader Ayatollah Khamenei in the late 1990s, is generally taken as the starting point for third-party donation (Inhorn 2006a; Clarke 2009; Tremayne 2009). However, prior to this *fatwa*, several Shia scholars had debated at length the legitimacy of third-party donation and had issued their views on it. One example, which proved an important landmark in influencing the decision-making process, was a conference organized by Dr. Mohammad Mehdi Akhondi, the Director of the Avicenna Research Institute and head of one of the leading fertility treatment centers, which resulted in the publication of its proceedings in *Modern Human Reproductive Techniques from the View of Jurisprudence and Law* (Akhondi 2001).[4] The book, the first in this field, includes several chapters by senior clerics and jurists in which they examine closely the legitimacy of third-party donation. Some of the chapters had been published a few years earlier and preceded the above conference. Indeed, those deliberations in the book which favored third-party donation themselves may have been the inspiration behind the late 1990s *fatwa*. Likewise, in addition to the views of the religious leaders of both convictions (for and against such practices), and long before the official decisions were announced in favor of such practices, experts from a variety of other disciplines in the legal, medical, and social sciences had also engaged in exploring the consequences of third-party donation and whether these breach any legal, religious, and social rules. The initial condition set for third-party donation was that it should take place between the married couple. A solution was found within the Shia practice of temporary marriage so that the gamete donor and recipient could get married temporarily to legitimize the donation.[5]

While debates on most aspects, hypothetical and real, of the implications of ARTs continued, and long before the supreme leader's *fatwa*, many clinics took their cue from those clerics who had endorsed them and started the practice of third-party gamete donation.[6] The 1990s *fatwa* proved very "liberal," to use Clarke's (2009) expression, and allowed the donation of both sperm and egg based on the religious edict[7] that "as long as no gaze or touch takes place between the donor and recipient, donation is allowed." Essentially, such endorsement served as the basis for all future forms of donation, such as embryo donation and surrogacy, and removed any suggestion of incest or adultery as long as no bodily contact took place between the two parties (Tremayne 2009: 148; see also Garmaroudi Naef 2012). While third-party egg donation did not provoke any fierce reaction, the approval of sperm donation met with such uproar among the majority of the *ulama* (Muslim legal scholars), as well as the general public, that its practice did not become widespread and only a few private clinics discreetly continue with sperm donation. Currently the majority of clinics practice egg donation only, though sperm donation does continue in some private clinics. Also, with the passage of time, temporary marriage is used to a lesser degree at the clinics.

The rationale behind the approval of ARTs was the stability and happiness they bring into the family by treating infertility. In legitimizing the use of ARTs, the initial deliberations by experts predominantly focused on issues concerning biological and social belonging and inheritance and their implications for donor children. But they did not address the long-term impact of the donor child on the dynamics of family relations, between the child and the parents, between the spouses and genders, and on the larger social group. Such a gap stemmed from the fact that the donor children had not yet reached the age to make a study of this kind possible, but, more importantly, the assumption behind the approval of third-party donation was that once lineage and other legal and practical matters are resolved and the child is born, a happy and stable family will be formed, which will function as any "normal" family (Tremayne 2009; Abbasi-Shavazi et al. 2008).

The hitherto limited research on donor families in Iran suggests that ARTs have saved thousands of marriages by helping couples conceive. However, no known in-depth research has been carried out to follow the life trajectories of the donor children and their families, to assess the actual outcome of their presence on their families and social group. This chapter will follow the life trajectories of a few selected cases who present the other side of the coin to the happy families. The cases presented here are extreme ones, and while the findings do not suggest that all donor cases are similar, they will try to demonstrate that focusing on the cases of happy families alone would be only a half-veiled truth about the full impact of ARTs. The findings and conclusion in this chapter are substantiated by tens of similar cases from a larger study carried out from 2004 to 2009.

ARTs in a State of Flux

The research that serves as the basis for this chapter started in 2004 in Iran. Third-party donation was still relatively new at that time, and donor children were few and far between and too novel to assess their impact. It was clear that the wider implications of third-party donations would be known only when the donor children come of age (Tremayne 2005). The follow-up research between 2004 and 2008 revealed that reproductive technologies have had so many unexpected and unintended outcomes that they seemed to remain in a constant state of flux (Tremayne 2009). The findings of one phase of research seemed to be overruled within six months, and new situations emerged frequently. For example, in

2004, according to the official figures, only twelve cases of surrogacy were known publicly, and the practitioners complained that due to cultural taboos it was difficult to find surrogate mothers. A year later, this number had gone up several fold. In 2004 many cases of same-sex sibling donation existed where sisters donated eggs to each other, but I did not come across siblings of the opposite sex who donated gametes to each other. Two years later, evidence came to the fore that many brothers and sisters had started donating gametes to each other and making embryos together following the *fatwas* that gave legitimacy to such donations, namely, that "as long as there is no touch or gaze third-party donation is allowed" (Tremayne 2009; Garmaroudi Naef 2008).[8]

In 2003 the law for embryo donation was approved and specified that embryo donation should come from a married couple and be donated as a gift. Three years later, in 2006, at a conference held in Tehran on gamete and embryo donation, one of the leading practitioners expressed his dismay publicly that some agencies had started selling embryos that were the result of prostitutes' eggs and unknown men's sperm, and that these agencies had tried to sell these embryos to his clinic. So, the changes are continuing in such unpredictable ways and at such speed that they leave the researcher in doubt as to the validity of his/her original findings. As Nancy Scheper-Hughes (2009: 4), in an editorial on a different topic, wrote: "One major obstacle to public anthropology is our [anthropologists'] reticence to describe events before we have gained a deep understanding of their context. By the time we finally feel we have something to say, the moment has passed into history. In a sense all ethnography is historical—a history of the present—always trailing well behind the moment."

However, in spite of the apparently rapid changes mentioned earlier, the present study shows that ARTs, which on first sight seem to have affected the landscape of kinship, have served to confirm and in some areas reinforce cultural values and practices. While the constant changes in the use of ARTs may be interpreted as confusing and paradoxical for their users, in reality these are mirroring a complex set of relations, which have their roots in cultural values but which, when faced with modern technologies, embrace them readily and gain strength from them. As Becker (2000: 236) puts it, "Because new reproductive technologies reflect cultural meanings and become a conduit for changing cultural practices, they signify both a challenge to and a reinforcement of the moral order."

Third-party donation of sperm and egg has been practiced for several years in Iran, and the donor children are now old enough to make it possible to assess their impact on their parents and the wider social group. In doing so, this chapter focuses on two different but related areas, and asks, first, whether conceiving through such modern technologies, and having received information on the scientific realities of procreation from the clinics, has really transformed the cultural values, beliefs, perceptions, and behavior of the users in a significant way. Second, whether it is correct to assume that proving their fertility and reproductive abilities to themselves and to their social group has resulted in the infertile users forming a "happy family," which, as mentioned earlier, has been the main driving force behind legitimizing third-party donation (Abbasi-Shavazi et al. 2008: 2; Tremayne 2009). Finally, I suggest that the wish for having a child, per se, is not limited to making a family happy or otherwise. It is seen as the duty of the individual to undergo the ritual of reproducing (see also Abbasi-Shavazi et al. 2008: 3), to contribute to the social reproduction of the group, before an adult is accepted as one of its members. To this end, I surmise that children become pawns in such cultural practices to be used for different purposes at different times, by different members of the social group.

Methodology

This chapter is based on two sets of data. The first were collected in Tehran and Yazd (central Iran), between 2004 and 2008 over the course of several field trips. Information from these data is used as the background to support the analysis and conclusion in this chapter. The second were data collected between 2007 and 2009 in the United Kingdom and were based on case studies of Iranian women refugees whom I had come across in my role as an expert witness to courts during their claims for asylum. These women had undergone third-party donation, and their donor children were old enough to allow an assessment of the long-term effect of their conceptions on their families and their wider social group. I have chosen two particular cases, from among several others, because they are representative of the large number of families whom I have come across who are users of third-party donation and whose stories remain untold. Although these two cases can be considered as "extreme," they epitomize the hidden lives of numerous families with similar social and cultural backgrounds, and can be considered the tip of the iceberg. They are exceptional in that these women have been able to leave Iran and tell their stories, and not because they are unique. One of the cases is that of third-party egg donation, and the other, sperm donation. The choice was made to examine whether and how the children who are conceived through gamete donation of egg or sperm differ in their impact on the families and community. Although these stories are written with the explicit permission of both women, I have tried to disguise their identity as much as possible.

Finally, as is clear from the above, the data presented in the case studies in this chapter have not been collected using the usual anthropological methods of fieldwork. For those of us who carry out research in fertility treatment clinics, we are less likely to encounter stories such as the ones told here. But, even when as anthropologists we live with our informants on a daily basis, as opposed to interviewing them at clinics, we are not always likely to be a party to the kind of stories the women in this chapter have recounted. I would have never been privy to these stories in such detail had it not been for the fact that, unknown to these women, I had read their stories and commented on them as an expert witness to the courts. The stories seemed to be so extreme that, to begin with, I doubted their veracity, but on cross-examination I was convinced of their being genuine and not fabricated to obtain asylum. The point is that these kinds of cases do not come to the fore frequently because those who are affected by them, especially women, are often willing parties to perpetuating and protecting the cultural values to which they belong by conforming to what is expected of them by their social group.[9] While such motivations do not reduce the emotional desire for having a child, it is above all the sense of belonging and identity that is the driving force for such submission and silent cooperation. Women in this study appear to have submitted of their own so-called volition[10] to the hardship of undergoing IVF treatment to contribute their shares to the social reproduction of the family and social group, and in doing so they have been greatly assisted by modern reproductive technologies. Unnithan-Kumar's (2010: 163) study of female-selected abortion in India shows that "[reproductive] technologies in themselves do not bring about social transformation but it is in how they are made socially meaningful that their power lies." Likewise, Thompson (2002: 52), in her analysis of feminists' theorization of infertility, illustrates the dilemma created by the modern infertility treatment technologies:

> On the one hand, the burden of involuntary childlessness is considered especially heavy for women, and prominent feminists call for it to be taken seriously as a feminist issue. On the other hand, feminists are also interested in disrupting the gendered role expectations and the essentialist connection between motherhood and women's identity that greatly intensify infertile women's suffering. Contemporary infertility and its treatment are conceptualized and structured on a strongly coupled, ultra-heterosexual, consumer-oriented, normative nuclear family scenario. When successful, treatment enables women to reinscribe themselves into that logic. The paradox of infertility for feminism, then, is this: feminists are well placed to understand the special burden of involuntary childlessness, but they are ambivalent about supporting women who seek infertility treatment because it seems to lend implicit support to conventional gender roles and gendered stratification.

As is clear from the above, ARTs can become a new form of coercion to which women submit willingly.

Creating a Culture (*Farhang Sazi*)

The health care system and the fertility clinics in Iran have taken a proactive role to educate infertile users of ARTs about the facts of procreation (Abbasi-Shavazi et al. 2008). In their view, this is the first step toward normalizing the use of ARTs by familiarizing infertile couples with the biological facts, as opposed to the common understanding and general beliefs about infertility and its causes. This education is generally referred to as "creating a culture" or "building a culture" (*farhang sazi*). The first time I came across such an educational program was in May 2004 when I walked into a private fertility clinic in Tehran. Around fifty men and women were sitting silently in the waiting hall, staring impassively at a giant television screen. At first, I did not pay any attention to what they were watching, assuming that it was the usual television program advocating the correct Islamic values. I was looking for the midwife, who was supposed to show me around. She was late, and while waiting for her, I turned my attention to the television screen. To my disbelief, I saw a live transmission of the fertilization of a woman's egg from the operating theater of the clinic, with the patient's name written on the screen and the doctor's voice explaining how Mrs. X's egg was being fertilized. I looked around anxiously, expecting a reaction from the crowd of men and women watching this.

Iran is a country where sex segregation is supposed to be enforced in theory. Here, at the fertility clinic, I see men and women watching the reproductive organs of a woman, who is being named, without any reaction. This was even more surprising because most of the couples seemed to come from conservative and, most likely, religious backgrounds.

The fertilization of the egg went on, and when the midwife finally arrived, I expressed my astonishment at such a demonstration. She did not seem particularly worried and just said, "Yes, we show these operations live for the patients to teach them what to expect." I then persisted, asking, "But what do the patients think of this?" She said, "We think it is good for them." I realized that my point was missed and did not continue. I then raised the question of why the clinic was called the center for the cure of *na-zai*, meaning the inability to give birth, which is the term used for female infertility. I wanted to know whether it implied that infertility is a uniquely female affliction, which seemed to be in direct contrast with the aims of the educational programs trying to explain that infertility could affect both men and women. The doctors looked blankly at me and then said, "This is a strange question, we have never thought about it in this way." But, they added, "Perhaps we should change this as we do try to tell men that they could be infertile, too."

Two years later, in 2006, I met with the director of a leading private fertility clinic. On my way to his office, I noticed the same giant television screen in the waiting hall with a similar large crowd of people sitting watching similar scenes of the fertilization of an egg. I raised the same question on the prohibition of women's bodies being displayed in such a public way. The director looked uncomfortable at first, then said, "Islam has said that the outside of women's bodies should not be seen, but it has never said that the inside cannot be displayed." Faced with the look of disbelief on my face and realizing that taking refuge behind an implicit religious explanation was not going to prove convincing, he laughed and said: "To tell you the truth, we have never thought about this aspect of the display. Our intention is to create/build a new culture (*farhang sazi*), so that people understand how babies are conceived and how infertility can be treated. We need to make these new techniques fit into the culture (*ja andakhtan*)." He went on, "Our intention is to teach these people scientifically that infertility should not be a stigma and to make them come forward without any shame about their infertility."

In 2008, during an interview with one of the practitioners, whom I had interviewed previously and who had proudly claimed that "we are building a new culture," I found him disillusioned and subdued and having second thoughts about "making a culture" and "creating babies." He mentioned that in starting his fertility clinic, he wanted to make happy families, allow people to have children, and save as many couples from their miseries of being infertile as possible. "What have I achieved?" he says in a low voice. "I have just come across brothers and sisters who have started making embryos together, some to help their siblings, but many for the purpose of making money. Is this what I have worked for so long and so hard? What have I managed to teach these people?" He mentions several cases whereby, in his judgment, norms have been breached and rules broken by both the donors and users of gametes. He repeats the story of the growing number of agencies that make embryos illegitimately (meaning from unmarried couples) and sell them.

Consequently, I heard similar stories from other practitioners. Such breaches seem to have led the clinics to try to take control of the process of donation, wherever possible, by minimizing contact between donors and recipients to prevent the "misuse" of gamete donation. As practitioners, the doctors are more concerned with the biological and genetic outcome of these breaches than the social and cultural rules, which they consider to fall outside their responsibilities. There are other instances whereby the education of users has produced opposite results too. For example, a counselor psychologist from a different private clinic mentioned: "We can familiarize our own users to these technologies, but the practice of ARTs is widespread now and we have no control over who learns in the right way about them. Doctors with minimum training are practicing IVF and third-party donation without any respect for the rules."[11]

From the limited research carried out among the successful recipients of gametes on the long-term effect of the education they have received, there are indications that the education has served the immediate interest of all parties involved to justify their resorting to ARTs. Beyond that, as soon as the baby is taken home, the "cultural education" fades into the background, and the new parents fall back into their "normal" lifestyle and behavior. However, this area remains under-researched and in need of further monitoring and verification.

Case Studies

The use of third-party donation among Iranian couples goes back many years before the technology reached Iran. Infertile Iranian couples used to come to the United Kingdom to seek IVF treatment, partly because these technologies did not exist in Iran, but mainly because they did not want anybody back home to find out that they could not conceive. In one case, I acted as interpreter for a couple and when, after long trials, the doctors told the husband that the problem was with him and not his wife, he started subjecting his wife to intolerable violence. When I asked the wife why she did not divorce him, she said that she had been married and divorced before, and a second divorce was simply not an option, "because even if my father and brothers don't kill me, they will not let me back into their house, and how am I going to live with my parents, neighbors and friends, all of whom will blame me? Divorce will be an added stigma to being infertile and one that I cannot live with." Research in Tehran's infertility clinics also highlights the stigma of infertility, especially male infertility (Abbasi-Shavazi et al. 2008: 14). Divorcing a violent husband who shifts the blame for infertility to his wife would "thrust them [divorced women] into an extremely vulnerable position" (Abbasi-Shavazi et al. 2008: 16).

Batoul's Story

The following case studies of two women form the second part of this chapter. Batoul is a 45-year-old woman who comes from a highly religious and conservative family. She was seventeen when her father forced her to marry a man several years older than herself. She had no say in the decision. Her husband was an engineer and went to work in the United Arab Emirates. In 1988, by the time she was twenty-two years old and had not conceived, her husband decided to take her to the United Kingdom for treatment. The couple received gamete intrafallopian transfer (GIFT) assisted reproduction. Batoul did not speak any English and did not understand anything about the procedures she underwent, so her husband took charge of the entire negotiations. The treatment proved successful, and she became pregnant. They returned to the United Arab Emirates, where she gave birth to nonidentical triplet girls in 1989. The triplets had blonde hair, two with brown eyes and the third with green eyes. It was obvious that the husband was not the biological father of the children. At such a finding, he accused

Batoul of having slept with the doctor in the clinic and became violent and started beating her.

They returned to Iran, where he told the members of his and her families that she had slept with the doctor and the children were bastards. Batoul's father and brothers sided with the husband and became abusive and threatened to kill her and the children because "they were not Muslims" and because "she had brought shame upon the family." Batoul was summoned by the security forces to account for what had happened at the clinic in the United Kingdom. During this time, she was subjected to extreme violence by her husband, who beat and injured her regularly. Over the years, in addition to the routine beatings, she suffered various fractures and burns, including: two broken legs; a sewing machine thrown at her head, which knocked her unconscious; burns with hot oil; and being frozen by having buckets of ice poured over her. The children were also beaten regularly and called bastards. Mina, the daughter with green eyes, developed a heart problem when she was eighteen months old and underwent an operation. After three years Batoul managed to get a divorce, but the court did not instruct the father to pay any maintenance for the "bastards." Legally, he could have claimed custody of the children, but did not do so and was happy for her to keep the children, but did not see it as his duty to contribute financially toward their upkeep.

Over the following five years, Mina had three heart operations. Every time Batoul had great difficulty in getting Mina admitted to the hospital, because no hospital would admit her without the father's permission and confirmation that she was his daughter. None of the members of the father's family were prepared to help with the "illegitimate" children. Batoul had to make a living by sewing and doing various jobs. As the children grew up, they were subjected to constant abuse at school because the father turned up and told the school that these girls were bastards and were Christians. The children were bullied, and once thrown out and told to go to a school for Christian children. The appearance of blonde hair and green eyes in Mina's case made it credible that they were not "Muslim" or from an Iranian father. Batoul kept changing location and moving from one school to another, only to find that her husband had turned up again and asked the school to throw them out. Eventually they moved to Batoul's native village, and Batoul managed to convince the head teacher that her children were Muslims. But the bullying continued by other children. Mina, whom I met recently in the United Kingdom, added that, in order to be allowed to stay at school, she even joined the Basij[12] at her school to prove that she was a Muslim. Finally, Batoul's husband told her that if she wanted his help with getting the children to schools or hospitals, she should remarry him. Batoul seemed to have little choice but to accept this. But, although she was now married to him, he refused to support the family financially. Throughout this time the only person who supported Batoul both financially and morally was her mother, despite the disapproval of her husband, Batoul's father.

After the renewal of the marriage, the husband did not live at home but came home occasionally and without warning. Batoul was lonely and miserable, and met another man with whom she fell in love and started an affair. One day, when he was visiting her, the husband came back home accompanied by three men from the security forces and caught Batoul and her lover in bed. The men were to be witnesses to adultery, and duly took photographs and took Batoul and her lover to their headquarters. She was held for two days in a dark cell, and while in custody was raped by the officers. Both she and her lover were sentenced to be stoned to death. By now, Batoul's father was dead, and her mother sold her house to pay a heavy bail for her temporary release while waiting to be stoned. Batoul hid two of her children and fled from Iran and came to the United Kingdom with Mina to allow her to have a fourth urgent operation for her heart. On arrival, she applied for asylum. At first, she and Mina were kept in a notorious detention center, where she attempted suicide twice and has suffered mental ill health since.

Soon after she left Iran, Batoul's husband started harassing her mother to discover Batoul's whereabouts. Mina is now twenty years old and is at university, while her two sisters are in Iran and still on the run from their social father. I heard recently that Batoul has gone back to Iran, clandestinely, to save her children from her husband, who was trying to sell them to some dealers in the United Arab Emirates. One of them was held at gunpoint recently by a man, who was employed by the husband to abduct them and take them to the United Arab Emirates. According to Batoul and Mina, the husband is still calling the girls "bastards" and wants to "wash this stain of shame from the family" by either forcing them into marriage or actually trafficking them as sex workers. Batoul said that she had no choice but to rescue her daughters, whose lives are in danger. She is still wanted by the courts in Iran, and if her husband finds her, he will make sure that she is arrested and that the death sentence is carried out. Her own brothers maintain their threat that they too will kill her. So, twenty-one years after Batoul underwent IVF treatment, her life, and that of her daughters in Iran, has gone from bad to worse, with no end in sight as yet. The two girls in Iran have now completed their secondary education, against all odds and with help from their grandmother. They wish to go to university, but do not have the financial means. The grandmother is old and frail and has run out of money, and the girls are still hiding from the father.

I met with Mina, to hear her side of the story. She is still under medical surveillance for her heart problems but is determined to make her life a success. She said that her maternal uncles are still telling the two sisters that if they ever catch Mina, they will kill her "because of her green eyes, because she, Mina, is the perfect testimony for our sister's shameful adultery." Mina told me: "I do not consider 'that man' to be my father. Apart from the fact that he is not my biological father, he never gave me any love or affection." To date, Batoul's brothers attack their own mother and abuse her verbally and throw stones at her house, where Batoul's two remaining daughters live. They are angry with their mother for helping Batoul. Batoul's relatives also reject the girls. On one occasion, when the two sisters ran away from their father's violence and took a bus to a town where their paternal aunt lived, they were cross-questioned by the police on the bus, asking what two young women were doing traveling by themselves and where were they going. The sisters gave their aunt's address and on arrival were delivered by the police to the aunt's house. She attacked them and beat them up and threw them out. One last remark from Mina was about her paternal uncle's youngest brother, who has married recently, and has realized that he is the infertile party. Since this discovery, his behavior has changed drastically toward Mina's sisters, saying that he now realizes that perhaps infertility runs in the family and, after all, it must have been his brother who was the infertile party.

In Batoul's case, the fact that her husband had been shown not to have been the biological father of the children dealt such a devastating blow to him, and made him lose face so seriously, that for the following twenty years he made Batoul and her three daughters' lives a misery and has kept them under constant threat. The recent investigations at the clinic that carried out the donation twenty years previously in the United Kingdom indicate that the clinic had explained fully to Batoul's husband about the procedure of third-party donation. The conclusion, therefore, must be that the husband was aware that Batoul's egg would be fertilized with another man's sperm, but that he had hoped to pretend that the child was his own as the result of the IVF treatment. Furthermore, what seems to matter more to him is to show his ability to reproduce, at all costs, even by secretly agreeing to use another man's sperm. Several other examples among the cases in this study show remarkable similarities. In one case the couple had gone abroad and on return claimed that the wife was pregnant. When the baby was born, he was black, and it became clear that they had undergone third-party donation. Or, in another case, the infertile man had made a deal with the doctor and his brother to receive the brother's sperm, without his wife's knowledge. In the latter case, I have previously argued that, whenever possible, infertile men and women resort to their families for gamete donation to keep the lineage intact (Tremayne 2009). At the same time, consistent with the stigma of infertility, if an infertile man can possibly hide his infertility even from his kin group, he will do so. Batoul's husband did not seek his brother's help for donation because the technologies did not exist in Iran then, but possibly also because he did not imagine that his "secret" would be revealed in such an unexpected way, or he might have resorted to his brothers for help. Data from previous research also testifies that even when men have willingly chosen to receive sperm from other men, after the children are born men find it hard to accept them, and in the case of those who do not resort to violence against their wives, some have been known to have developed serious psychological problems themselves and have had to resort to treatment and counseling. One such man told his psychologist, "I cannot help looking at him and thinking that he is not my child. I cannot stand having him around." Inhorn (2006c) also provides substantial evidence of such deeply ingrained adversity elsewhere (see also Tremayne 2009).

Sahar's Story

Sahar's story is a contrast to that of Batoul in some respects. She is fifty-three years old and comes from a wealthy and moderately religious and conservative family. When she was thirteen, she was given in marriage to a man who raped her before the marriage ceremony had taken place. As a result, she became pregnant, and gave birth to a disabled child; her family made her divorce the man and give the child to the husband's family. Sahar never saw her son again. A few years later, she married a wealthy man who told her that he was impotent and could not satisfy her sexual needs.

"But, he was a fair man and told me that I could have lovers if I wanted to, but I was so traumatized by my past experience that I was content living with him." Sahar lived in "real style," as she puts it, traveling everywhere with her husband, owning several homes, and employing an army of helpers. The marriage lasted a few years, but he was posted to other countries and she did not want to leave Iran. So, they separated. She started a property management business that became very successful, and she purchased several homes for herself, including some in the United Kingdom. She then married her third husband, who came from a highly conservative background, and had a senior position as the mayor of a district in a major city in Iran. Soon after they were married the husband became violent and started beating her severely. As a result, she had a miscarriage, two broken legs, and is lame in one leg and deaf in one ear.

By the time Sahar was forty-one years old, in 1997, she thought that having a child might help improve the marriage and reduce her husband's violent behavior. Due to her age, she resorted to third-party egg donation. To do so, a temporary marriage[13] arrangement was used between the donor and Sahar's husband at the fertility clinic. The egg donor was married to Sahar's husband for three days, until the doctor was satisfied that the egg was fertilized. Sahar became pregnant with twins, but during one of the severe regular beatings from her husband, she had a miscarriage and lost one child and only just managed to keep the second one. She gave birth to a son in 1998. But giving her husband a son did not improve his behavior, and after five years she was forced to separate from him and live on her own with her son. Her husband then came to the United Kingdom to seek asylum, claiming that he had converted to Christianity. Their son was desperate to see his father, and Sahar brought him to the United Kingdom. While visiting her husband, he asked her to give false evidence to the courts about his conversion to Christianity, which she refused to do. He beat her up so badly that she needed hospital treatment. Her injuries were so severe that the authorities in the United Kingdom, realizing that she was the victim of domestic violence, offered her asylum. But she refused this offer and returned to Iran.

The husband, having had his asylum turned down, returned to Iran too. Once in Iran, he banned Sahar and their son from leaving the country, since a woman needs her husband's or father's permission to leave the country. He then took the son away to live with him in a town 1,200 kilometers away. Since legally the child belongs to the father, she could not protest and was given visitation rights of thirty-six hours every three months. He started using the son to blackmail Sahar financially and managed to obtain some of her properties but refused to return the child. In effect, the child had become a bargaining chip in the relationship between Sahar and her husband.

The husband then complained to the courts that she had falsified papers to implicate him as having sought asylum in the United Kingdom on the grounds that he had converted to Christianity. This is a very serious accusation since conversion from Islam in Iran carries a death sentence. The husband and his father also attempted to kill her by driving a car toward her and trying to run her off the road. At this point, Sahar, who had succeeded in getting a divorce but whose court case on her husband's accusations was still pending, left the country for the United Kingdom and sought asylum. In the meantime, the husband had taken the son away to an unknown location. In spite of appealing to international agencies to track the child down, she has not been able to find him and is thinking of returning to Iran even at the risk of having to face the Revolutionary Courts. She says that "life without my son is meaningless." Unlike Batoul, Sahar's parents and relatives are supportive of her, but her in-laws, especially her mother-in-law, have gone to great lengths to make life difficult for her.

Discussion

In this chapter I have examined the implications of the use of third-party donation of sperm and eggs on the lives of some families who have gone home with children. I have considered whether the use of the state-of-the-art reproductive technologies has altered the values that are the driving force behind the reproductive decisions infertile couples make. The effect of the donor child on the parents and the wider social group was also considered. To this end, two cases were selected on the basis that they reflected the "other side of the coin" to the successful cases and happy families. These cases are extreme ones, but by no means unique or even rare. The findings presented in this chapter are supported by a larger study of donor technologies, which include tens of other cases and which serve as the main source for the analysis in this chapter. Other studies also support some of the findings in this chapter (see for example Abbasi-Shavazi et al. 2008).

Several points emerge from the combination of the studies mentioned above. In general, men's and women's approaches to ARTs have been shown to differ, and the way donor children are treated depends upon whose biological child they are in the family. Women seem to have invariably welcomed egg donation and have submitted to the treatment and cherished the child afterward. In some of the cases of egg donation, the couple returned with the same donor to have another child. Such reactions, viewed in their cultural context, support the suggestion that the way the ARTs have been used reflect the users' understanding of what constitutes kinship, families, lineage, and relationships (Inhorn 1996, 2006a, 2006b; Inhorn and Van Balen 2002; Becker 2000). In the case of Iranian donor parents and children, although in Shia Islam a child takes its lineage from both parents, it belongs to the father whose lineage takes precedence over that of the mother (Mir-Hosseini 1993; Ebadi 2003a). It is therefore understandable why the clerics and jurists went to such trouble to establish the lineage of donor children before allowing third-party donation. However, the prevailing cultural values have proved more powerful and have undermined the legal and religious endorsements.

The use of third-party donation provides ample scope for a reinforcement of the patriarchal values in relation to reproduction. This mirrors the experience of infertile Iranian women and is highlighted in the practice of third-party donation, more specifically that of sperm donation, which has been shown to result in further widening an existing gender gap depending on who the infertile party is. In the case of egg donation, society's reaction has proved, by and large, to be consistent with patriarchal values. No hostile reaction is known to have been provoked in such instances toward the mother and child on the grounds that the child is a donor child. But third-party sperm donation does not follow a symmetrical pattern. In spite of the initial legitimization of sperm donation, this remains frowned upon, the approval or disapproval of religious leaders notwithstanding. Having a donor child who is the result of sperm donation often leads to the child's rejection by the social father and often other male members of the social group, or, at its best, does not lead to the "happiness" and "stability" of the family, which are considered as the two cornerstones for a "perfect" family.

It follows, therefore, that the donor children's future depends on whether they are the result of egg or sperm donation. In both of the cases studied, not only had the donor children not brought happiness to the couple, or reduced the violence inflicted on the women who bore them, they had increased the violence to an intolerable level. To use Inhorn's (1996) argument (cited in Abbasi-Shavazi et al. 2008: 21), in the case of infertile Egyptian women, "infertility experience is a form of 'lived patriarchy.'" Finally, the use of third-party gamete donation, which aims at improving the quality of life of the couple and ensuring the stability of the family, has so far also resulted in reinforcing the patriarchal family where gender inequality remains a social reality. In reproducing in a patriarchal culture, men and women are expected to fulfill different duties, which Inhorn (2003: 221), citing from others, calls "infertility: his and hers" (Greil, Leitko, and Porter 1988).

The intervention of reproductive technologies has been shown in various studies to increase the collective social control over women's bodies (Unnithan-Kumar 2010; Martin 1987; Petchesky 1995; Thompson 2002; Inhorn 2006c). In general, in Middle Eastern countries, pressure on married couples to have children starts from the first day of marriage. Iran is no exception to this, and while a woman's personal desire to have a child is not disputed, studies at clinics in Iran show time and again that women undergo third-party donation under immense pressure from the kin group, predominantly that of their in-laws. To find out at what stage of marriage women are forced to seek infertility treatment, during one of my visits to a fertility clinic in Tehran I asked whether any of the infertile women were under the age of fifteen.[14] The clinic's record showed that it had received several females below the age of fifteen. These girls must have been at least thirteen years old, if not younger, at marriage, and when they had failed to produce children, their husbands and in-laws had brought them to the clinic to seek treatment.[15] Abbasi-Shavazi et al.'s (2008: 14) study of Tehran's fertility clinics also confirms the extent of coercion by in-laws on women to seek fertility treatment. Finally, as Unnithan-Kumar's (2010: 162) study of the case of lack of choices for female selective abortions in India explains: "Their choice . . . is not an autonomous choice at all. But, by focusing on the freedom of choice alone, we are foreclosing the ability to understand the more complex aspects of how women's agency works in collectively oriented patriarchal contexts."[16] Unnithan-Kumar (2010: 163) continues:

> The salience of this perspective is clear when we consider the wider social, marital, and, especially, conjugal context where notions of self and control over one's body are both collectively constituted as they are individually desired, crafted, and experienced. The responses of

> lower- and middle-class women to technological intervention ... reflect a wider interactive social process in which women continually participate, which serves their own interests as well as those of the wider social group to which they belong.

This kind of participation is what Lock and Kaufert (1998), cited in Unnithan-Kumar (2010), refer to as "pragmatic agency," whereby individuals do not necessarily either comply with or resist the "disciplining" that accompanies technological interventions but often act in accordance with pragmatic considerations. Accordingly, the donor children, in turn, become a tool to exercise control over women by the male members of the larger family. Batoul's example shows how all the male members of her own family took sides with her husband. The support for the husband was so strong that, as long as her father was alive, her mother helped her secretly, and it was not until he died that she openly supported her. The case of Sahar epitomizes the lives of several other women among the cases studied and shows a different kind of control exercised by men, by using the donor children as a pawn to retain control over the family and women in particular.

Previous studies on the causes of rejection of donor sperm by infertile men have convincingly argued that in the Middle East, with predominantly patriarchal values in relation to reproduction and fertility, men have a strong desire to maintain their *nasab* and reject the idea of sperm donation (Inhorn 2006c; Tremayne 2009; Clarke 2009). However, the combination of research from the larger study of third-party sperm donation carried out between 2004 and 2009 and from the present study provides unexpected insights into the behavior of infertile men who resort to donor sperm. They raise the question of whether in reality it is the biological infertility that matters more to infertile men, or the fact that they are seen to be infertile and not fulfilling their social role and losing their identity and status in society. Key to such use, however, remains anonymity. As long as the "secret" is not revealed, men with strong conservative values in this study seem to have been willing to compromise the "purity" of their biological lineage when faced with having to choose between remaining childless or using a stranger's sperm.

ARTs in cases of sperm donation have generated two kinds of responses by infertile men. There are those who have chosen openly to opt for donor sperm. Most of these men come from the more-educated and less-conservative layers of society. Even some of these men have rejected the donor child later as they "could not bear to see another man's child roam around their home." This rejection has taken various forms, from violence toward the mother and child to falling into depression by the social father, who could not blame anybody else but himself (Tremayne 2009). Often conceiving through sperm donation transcends the boundaries of fertility and reproduction and becomes a form of symbolic sexual transgression in the mind of these infertile men. Such reactions, however, are predictable and do not come as a real surprise. It is the unanticipated responses of the second group of infertile men, who come from highly conservative layers of society and who have decided to use donor sperm, which challenge the previous findings that mention that "men refuse to compromise their lineage by resorting to donor sperm." Infertile men in this study, who have used donor sperm, seem to have overcome their dilemma of keeping their purity of lineage intact or having to live the life of a barren man with all its ramifications, and have opted for donor sperm to prove their fertility, fulfill their duty to their social group, and maintain their social status, masculinity, and identity. While such solutions have existed historically, and examples are known of infertile men who have resorted to their brothers to impregnate their wives, the emergence of new possibilities in the form of ARTs has made it possible for infertile men to hide their infertility more easily and pass off another man's sperm as their own.

What is emerging strongly from this analysis is the interface between reproduction as a means of personal achievement and love of one's own biological child, against one's sense of social identity as a member of the social group. Clearly, the importance of reproducing socially is paramount for individuals, who are prepared to go to any length to demonstrate that they have fulfilled their reproductive duties and to secure their rightful place in society. For those who do not wish to reveal their infertility, even to the close members of the kin group, ARTs have provided the perfect way out, and it is not until something goes wrong that the true extent and implications of such practices become evident.

Conclusion

The data in this chapter have shown that the use of ARTs has led to a reinforcement of cultural values among infertile couples rather than altering them. Further, ARTs have been a contributory factor in the broadening of the gender gap among infertile couples of a certain social group. The findings of the earlier data clearly indicated that the efforts of the practitioners to break some of the cultural molds and alter attitudes toward infertility have had limited effects on the recipients, especially in the case of men. The deeply rooted values on fertility/infertility, acting as cultural barriers to further penetration and acceptance of ARTs, were shown not to have been dislodged beyond their immediate use. To date, infertile men seeking treatment seem to be so imbued with their cultural understanding of what constitutes masculinity that the clinic's education has little significant effect on them. The use of reproductive technologies, and the information that goes with them, become a medium that may help these men achieve "their" ideas of masculinity, rather than transform them.

In addition to highlighting the role of ARTs in deepening the gender gap among certain layers of society, some unanticipated facts in cases of third-party gamete donation have also emerged. One such finding shows that the ground is beginning to shift for many infertile men to move toward a compromise on the "purity" of their lineage in favor of being "seen" to be fertile, by resorting to reproductive technologies to make them be, or appear to be, fertile. ARTs provide the perfect "secrecy" they need to disguise their infertility, something that the traditional method of resorting to one's brother could not. Infertile men's reluctance and hostile reactions to publicizing their infertility (by being seen to receive another man's sperm) stems not just from feelings of humiliation or inadequacy, but also from deeper cosmological and metaphysical beliefs in relation to procreation. Furthermore, while the resistance of infertile men toward sperm donation has been understood all along to derive from a lineage, gender, and "face" issue, in reality it also lies, in great part, in the fact that in resorting to other men's donated sperm to gain progeny, men become passive spectators, watching their wives being impregnated by what they may view as a "symbolic act of sexual transgression" without playing any role in such a process themselves. The consequent feeling of alienation is what often drives the infertile men to violence toward women or self-deprecation. For women, on the other hand, the IVF treatment takes a totally different meaning since they take an active part throughout the process of procreation. Third-party donation for women, to use Hadolt's (2009) expression, "is a process which is an ensemble of body parts, machines, techniques to which women unavoidably make a corporeal contribution," and in which they fully participate. In this sense, women's relationships with their donor children differ too from that of men, and make them cherish and treat the children as their own even though such children may be the result of donor eggs.

The future of men and women users of third-party gamete donation and that of their children will therefore continue to be shaped by the fragile balance between disempowered infertile men and their wives who are at the receiving end of their husband's shortcomings. It must be expected that as these technologies continue to reach a higher number of users and the range of class, education, and generation of their users continues to broaden, further research will be needed to assess their impact on kinship, gender relations, donor children, and family, and on the ongoing dialogue between these technologies and their users.

Acknowledgments

This chapter was published originally as "The 'Down Side' of Gamete Donation: Challenging 'Happy Family' Rhetoric in Iran." In *Islam and Assisted Reproductive Technologies: Sunni and Shia Perspectives*, ed. Marcia C. Inhorn and Soraya Tremayne, 130–156. New York and Oxford: Berghahn Books (2012).

Notes

1. Opening speech given at Reproductive Disruptions Conference, Ann Arbor, MI, 2005.
2. For a clarification of the meaning of *nasab*, see Clarke (2009: 40). As he explains, *nasab* refers to agnatic and uterine relations of filiation in legal discourse. It is also commonly used as "genealogy," i.e., purely agnatic descent, projected backward in time. In Shia Islam, a child can take his *nasab* from both his parents but belongs to the father and his lineage. For details of this see Mir-Hosseini (1993) and Ebadi (2003b).
3. Also see Abbasi-Shavazi et al. (2008).
4. The conference was organized by one of the two major leading clinics, the Avicenna Research Center (the other being the Royan Institute), and has paved the way for the legitimization of several ARTs by engaging some of the more "progressive" clerics to openly debate and endorse ARTs.
5. The practice of temporary marriage is a form of marriage whereby a man and a woman agree to get married for a fixed length of time

between one hour and ninety-nine years (Haeri 1989; Tremayne 2009: 148–149). In the case of the wife's infertility, the husband would marry the egg donor without any sexual contact, to receive her egg to be fertilized with his sperm. Polygyny being allowed in Islam, this would not necessarily cause any complications. But, in the case of the husband's infertility, the wife, not being able to be married to two men at the same time, would divorce her own husband, marry the sperm donor without any sexual contact taking place, receive his sperm, and remarry the first husband. In both cases the embryo is fertilized outside the womb and planted in the uterus.

6. When I first started my field research on third-party donation in 2004, I came across couples who had used temporary marriage before the Supreme Leader's *fatwa* and had children who were three or four years old.
7. See Tremayne (2009).
8. This data also came from personal interviews conducted between 2006 and 2008.
9. Cases of women in Tehran clinics who help cover up their husbands' infertility are documented in Abbasi-Shavazi et al. (2008: 14). According to the study, some of the women interviewed mentioned that they were infertile, but "they soon disclosed that their husbands were the infertile ones; both had been threatened with divorce if they disclosed the male infertility or refused to shoulder the blame."
10. What may appear to be a voluntary act to undergo treatment often turns out to have been coerced, on close examination.
11. This information is based on personal interviews that took place in 2006.
12. Basij is the paramilitary volunteer militia working under orders from the Revolutionary Guards. Basij have local organizations in every town, government offices, and schools.
13. Temporary marriage is used by Shia only and is an arrangement for marriage between a man and a woman with a time limit on it (see Note 5). Temporary marriage has been used as a solution to legitimize third-party donation of sperm and eggs in Iran. For more details on temporary marriage see Haeri (1989).
14. The minimum age of marriage in Iran is thirteen for girls and fifteen for boys. Following the Islamic law (*sharia*) the minimum age of marriage used to be nine for girls, but, in 2003, under pressure from female members of the Iranian Parliament, the age was increased to thirteen for girls. This remains conditional to date. If the girl's father or her guardian or a medical doctor judges her ready to be married earlier, this can be done.
15. For more details on links between age, marriage, sexuality, family, and Islam see Moghadam (1994) and Tremayne (2004). As Moghadam argues, traditionally marriage and the formation of the marital union in

patriarchal Muslim societies were viewed as a transaction, with female sexuality as a commodity traded by men. She argues that the legal commoditization of female sexuality should be incorporated in the analysis of gender economics in Muslim societies.

16. Although the Iranian family is moving toward the nuclear family form, the essence of family and kin relations has not changed accordingly. The assumption that an educated, secular couple seeking to have a child is an independent unit and free from the influence of its social group is untrue. The collective involvement of the larger social group prevails, regardless of the lifestyle or physical distance of the couple from its larger social group. The influence of the kin group remains so strong that the educated and secular as well as the less-educated and conservative layers of society, alike, conform to its will. Young Iranian men, who have grown up in the West, come back to Iran often "because I want to marry a virgin and have children by an innocent [presumably meaning sexually inexperienced] girl." To do so, their families in Iran find the right girl in advance and arrange for him to return, marry her, and take her back with him. The influence of the family, however, continues from across the oceans, and firm control is exercised over most of the couple's decisions through daily contact by telephone, for both sides of the families. In this sense, having a child for a couple goes beyond the mere fact of biological reproduction between them and remains a matter for the social group. Having a child becomes an obligation and a necessity toward the social reproduction of the group and the continuity of the lineage. It is clear that unless the way donor children are conceived fits into the cultural understanding of what constitutes parenthood, their presence creates hostilities and proves disruptive for the family and the wider social group.

References

Abbasi-Shavazi, Mohammad Jalal, Marcia C. Inhorn, Hajiieh Bibi Razeghi-Nasrabad, and Ghasem Toloo. 2008. "The 'Iranian ART Revolution': Infertility, Assisted Reproductive Technology, and Third-Party Donation in the Islamic Republic of Iran." *Journal of Middle East Women's Studies* 4(2): 1–28.

Akhondi, Mohammad Mehdi, ed. 2001. *Modern Human Reproductive Techniques from the View of Jurisprudence and Law.* In Persian. Book based on papers presented in a symposium of the same title. Tehran: Avicenna Research Institute, Academic Publishing House for the Social Science.

Becker, Gay. 2000. *The Elusive Embryo: How Women and Men Approach the New Reproductive Technologies.* Berkeley: University of California Press.

Clarke, Morgan. 2006a. "Islam, Kinship and New Reproductive Technology." *Anthropology Today* 22(5): 17–20.

———. 2006b. "Shiite Perspectives on Kinship and New Reproductive Technologies." *ISIM Review* 17: 26–27.

———. 2009. *Islam and New Kinship: Reproductive Technologies and the Shariah in Lebanon*. New York and Oxford: Berghahn Books.

Ebadi, Shirin. 2003a. *Women's Rights in the Laws of the Islamic Republic of Iran*. In Persian. Tehran: Ganje Danesh Publishers.

———. 2003b. Interview with *Yas-e-No*. In Persian. 10 October.

Garmaroudi Naef, Shirin. 2008. "Sibling Intimacy in the Age of Assisted Reproduction: An Ethnography of New Reproductive Technologies in Iran." Master's thesis, University of Berne.

———. 2012. "Gestational Surrogacy in Iran: Uterine Kinship in Shia Thought and Practice." In *Islam and Assisted Reproductive Technologies: Sunni and Shia Perspectives*, ed. Marcia C. Inhorn and Soraya Tremayne, 157–194. New York and Oxford: Berghahn Books.

Greil, Arthur L., Thomas A. Leitko, and Karen L. Porter. 1988. "Infertility: His and Hers." *Gender & Society* 2(2): 172–199.

Hadolt, Bernard. 2009. Seminar on "Age and Reproduction," Fertility and Reproduction Seminars, Institute of Social and Cultural Anthropology, University of Oxford, 30 November.

Haeri, Shahla. 1989. *Law of Desire: Temporary Marriage in Shi'i Islam*. Syracuse, NY: Syracuse University Press.

Inhorn, Marcia C. 1996. *Infertility and Patriarchy: The Cultural Politics of Gender and Family Life in Egypt*. Philadelphia: University of Pennsylvania Press.

———. 2003. *Local Babies, Global Science: Gender, Religion, and In Vitro Fertilization in Egypt*. New York: Routledge.

———. 2004. "Middle Eastern Masculinities in the Age of New Reproductive Technologies: Male Infertility and Stigma in Egypt and Lebanon." *Medical Anthropology Quarterly* 18(2): 162–182.

———. 2005a. "Religion and Reproductive Technologies: IVF and Gamete Donation in the Muslim World." *Anthropology News* 46(2): 14–18.

———. 2005b. "Reproductive Disruptions." Paper presented at the International Conference on Reproductive Disruptions: Childlessness, Adoption, and Other Reproductive Complexities, 19 May, University of Michigan, Ann Arbor.

———. 2006a. "Making Muslim Babies: IVF and Gamete Donation in Sunni versus Shia Islam." *Culture, Medicine and Psychiatry* 30(4): 427–450.

———. 2006b. "A More Open Mind toward Iran." *Chronicle of Higher Education* B12.

———. 2006c. "He Won't Be My Son." *Medical Anthropology Quarterly* 20(1): 94–120.

Inhorn, Marcia C., and Frank Van Balen, eds. 2002. *Infertility around the Globe: New Thinking on Childlessness, Gender, and Reproductive Technologies*. Berkeley: University of California Press.

Lock, Margaret, and Patricia Kaufert. 1998. *Pragmatic Women and Body Politics*. Cambridge: Cambridge University Press.

Martin, Emily. 1987. *The Woman in the Body: A Cultural Analysis of Reproduction*. Milton Keynes: Open University.
Mir-Hosseini, Ziba. 1993. *Marriage on Trial: A Study of Islamic Family Law*. London: I.B. Tauris.
Moghadam, Fatemeh. 1994. "Commoditisation of Sexuality and Female Labour Participation in Islam: Implications for Iran 1960–90." In *In the Eye of the Storm: Women in Post-Revolutionary Iran*, ed. Mahnaz Afkhami and Erika Friedl. London: I.B. Tauris.
Petchesky, Rosalind. 1995. "The Body as Property: A Revision." In *Conceiving the New World Order: The Global Politics of Reproduction*, ed. Faye D. Ginsburg and Rayna Rapp. Berkeley: University of California Press.
Scheper-Hughes, Nancy. 2009. "Editorial." *Anthropology Today* 25 (August): 4.
Serour, Gamal I. 1993. "Bioethics in Reproductive Health: A Muslim Perspective." *Middle East Fertility Society Journal* 1: 30–35.
Thompson, Charis M. 2002. "Fertile Ground: Feminists Theorize Infertility." In *Infertility Around the Globe: New Thinking on Childlessness, Gender, and Reproductive Technologies*, ed. Marcia C. Inhorn and Frank Van Balen. Berkeley: University of California Press.
Tremayne, Soraya. 2004. "'And Never the Twain Shall Meet': Reproductive Health Policies in the Islamic Republic of Iran." In *Reproductive Agency, Medicine and the State: Cultural Transformations in Childbearing*, ed. Maya Unnithan-Kumar, 181–202. New York and Oxford: Berghahn Books.
———. 2005. "The Moral, Ethical and Legal Implications of Egg, Sperm and Embryo Donation in Iran." Paper presented at the International Conference on Reproductive Disruptions: Childlessness, Adoption, and Other Reproductive Complexities, 19 May, University of Michigan, Ann Arbor.
———. 2006a. "Whither Kinship? New Procreative Practices, Authoritative Knowledge, and Relatedness: Case Studies from Iran." Paper presented at the Conference on Gamete and Embryo Donation for Infertility Treatment, 2 March, University of Tehran, Iran.
———. 2006b. "Not All Muslims Are Luddites." *Anthropology Today* 22(93): 1–2.
———. 2009. "Law, Ethics and Donor Technologies in Shia Iran." In *Assisting Reproduction, Testing Genes: Global Encounters with New Biotechnologies*, ed. Daphna Birenbaum-Carmeli and Marcia C. Inhorn. New York and Oxford: Berghahn Books.
Unnithan-Kumar, Maya. 2010. "Female Selective Abortion—Beyond Culture: Family Making and Gender Inequality in a Globalising India." *Culture, Health and Sexuality* 12(2): 153–166.

Chapter 8

GENDER AND REPRODUCTIVE TECHNOLOGIES IN SHIA IRAN

The abundant contemporary Middle East scholarship on Islam and gender has been instrumental in undoing the myth that Islam is a rigid religion not open to change.[1] Over the past three decades, the profusion of information emerging from Muslim countries, especially on women, has thrown light on the dynamics and intricacies involved in the relationship between men and women. Research also has demonstrated the shift in the balance of gender relations as a result of the encounter between the persisting old norms and values and modernity and globalization.[2] In those countries where Islam is taking an increasingly prominent role and religious leaders are getting more involved in the political aspects of governance, gender relations have taken many turns and twists. Modernity and globalization, combined with cultural practices and religious beliefs, have redefined the boundaries of the interaction between men and women in unexpected ways. In what follows, I propose to use the example of the theocratic state of Shia Iran to illustrate the extent to which the involvement of the ruling religious leaders in policies has left a lasting impact on gender relations at all levels in society, both inter- and intra-generationally.

Following the Islamic Revolution of 1979 and the establishment of a theocratic regime in Iran, one of the main aims of the ruling religious authorities became the revival of the old values and norms which had been threatened under the previous regime. Among the priorities was to ensure that Islamic law (*sharia*) became the basis of the civil code, especially with regard to women's rights and position in society. Under the renewed *sharia* women were considered mothers and custodians of the family above all and their rights were limited accordingly (Kashani-Sabet 2011: 215–217). At the same time, in the early years after the revolution the regime was faced with fundamental social and political problems which, if unaddressed, would have threatened its very foundation. These included rapid population growth and an eight-year war with Iraq, which resulted in an economic crisis, testing all the country's resources (Hoodfar 1995; Mehryar 1998). The regime found itself in a conundrum. On the one hand, it had to respond to the country's sociocultural and economic problems by adapting to change and modernity and developing an all-encompassing socioeconomic plan, and on the other it had to do so within a strictly Islamic framework. Some of the policies introduced subsequently concerned women, whom the regime had to acknowledge and include in its reforms. The recognition of women's role in development programs had a major impact on gender relations, altering them in unexpected and unintended ways. The outcome of the interaction between Islamic law, the government's modernizing policies, and men and women's responses to them, worked in women's favor in some instances and to their disadvantage in others. However, the dynamics generated by these reforms inadvertently opened the gateway to greater freedom and aspirations for women and proved irreversible. It was a double-edged sword for the authorities. To illustrate these points, I have chosen to examine two examples from the area of reproductive technologies introduced with the approval and full support of senior religious leaders, and to explore their implications for gender relations.

The first example is that of population policies (*barnameyeh tanzim khanevadeh*) and their major and long-term impact on society. The second area is that of assisted reproductive technologies (ARTs), more specifically the third-party gamete donation of sperm and egg for the treatment of infertility. Although the religious leaders' endorsement of the infertility treatment is not official policy, it did require religious approval before the practice was allowed. The latter example is much smaller in scale compared with the population policies, as it only affects the infertile population. Nevertheless, the infertility rate in Iran seems to be higher than the global rate given by the World Health Organization (WHO), which puts the average infertility rate at around 15 percent. A recent survey of 17,000 households in Iran carried out by the Avicenna Research Center showed that the infertility rate among the population surveyed was between 20 to 22 percent for urban and rural areas respectively.

Therefore, in spite of the difference in scale between the population policies and ARTs, the significance of the latter is clear, as it concerns some of the most important institutions in society, namely, those of reproduction, kinship, and the family. The legitimization of both these reproductive technologies was justified in the interests of the family, which is the most fundamental institution in a Muslim society and which the Islamic regime in Iran is anxious to protect. The legitimization of both reproductive technologies has led to major transformations in the structure of the family and kinship, albeit to different degrees.

Methodology

The data presented in this chapter are drawn from a longitudinal study focusing on the dynamics of reproduction in Iran across three generations. The research started in 1997 and continues to date. It includes several field trips in 2000 in Tehran and Ardebil (northwest Iran) to study the links between gender and development, in 2004 in Yazd (central Iran) to study the impact of education on early marriage, and in Tehran and Yazd on ARTs. The follow-up studies were carried out in 2006, 2008, 2011, and 2012. Since 2003, I have also carried out research among Iranian women refugees in the United Kingdom who had fled from family violence. The main method used throughout has been the anthropological technique of participant observation. In addition, extensive in-depth interviews on early marriage and early pregnancy, and on ARTs, were carried out with medical practitioners and infertile couples at the clinics. The data presented in this chapter are based on 150 cases and also include the larger network of the kin group of several of the individuals studied.

Iran's Population Policies

The history of Iran's population policies predates the Islamic Revolution and goes back to the creation of the Ministry of Women's Affairs and the inception of a government-sponsored family planning program in 1967. These policies aimed to reduce population growth, which was at 3.8 per annum. But because of their top-down and paternalistic style of implementation that bore little relation to prevailing cultural norms among the target population, they were not as successful as they might have been (Hoodfar 1996; Makhlouf-Obermeyer 1994). However, Iran remained committed to implementing its population policies and participated in the first world population conference in Bucharest in 1974. At that conference, the critical role of women in population policies was acknowledged and links were made between fertility and women's status, associating women's high status with factors such as female education, female literacy, and female labor participation. The assumption was that improving women's conditions would automatically lead to low fertility, smaller families, later age of marriage, and contraceptive use. The literature of the period indicates that women's development was bound up with demographic objectives and was not concerned with the well-being of women as such (see Tremayne 2001).

After the Islamic Revolution, the family planning program of the previous regime fell into disarray and the new regime did not formulate an explicit policy, the religious authorities arguing against controlling population growth on religious and political grounds. For example, they claimed inter alia that high population growth was the sign of a strong nation; for this reason, the family planning clinics were subsequently dismantled. After the war with Iraq began in 1980, Ayatollah Khomeini encouraged people to have large families and mentioned the need for "the army of 20 million," referring to the human loss caused by the war. The new regime also lowered the age of marriage from sixteen to nine years for girls, and from eighteen to fourteen years for boys, following the *sharia*'s instructions (see Tremayne 2004). Thus, the population continued to grow and its magnitude raised an alarm when the National Census of 1986 was carried out. It showed that the population had almost doubled in two decades, from 25.7 million to over 50 million. Policymakers realized the enormity of the problem and appealed to the senior religious leaders for their intervention, pointing out that such rapid population growth could pose a major threat to the stability of the regime, which would not be able to fulfill its promises nor meet the demands of the population. Senior politico-religious leaders believed that the population growth had become a strategic challenge and its outcome was too important to be left to individual whim. They showed real commitment and played an active part in the introduction and implementation of new population policies. These well-coordinated policies proved so successful that within a space of ten years the rate of growth dropped from 3.8 in 1986 to below 2 percent in 1996. Iran was awarded the UN Population

Award in 1998 for its achievements. World Bank figures show that in 2010 the rate of population growth stood at around 1.5 percent, with variations among rural and urban families. Although many factors were responsible for this success in addition to the support of religious leaders, the role played by the latter proved crucial in the initial stages of implementation. Without their endorsement, the policies would probably have encountered fierce resistance from conservative quarters, as they did under the Pahlavi regime.[3]

The details of the implementation of the family planning policies and the role played by religious leaders have been fully addressed by other scholars and are beyond the remit of this chapter. Here, I want to mention only the effectiveness of the special attention the policies paid to people's sensitivities on matters of procreation. With help from Islamic scholars, the planners presented convincing alternative explanations that questioned the general belief that Islam favors large families and is a pronatalist religion. Religious sermons emphasized that having fewer children and bringing them up as healthy and happy citizens was more in line with what Islam advocates than having too many children who would live in poverty and suffer from ill health. The history of Islamic family planning was included in the national curricula at schools, in adult literacy classes, and special family planning sessions were organized in mosques and factories. Medieval religious texts by leading Muslim scholars such as al-Ghazali were produced, showing that Islam did not forbid family planning.[4]

One of the key factors in the success of the family planning programs was the realization that women's cooperation and willing participation in birth control were essential if the policies were to succeed. The planners therefore addressed women directly and included them in their programs from the start. Women responded to this invitation with open arms. They welcomed the endorsement of birth control by the religious leaders and used it to make their own reproductive decisions and counteract resistance from their husbands to the use of contraceptives. Even several years after the implementation of the family planning measures, many men showed their strong disapproval of birth control. For example, in Yazd and Ardebil, two of the most conservative cities in Iran, I heard women whose husbands objected to their taking the pill, telling them, "*Agha* (referring to Ayatollah Khomeini) himself has said that we should not have too many children." Health workers, who were responsible for the distribution of contraceptive pills to women in rural areas, also reported encountering male resistance and husbands even inflicting violence on their wives to force them to give up the pill. Many men from more conservative and/or religious groups resorted to coercive measures to prevent their wives from using the contraceptive pill. In Yazd, I came across instances of pregnant women who had come to the maternity clinics asking for abortions because their husbands had found their pills and forced them to give them up, and/or had raped them to make them pregnant. There were also women who had given up their pills voluntarily and had several children in order to prevent their husbands from marrying second wives. However, among the more educated and secular groups both men and women were in favor of having fewer children and had either reduced the number of children before the family planning program started or welcomed its introduction and responded positively.

In addition to and in tandem with these policies, an elaborate literacy campaign was also launched. Soon after the establishment of the Islamic regime, coeducation was banned, and sex segregation was imposed in keeping with Islamic principles. Contrary to the expectation of a drop in girls' attendance at schools, parents from rural areas and the conservative sectors of society showed great willingness to send their daughters to single-sex schools, and the attendance rate of girls rose considerably. Following such an increase, the need arose for more qualified female teachers and health workers and thousands of new female teachers and health workers had to be trained. However, one of the original reasons for encouraging female education was to educate girls in the Islamic ideals of womanhood. As Golnar Mehran (2003/4), a professor of education at Al-Zahra University in Tehran, explains:

> One can see a cycle in female education in Iran in which the ruling elite seeks to educate the ideal female citizen according to the dictates of an Islamizing and revolutionary society, thus creating a generation of educated women who, in turn, influence their society and act as role models for young girls, who then seek education as a means of equality and empowerment.

But the generation of educated young women did not turn out to be the ideal role model, as anticipated. In Mehran's (2003/4) words: "The educated women of Iran are pushing the boundaries due to their growing tendency to delay marriage and have fewer children, coupled with their active search to transform the traditional role of women in the family and society, leading to growing female expectations that need to be met sooner or later." Not only did the state policies not succeed in producing the ideal Muslim woman, but their impact on gender relations was profound and definite. Girls did not stop at secondary education. Instead, they went on to higher education, and by 2011 the ratio of female students had increased to over 60 percent. The result of the rise in female education has meant the emergence of new aspirations among young women. They are no longer prepared to fit into the ideal Muslim woman's mold of being mothers and wives, but demand that they be treated as individuals. Another major impact of education has been a rise in the age of marriage, although other factors are also responsible for the change in marriage patterns. Many young, educated women who wish to establish their identity through means other than motherhood do not consider having children a prerequisite to womanhood. A number of scholarly studies point to an emerging trend among young women not to marry and/or have families.[5] So far, this is the case among a minority of women, but they usually spread out from Tehran or one of the major cities in Iran to other parts of the country. Although women in smaller localities are not yet part of this trend, which is often decontextualized and does not translate into local practice, the issue is deemed serious enough to have raised an alarm and has provoked a strong reaction among senior clerics. The ruling clerics are concerned about the social "side effects" of rising educational standards among women and blame the declining birth and marriage rates, which in their view leads to the destruction of the foundation of the family, on women's high level of education. The effect of higher education is viewed as such a threat that in 2011 thirty-six universities across the country decided to ban women from studying seventy-seven subjects due to government pressure. As Shirin Ebadi, the Iranian winner of the Nobel Peace Prize, explains, "The Iranian government is using various initiatives to restrict women's access to education, to stop them being active in society, and to return them to the home."[6] A further recent reaction to both the delay in the age at marriage as well as a drop in the rate of marriage is reflected in the debates in the Iranian parliament, which is proposing to drop the minimum age at marriage from its current limit of thirteen for girls back to nine years, so that it is "fully within Islamic law." Under President Khatami's reformist regime (1997–2005) the minimum age at marriage was increased in 2003 from nine years for girls to thirteen (Weir 2012). Furthermore, in July 2012 the government announced that it would no longer fund family planning programs and Ayatollah Khamenei, the Supreme Religious Leader, called on women to have more children (Madsen 2012). However, in spite of new restrictions being reintroduced, Iranian women's increasing awareness of their rights has turned out to be an irreversible process and is acting as a gateway to future choices for women. The process triggered by the government's population and educational policies has fueled women's determination to continue to challenge both the state and their men to expand their freedoms and goes beyond mere protest.

The advocacy of the family planning program and the campaign for literacy resulted in a shift in reliance on "God's will"[7] and allowed women to make their own reproductive decisions. But as the goals of family planning were being achieved, the initial direct involvement by clerics in population policies gradually diminished and public acknowledgment of women's prominent role as important agents and decision makers moved out of the limelight. Once implementation of the population policies was on track, policymakers turned their attention to maternal and child health, and areas such as the sexual health of young people were limited to basic education and applied within an Islamic framework. A review by the United Nations Population Fund (UNFPA) in 2007 of two decades of government implementation of these policies shows that the only area which has benefited from strong support by the regime has been that of maternal and child health. It became clear that, although women could potentially benefit from the progress made through many reproductive health policies, laws which constrain their rights have not been amended accordingly and have left women in a vulnerable situation vis-à-vis their fathers and husbands.

In spite of their empowerment of women, these policies also proved a double-edged sword in many respects. Women found themselves being able to control their fertility, but at the same time powerless vis-à-vis the Islamic law of marriage, child custody, and other matters. Although women used their newfound ability to make their own reproductive decisions as a bargaining tool to negotiate and gain control in other spheres, this power remained intermittent and lost its effectiveness once they had passed their reproductive years. The areas in which they gained power included the ability to work and become financially independent, and to enforce better conditions for their daughters' educations and future, including the choice of marriage partners.[8] Also, smaller family size combined with rapid urbanization and living away from their hometowns allowed a considerable number of women to reduce the involvement and interference of the larger kin group, especially their in-laws, in family decisions and thus strengthened their position within the household. However, for most women the exercise of power and control remained tentative during the implementation of the population policies. The real impact of these policies was witnessed in the next generation because their children had become involved in their reproductive decision making. Many women were told by their young children that they should not have more than two children because they (the children) were ashamed to go to school and tell others that there were more than two children in their family. Several women whose case studies I collected recounted their personal experiences of being confronted by their children when they began to expect yet another child. One mother told me that when her teenage daughter heard that she was pregnant again, she said, "You are not a battery hen; why are you having more than two children?" These were not isolated examples. Several of the teachers and rural and urban health workers had similar stories, confirming the role being played by children in preventing their parents from having too many children. The focus of this chapter is therefore on the effect of the population policies on this younger generation who grew to adulthood in the "post-population policy" period.

As I have argued elsewhere, although women gained some powers in specific areas, their empowerment was effectively reduced to a selective reinforcement of capabilities by the regime. For example, the dramatic expansion in women's literacy has been clearly—but not necessarily successfully—used as a tool for inculcating the values and strength of the regime. Yet as Hoodfar (1996) has argued, the government failed to introduce any measures to address a key demand of the women's movement: namely, access to employment. Thus, despite the record decline in fertility in Iran and a drastic increase in the literacy rate, women's participation in the labor force, for example, has not followed at the pace women desired, as it has elsewhere in the region (Hoodfar 1996). Likewise, on the one hand the government's reproductive health policies paved the way for women to negotiate some form of reproductive autonomy and improved health. On the other hand, the same policies were also used by the theocratic regime to reinforce its Islamic ideology. Thus, although women have remained the focus of government policies throughout, change has occurred within the bounds determined by the *sharia* and women's role as mothers and custodians of the family. Improvement has therefore been selective, framed by Islamic values, which have at the same time been used to constrain their rights in other spheres such as women's legal rights, women's employment, and their ability to organize politically.

Assisted Reproductive Technologies

The second area where the intervention of religion has played a significant role in gender relations is in the treatment of infertility through the use of modern assisted reproductive technologies (ARTs), especially that of third-party gamete donation of sperm and egg. As the implications of third-party gamete donation for family and kinship have been documented extensively, I shall not elaborate on them in this chapter.[9] As studies have shown, the legitimization of global reproductive technologies and the local responses to them are as varied as the societies themselves. While in many countries where the state is secular the legitimization of ARTs has been the responsibility of legal and ethical committees and religion has played a marginal or even negligible role, in the Muslim Middle East religious leaders have played a prominent role in the legitimization of ARTs to overcome infertility. Their involvement is not surprising, considering that reproduction is one of the most important aspects of an individual's life in Islam, which views it as the duty of every individual to reproduce to ensure the continuity of his or her lineage, kin, and community. Throughout the history of Islam, Muslim scholars and clerics have taken an intense interest in reproduction, especially the female body, as the vehicle for reproduction. Religious scholars' deliberations on the sexual and reproductive life of women are abundant, as Marion Katz's (2014) work on menstruation in this volume demonstrates. Katz's (2014) discussion of the involvement of Muslim scholars in women's menstrual problems testifies that women are not considered fit to pass judgment on their own bodies. But it also shows that reproduction is not a private matter to be decided solely by the individuals involved, but it is also of interest to the larger community. It requires the intervention of people with higher expertise to oversee the proper functioning of reproductive bodies. Muslim scholars, as the custodians of Islamic values, consider it their duty to attend to women's reproductive health and control their sexuality to ensure the sanctity of the family and the purity of the lineage, which they view as paramount for the stability of society.

With the introduction of ARTs in Muslim countries in the Middle East, Sunnis, who constitute the majority of Muslims, allowed the treatment of infertility among married couples. But no form of third-party gamete donation of sperm, egg, embryo, or surrogacy was permitted. As Marcia C. Inhorn (2006), the leading anthropologist on ARTs in Arab Muslim countries, explains, the main reasons for such a ban are that third-party gamete donation is viewed as equivalent to adultery and as interfering with and confusing lineage and inheritance issues. In his book *Islam and New Kinship*, Morgan Clarke (2009: 47) explains the importance of establishing the lineage through procreation as follows: "According to the vision of the Islamic legal establishment, relations of filiation (*nasab*), are not mutable or fluid, but are given, paradigmatically—but not exclusively—through procreation. Relation through procreation is not, however, a sufficient condition for the establishment of *nasab* in Islamic law. *Nasab* accrues to those conceived within a union of marriage."[10] Sunnis therefore have consistently argued that no third-party donation is allowed in the treatment of infertility. Senior Shia religious leaders in Iran, on the other hand, have allowed the use of ARTs in all its forms, from the practice of IVF between a married couple, to third-party donation of sperm, egg, and embryo, surrogacy, stem cell research, and sex selection, without breaching any Islamic rules. Soon after IVF became available in the West, Iranian medical practitioners introduced it in Iran. The introduction of IVF between a married couple was considered a medical technology, and Ayatollah Khomeini issued a *fatwa* allowing masturbation, which is considered *makruh*—that is, disliked or not approved of—in Islam, for the purpose of semen collection. As these reproductive technologies advanced and third-party donation of sperm and egg became available, Iranian jurists were faced with the problem of justifying using a stranger's gamete to treat a married infertile person. The responsibility for allowing or refusing the use of third-party gamete donation fell on the senior clerics, who agreed with their Sunni counterparts that third-party gamete donation was similar to incest or adultery and that donation should take place only between a wife and husband. These clerics, who were sources of emulation (*marja*), resorted to independent reasoning (*ijtihad*) to decide whether to allow or ban third-party gamete donation.[11] Although they have never reached a consensus and they remain divided to date, the approval of *marjas* who were in favor of third-party donation opened the way for the practice. However, the fact that the leading medical practitioners took the initiative of involving clerics in the public debates concerning third-party donation has been widely overlooked.[12]

The deliberations by clerics and Islamic jurists to legitimize third-party donation within the marital union initially led to the use of temporary marriage. Although there is no record of when or how, or even who, first introduced the idea of temporary marriage, the suggestion was welcomed and by the mid-1990s temporary marriage was being extensively practiced at clinics.[13] This practice meant that if a woman was infertile, her husband entered into a temporary marriage—usually for a short time—with the egg donor (Islam permitting polygyny), until the egg was fertilized. Thus, the husband received the donor's egg, which was legitimately fertilized with his sperm outside his infertile wife's womb. The fertilized egg was then transferred into the wife's womb. No sexual act took place between the egg donor and the husband at any stage. If the husband was infertile, the process was reversed. The fertile wife divorced her infertile husband, as she could not be married to two men at the same time, and entered into a temporary marriage with the sperm donor to receive his sperm. The practice of sperm and egg donation started in the mid-1990s and in 1999 the supreme religious leader, Ayatollah Khamenei, gave his opinion on third-party gamete donation, endorsing both sperm and egg donation subject to "no touch or gaze taking place." Although third-party donation had been practiced for some years by that time, it was his approval which gave gamete donation "official" legitimacy. Ayatollah Khamenei's *fatwa* did not even refer to temporary marriage as a condition for donation and only emphasized the avoidance of "touch" and "gaze." To date, it remains unclear as to who should avoid "touch" and "gaze," the donor and recipient or the medical practitioner and the infertile person, and the phrase is interpreted differently depending on who uses it and to what purpose. However, Ayatollah Khamenei's endorsement made it easier for medical practitioners to engage in third-party donation openly. While the approval of egg donation did not cause any problem, that of sperm donation led to a great deal of protest and anger among more conservative segments of society, and there was also strong protest by some conservative clerics and even members of parliament.[14] To this day, religious and conservative medical practitioners do not allow sperm donation. As a result, semi- or fully funded government clinics only practice egg donation, and sperm donation takes place only in select private clinics. The practice of temporary marriage has gradually diminished, and currently (in 2014) most clinics practice third-party donation without going through this ceremony. The third-party donation of sperm and egg was not regulated by any laws and followed Islamic ethics alone. As a result, numerous ethical and legal problems have arisen for both medical practitioners and infertile couples, which they resolve as best they can in the absence of a law enforcement body.[15] When embryo donation was introduced in Iran, the clerics could not find any justification in the Qur'an to allow it. A law was passed permitting embryo donation in 2003, but it remains vague in several areas and leaves medical practitioners, donors, and the recipients of embryos in limbo.

The official involvement of the religious authorities aside, religion plays an important role among infertile individuals themselves, especially those from conservative and religious social groups. In seeking fertility treatment, many still refer to their *marja* for his approval, while some refrain from seeking treatment altogether on the grounds that it was God's will that they should be infertile. Interestingly, interviews with infertile couples reveal that they are not always aware of the *fatwas* and views of the higher religious authorities and act on their own beliefs or follow the opinion of their sources of emulation or *marjas*.[16]

Having discussed the jurisprudential aspects of third-party donation, in what follows I examine some of the consequences of third-party donation on gender relations. In discussing the link between infertility and gender, three factors must be taken into consideration. Most infertile couples who seek treatment come from the conservative segments of society and are religious; infertility remains a major stigma; and male infertility is still denied by many men and dismissed as impossible. For many infertile couples, the first step is to satisfy themselves that they are not breaching any religious taboos. As Inhorn (2008) puts it, "Muslim couples want to make sure that they are making their babies in an Islamic way." Interestingly, a visit to the website of some fertility clinics in Iran shows that some Shia couples, whether Iranian or Shia from other parts of the world seeking treatment in Iran, emphatically ask for "a Shia egg."[17]

Cases in my study show that most of the infertile individuals had consulted with their *marja* before coming to the clinic. However, some couples mentioned that they had first gone to their own *marja*, who had advised them against the treatment. "But we thought of going to another *marja* and asked around to find out which one approves of ARTs, and went to him and he gave his approval. We now know that we are not breaching any Islamic rules." The importance of religious approval for those seeking fertility treatment is also shown by other studies, such as the following:

> Many women in the study considered infertility to be beyond their control—i.e. their "fate" and "the will of God." They argued that if they were not able to "bring children" into the world, this was God's wish, and they referred to Qur'anic verses to support their contention. Accordingly, if God does not will a woman to be fertile, no treatment will ever be able to help her. Nonetheless, God also expects women to seek solutions to their suffering; thus, searching for infertility treatment is meritorious and is conceived of as part of God's test of an infertile woman's patience and endurance. (Abbasi-Shavazi et al. 2008: 13)

These beliefs are shared by couples in need of surrogate mothers. A study carried out on 238 women in the infertility clinic in Tabriz (eastern Azerbaijan) shows that 15 percent of the women were against the practice of surrogacy because of their religious beliefs. The study concludes that "in spite of the positive attitude of the women in the study, further efforts are needed to increase the acceptability of surrogacy." A considerable majority also thought that religious matters should be dealt with before legal ones.

Infertility, especially male infertility, remains a major stigma in Iran, as in many other parts of the world, and the blame often falls on women. Even when it is clear that the man is the infertile party, he tries to hide it and asks his wife to pretend to be the one who is infertile. Many women agree willingly. For example, in an article about the "Iranian ART Revolution," women confided that their infertile husbands had threatened them with divorce if they did not agree to take the blame for the couple's infertility (Abbasi-Shavazi et al. 2008). Infertility is thus generally viewed as a woman's failure to reproduce. Although there has been no follow-up research to study the life stories of couples who have conceived and gone home with babies, the general assumption is that these technologies have made families happy and have improved the status of women within the family and among kin. Pictures of such parents with their children cover the walls of fertility clinics together with thank you notes from the parents.

A further contribution of ARTs has been to allow infertile couples to seek treatment secretly and be spared the stigma of infertility, although this is still difficult to do in practice. In theory an infertile couple can go to the clinic and seek treatment without anybody finding out. However, close contact with one's kin group is often unavoidable in Iranian society, and relatives tend to get involved, especially in matters relating to reproduction. So the couple can only resort to ARTs discreetly if it can get away from the close network of the kin group. Another difficulty is that in cases of third-party donation many infertile parties resort to their siblings or close relatives for gamete donation, which makes it impossible to hide the facts.

In general, sperm and egg donation have resulted in a host of moral, religious, and legal problems, in addition to social and cultural ones. These problems were not foreseen by the religious authorities who approved them. Gender relations are no exception. While in cases of female infertility women have submitted to the treatment willingly, male infertility provokes strong negative reactions in men. When they find out that they are infertile, men's ideas of manhood and masculinity are shattered and, in some extreme but not rare cases they resort to violence to compensate. Among some of the cases in this study, even those infertile men who had initially agreed to resort to donor sperm rejected the child later, either by actually dissociating themselves from him, becoming indifferent toward him, or falling into depression and suffering ill-health themselves. Violence among infertile men is so widespread that the two leading fertility clinics in Iran have launched their own research projects on violence. The Avicenna Research Center has made a film based on the life story of one of its infertile patients, and the Royan Institute has carried out research on violence among its infertile patients. Women seem to be at the receiving end of violence from their husbands regardless of which party is infertile. The two following cases, which I have discussed at length elsewhere,[18] demonstrate some of the negative aspects of third-party donation and its impact on gender relations. While by citing these stories I do not mean to suggest that all infertile men turn to violence, several cases of male infertility in this study confirm that men had used some form or degree of violence toward their wives.

The first case is that of an infertile couple who sought treatment in the United Kingdom soon after third-party donation became available. The treatment was successful, and the wife gave birth to triplet girls, one of whom had green eyes and all three of whom had blonde hair. It became obvious that one of the parents was not the biological parent and that a third-party gamete had been used. On their return to Iran, the husband, who had carried out the negotiations with the clinic but had not revealed that he was the infertile party, lost face in such a way that he blamed his wife, accusing her of having slept with the doctor at the clinic, and subjected his wife and the children to extreme violence for twenty years. The violence ranged from regular severe beatings to asking schools to expel the "bastard," "Christian" children. The wife's father and brothers also sided with her husband, stating that infertility is a female problem and that he could not have been infertile. After several years of abuse, she divorced her husband and found a boyfriend. But her ex-husband caught her in bed with her boyfriend and called the police. She was arrested for having a sexual relationship with a man to whom she was not married, raped while in police custody, and sentenced to stoning for adultery. At that point she ran away and sought asylum in the United Kingdom, where I met her. A few years later all three of the husband's brothers found out that they were infertile too and agreed that it must have been their brother who had been the infertile party.

The second case is one of third-party egg donation involving another woman refugee in the United Kingdom. She was married to a violent man and thought that having a child would make him less violent. But she was nearly forty years old and needed fertility treatment to conceive. After consulting with her *marja*, she resorted to a donor egg and conceived twins, one of whom was aborted after her husband beat her, as he regularly did. Soon after the birth of the child, her husband, knowing how attached she was to the child, abducted the child and started blackmailing her for money. When she refused, he reported her to the Revolutionary Courts for having converted to Christianity, an act which is punishable by death in Iran. At this point she ran away and became a refugee. She has not seen her child for several years and even when she found him, he did not want to see her, having lived under his father's influence for years.

Conclusion

In discussing the interaction between religion and gender in Islam, I have chosen two examples from Iran, which is a Shia country and a theocracy. Both examples involve modern reproductive technologies, which have been practiced with the full endorsement of the senior ruling clerics. The clerics fully supported the population policy programs, which aimed at reducing population growth, and approved assisted reproductive technologies for the treatment of infertility. Although the purposes of these technologies seem to be opposed to one another, both formed part of the same agenda which, it was emphasized, was not just about reducing population growth but also about helping infertile couples receive treatment.[19]

In this chapter, I have shown that without the endorsement of the senior clerics these technologies could not have been applied, well received, or even accepted by their users. I have also argued that the successful application of these technologies has had significant unintended and unanticipated consequences and has led to profound transformations in the structure of the family and in gender relations.

For women, their liberation from uncontrolled and multiple pregnancies and childbirth, combined with better health and greater access to education and employment, opened up new possibilities allowing them to go beyond their traditional female roles and aspire to equality with men, and even break into areas which had been traditional male preserves.[20] Rapid socioeconomic development also resulted in urbanization and mobility, and many families moved away from their hometowns and formed smaller families. This freed women from the relentless interference of their kin groups, especially their in-laws, and strengthened their positions vis-à-vis their husbands and families. The overall outcome for women has been an outwardly liberated and "modern" woman, seeking recognition not as a mother or wife, but as a person in her own right. These aspirations are not limited to young women from secular and highly educated backgrounds, but include women from all social groups, including conservative and religious ones.

I have shown that the real impact of these changes became evident among those, especially the women, who were either born or grew up during the implementation of the population policies, between 1986 and 1996. The aspirations of these women had not been anticipated by the Islamic regime, as they went in the opposite direction from its expectation of reproducing the ideal Islamic female role model. However, in spite of such profound changes the Islamic regime has not altered its legal and political structures. In fact, the authorities have taken a retrograde step by trying to restrict women's freedom further to make them fit into the mold of mothers and wives, as opposed to giving them recognition as individuals outside the family. The ongoing struggle between the state attempting to harness women, and women's provocative responses, has become the defining factor in dictating the state's next move toward them. In other words, regardless of the negative or positive actions of the state, young Iranian women are chipping away at the restrictions imposed on them and in so doing evoke the Old Persian saying that "rights are to be taken, they are not given" (*haq gereftanist na dadani*).

As a result of the ongoing tensions between young people and the state, a generation of women has emerged which, in the quest for recognition of their womanhood, seems to have violated many cultural and religious rules from sexual taboos to the sanctity of marriage and family. At the same time, the analysis of the data in this study also points to another reality, which reveals a different perspective on the identity and aspirations of women. While the relationships between the genders and with the state may have changed, when women come face-to-face with making decisions about some of the most fundamental core cultural values, for example marriage or reproduction, their modernity and individuality can be put to the test and proven skin deep. This is particularly true of a great number of women for whom change is more form than substance. Regardless of their level of education and degree of modernity, for most women being married and having children remains key to their identity, social status, and womanhood. This persistence of cultural values can be observed nowhere better than among cases of infertility, where infertile women comply fully with cultural norms. Even for highly educated and those who might be considered "modern" infertile men and women, the stigma of infertility seems as strong as it is for the older generation or for their less educated and more conservative counterparts. To date, regardless of how successful and independent a young woman may be, her status as a mother prevails over that of the professional in society. While marriage patterns and attitudes toward fertility and childbearing may have changed, the actual values attached to the status they provide for women remain firmly anchored in old norms and values.[21] As research in fertility clinics shows, a considerable number of women seeking fertility treatment are highly educated, are professional, have married late, and are past their reproductive age, which is why they are resorting to fertility treatment. There are also older women who have been divorced and have remarried and need to secure their marriages by having a child.[22]

Finally, the two reproductive technologies discussed in this chapter, which were intended for contrary purposes, have also led to contrary outcomes as far as gender relations are concerned. While population policies empowered the younger generation of women and led to a narrowing of the gender gap, the endorsement of third-party fertility treatment has widened the gap between infertile men and women. In cases of infertility, regardless of who is infertile, women have had to comply with the expectations of their husbands and often those of other close male relatives, to maintain their positions in society. Even the scientific proof that men can also be infertile has not changed men's behavior toward their wives. On the positive side, however, ARTs have provided some choices for women, for example by allowing them to delay marriage and childbearing, knowing that they can have a child through the preservation of their eggs. However, this remains more of an ideal than a reality for most women, who are under intense pressure from their husbands and/or kin group and in-laws to reproduce soon after getting married.

As the women of post-population policies strive to establish their identities as women rather than as mothers and wives, and in the process also define the boundaries of gender relations, the question arises as to whether these young women's resistance and new aspirations are a passing "rebellion" or a profound and lasting "revolution."

Acknowledgments

This chapter was published originally as "Gender and Reproductive Technologies in Shia Iran." In *Gender in Judaism and Islam: Common Lives, Uncommon Heritage*, ed. Firoozeh Kashani-Sabet and Beth S. Wenger, 126–149. New York: New York University Press (2015).

Notes

1. See, for example, inter alia, Kandiyoti (1996), El-Solh and Mabro (1994), Okkenhaug and Flaskerud (2005), and Tremayne (2006).
2. See, for example, Tadros (2010).
3. See, for example, Mehryar (1998), Abbasi-Shavazi (2001), Hoodfar (1995), Tremayne (2004), and Kashani-Sabet (2011).
4. For more on the medieval Islamic debates on family planning, see Makhlouf-Obermeyer (1991: 42–43). As Makhlouf-Obermeyer explains, "A clear consensus exists among schools of Islamic law that family planning is permissible. This is based on the absence of any prohibition against birth control in the [Qur'an] and on general statements in the [Qur'an] that God does not want to burden man but wishes to improve his life. More specifically, statements in the Hadith indicate that withdrawal (*azl*) was practiced in Mohammad's time and that he did not discourage his followers from the practice." As Makhlouf-Obermeyer points out, the Sunni and Shia positions on birth control are the same in substance. They derive from the work of

al-Ghazali, the most celebrated theologian of Islam, who establishes five reasons for which birth control may be allowed.

5. Interview in September 2012 with Dr. Amir Ebrahimi, an Iranian urban sociologist and geographer working mainly in Tehran on women and the public space. Also see Torabi and Baschieri (2010).
6. Interview given to BBC on 2 September 2012. I heard the program myself on BBC Radio 4, Today Program between 8 and 9 a.m., but I am not sure that there is a link or whether it is still functioning.
7. In 2009 the Iranian president, Ahmadinejad, announced that the number of children in a family is in the hands of God and therefore people must stop family planning and start having more children. As an incentive to do so, he proposed to open bank accounts, depositing a considerable sum of money for each new child being born. However, this was not well received by people. In 2011 the Iranian parliament reversed the decision and put a stop to the payments.
8. See, for example, Salehi-Isfahani and Taghvatalab (2009).
9. The following scholars have written extensively about Islam and ARTs: Marcia C. Inhorn (2003, 2006), Marcia C. Inhorn and Soraya Tremayne (2012), Soraya Tremayne (2005, 2006, 2009, 2012), Morgan Clarke (2009: 45–48).
10. See also Inhorn and Tremayne (2012: 6).
11. According to the nineteenth-century development of the concept of "sources of emulation" (*marja-e taqlid*), or Shia religious scholars who are to be followed for their learnedness, the Shia emphasize independent reasoning (*ijtihad*) to find new answers to new problems. However, the interpretations of these texts have not been monolithic; differences of opinion have emerged among the four Sunni legal schools (*madhhab*) and on basic principles, such as what constitutes lineage or who can be considered the legitimate parent or child in a family. Likewise, Shia leaders are not unanimous in their views and remain divided in their interpretations and verdicts on the extent to which the ARTs can be applied. See Inhorn and Tremayne (2012: 6).
12. Two leading institutions have pioneered ARTs in Iran, namely, the Avicenna Research Center and the Royan Institute. The Avicenna Research Center, headed by Dr. Akhondi, has pioneered the opening up of debates at conferences and has published extensively on the religious, legal, and social aspects of ARTs. See Avicenna Research Center (2001, 2007).
13. Temporary marriage is a form of marriage unique to the Shia school, whereby a man and a woman agree to get married for a specified length of time, which can be anywhere between one hour and ninety-nine years (see Haeri 1989).
14. For a fuller discussion of the *fatwas* given for and against third-party gamete donation, see the Avicenna Research Center (2001, 2007). Also, for *fatwas* on surrogacy, see Garmaroudi Naef (2012).

15. For a discussion of ARTs and Islamic ethics in Iran, see Tappan (2012).
16. See, for example, Abbasi-Shavazi et al. (2008) and Garmaroudi Naef (2012).
17. See, for example, "IVF Cost at Dr. Erfanian Clinic, Iran." Retrieved 26 September 2013 from www.ivfcost.net/ivf-cost/ivf-cost-at-dr-erfanian-ivf-clinic-iran.
18. See Inhorn and Tremayne (2012: 130–157).
19. For more details on this, see Tremayne (2004).
20. For further information on links between education and delay in marriage, see Salehi-Isfahani (2010). The percentage of women married by age twenty has fallen from 60 percent for the 1964 birth cohort to under 30 percent for the 1984 cohort (Egel and Salehi-Isfahani 2010: 27). Also, according to this report:

    > Delayed marriage clearly has some positive effects such as an increased opportunity for accumulation of human capital, particularly among women. However in a culture where it is difficult to socialize and interact with the opposite sex before marriage and where marriage is typically a prerequisite for being accepted as an adult, delayed marriage can have deleterious effects (Gregg 2005). The importance of marriage in the lives of these youth is illustrated by the responses to a question in the [survey] regarding the most important goal in their lives where "having a good family life" was the most popular response among both men and women. This response was favored over the next most popular response, "being successful in work," by 50 percent over 14 percent for women and 31 percent over 28 percent for men (Statistical Center of Iran 2006). (Egel and Isfahani 2010: 27)

21. The social, political, and individual value of motherhood is also shown by Kashani-Sabet (2011) in her groundbreaking study of the meaning of motherhood.
22. Clear evidence of the persistence of old cultural norms and values can be found in the importance attached to female virginity by both men and women. The number of young, liberated women secretly seeking hymenoplasty to restore their virginity is so high that it has once more engaged the clerics, and one of the Grand Ayatollahs, Sadeq Rohani from Qom, among others, has issued a *fatwa* permitting the operation. If a woman loses her virginity, her fear of rejection by her future husband, who could be an educated and modern man, and the negative reactions of his or even her own family, drives her to have her hymen repaired so that she can get married as a respectable girl. On virginity in Iran, also see Afary (2009a, 2009b) and Azal (2011).

References

Abbasi-Shavazi, Mohammad Jalal. 2001. "La fécondités en Iran: L'autre révolution" [Fertility in Iran: The other revolution]. *Population et Sociéte* 373(November): 1–4.

Abbasi-Shavazi, Mohammad Jalal, Marcia C. Inhorn, Hajiieh Bibi Razeghi-Nasrabad, and Ghasem Toloo. 2008. "The 'Iranian ART Revolution': Infertility, Assisted Reproductive Technology, and Third-Party Donation in the Islamic Republic of Iran." *Journal of Middle East Women's Studies* 4(2): 1–28.

Afary, Janet. 2009a. "Recreating Virginity in Iran." *The Guardian*, 12 May. Retrieved 26 September 2013 from http://www.guardian.co.uk/com mentisfree/2009/may/12/virgin-hymen-repair-iran.

———. 2009b. *Sexual Politics in Modern Iran*. New York: Cambridge University Press.

Avicenna Research Center. 2001. *Essays on Modern Human Reproductive Techniques from the View of Jurisprudence and Law*. In Persian.

———. 2007. *Essays on Gamete and Embryo Donation in Infertility Treatment: From Medical, Theological, Ethical, Psychological and Sociological Approaches*. In Persian.

Azal, Ahmadi. 2011. "Reconstructing Virginity in Iran: Hymenoplasty as a Form of Resistance," M.Phil. thesis [published in *Medical Anthropology Quarterly* in 2015].

Clarke, Morgan. 2009. *Islam and New Kinship: Reproductive Technologies and the Shariah in Lebanon*. New York: Berghahn Books.

Egel, David, and Djavad Salehi-Isfahani. 2010. "Youth Transitions to Employment and Marriage in Iran: Evidence from the School to Work Transition Survey." Middle East Youth Initiative Working Paper 11. June. Wolfensohn Center for Development, Dubai School of Government.

El-Solh, Camillia, and Judy Mabro, eds. 1994. *Muslim Women's Choices: Religious Belief and Social Reality*. Providence: Berg.

Garmaroudi Naef, Shirin. 2012. "Gestational Surrogacy in Iran: Uterine Kinship in Shia Thought and Practice." In *Islam and Assisted Reproductive Technologies: Sunni and Shia Perspectives*, ed. Marcia C. Inhorn and Soraya Tremayne, 157–194. New York and Oxford: Berghahn Books.

Gregg, Gary S. 2005. *The Middle East: A Cultural Psychology*. Oxford: Oxford University Press.

Haeri, Shahla. 1989. *The Law of Desire: Temporary Marriage in Shi'i Iran*. London: I.B. Tauris.

Hoodfar, Homa. 1995. "Population Policy and Gender Equity in Post-Revolutionary Iran." In *Family, Gender and Population in the Middle East: Policies in Context*, ed. Carla Makhlouf-Olbermeyer. Cairo: American University in Cairo Press.

———. 1996. "Bargaining with Fundamentalism: Women and the Politics of Population Control in Iran." *Reproductive Health Matters* 4(8): 30–41.

Inhorn, Marcia C. 2003. *Local Babies, Global Science: Gender, Religion and In Vitro Fertilization in Egypt*. New York: Routledge.

———. 2006. "Making Muslim Babies: IVF and Gamete Donation in Sunni versus Shia Islam." *Culture, Medicine, and Psychiatry* 30(4): 427–450.

———. 2008. "Local Babies, Global Science." Paper presented at the Embryo and Gamete Donation Conference. Tehran: Avicenna Research Center.

Inhorn, Marcia C., and Soraya Tremayne, eds. 2012. *Islam and Assisted Reproductive Technologies: Sunni and Shia Perspectives*. New York and Oxford: Berghahn Books.

Kandiyoti, Deniz. 1996. *Gendering the Middle East*. Syracuse, NY: Syracuse University Press.

Kashani-Sabet, Firoozeh. 2011. *Conceiving Citizens: Women and the Politics of Motherhood in Iran*. New York: Oxford University Press.

Katz, Marion. 2014. "Scholarly versus Women's Authority in the Islamic Law of Menstrual Purity." *Gender in Judaism and Islam: Common Lives, Uncommon Heritage*, ed. Firoozeh Kashani-Sabet and Beth S. Wenger, 73–105. New York: New York University Press.

Madsen, Elizabeth Leahy. 2012. "Iran's Surprising and Shortsighted Shift on Family Planning." *New Security Beat*, 8 August. Retrieved 24 September 2013 from http://www.newsecuritybeat.org/2012/08/irans-surprising-and-shortsighted-shift-on-family-planning/.

Makhlouf-Obermeyer, Carla. 1991. "Women, Islam and Population: Is the Triangle Fateful?" Working Series Paper No. 6, Harvard School of Public Health, Harvard University.

———. 1994. "Reproductive Choice in Islam: Gender and State in Iran and Tunisia." *Studies in Family Planning* 25(1): 41–51.

Mehran, Golnar. 2003/4. "Gender and Education in Iran." Paper commissioned for the EFA Global Monitoring Report, *Gender and Education for All: The Leap to Equality*. Retrieved 19 September 2021 from http://unesdoc.unesco.org/images/0014/001468/146809e.pdf.

Mehryar, Amir. 1998. *Country Population Assessment Report*. Plan Organization of Islamic Republic of Iran, unpublished draft with limited circulation.

Okkenhaug, Inger Mari, and Ingvilid Flaskerud. 2005. *Gender, Religion and Change in the Middle East: Two Hundred Years of History*. Oxford: Berg.

Salehi-Isfahani, Djavad. 2010. "Iranian Youth in Times of Economic Crisis." Brookings Institution, 10 October. Retrieved 23 September 2021 from https://www.brookings.edu/research/iranian-youth-in-times-of-economic-crisis/.

Salehi-Isfahani, Djavad, and Golnaz Taghvatalab. 2009. *Marriage Squeeze and the Changing Pattern of Marriage in Iran*. Working Papers Series. Retrieved 19 September 2021 from http://iussp2009.princeton.edu/papers/93356.

Statistical Center of Iran. 2006. "School-to-Work Transition Survey for

Islamic Republic of Iran." Technical report, Statistical Center of Iran, Technical Designs and Statistical Methods Research Group, Statistical Research Center.

Tadros, Mariz, ed. 2010. "Religion, Rights and Gender at the Crossroads." *Institute for Development Studies Bulletin* 42(1) December.

Tappan, Robert. 2012. "Ethical Decision-Making in Iranian Fertility Clinics." In *Islam and Assisted Reproductive Technologies: Sunni and Shia Perspectives*, ed. Marcia C. Inhorn and Soraya Tremayne, 103–129. New York: Berghahn Books.

Torabi, Fatemeh, and Angela Baschieri. 2010. "Ethnic Differences in Transition to First Marriage in Iran: The Role of Marriage Market, Women's Socio-Economic Status, and Process of Development." *Demographic Research* 22, article 2 (8 January): 29–62.

Tremayne, Soraya. 2004. "'And Never the Twain Shall Meet': Reproductive Health Policies in the Islamic Republic of Iran." In *Reproductive Agency, Medicine and the State: Cultural Transformations in Childbearing*, ed. Maya Unnithan-Kumar, 181–202. New York: Berghahn Books.

———. 2005. "The Moral, Ethical, and Legal Implications of Egg, Sperm and Embryo Donation in Iran." Paper presented at the International Conference on Reproductive Disruptions: Childlessness, Adoption and other Reproductive Complexities, University of Michigan, 19 May, Ann Arbor, Michigan.

———. 2006. "Not all Muslims Are Luddites." *Anthropology Today* 22(93): 1–2.

———. 2009. "Law, Ethics, and Donor Technologies in Shia Iran." In *Assisting Reproduction Testing Genes: Global Encounters with New Biotechnologies*, ed. Daphna Birenbaum-Carmeli and Marcia C. Inhorn, 144–164. New York and Oxford: Berghahn Books.

———. 2012. "The 'Down Side' of Gamete Donation: Challenging 'Happy Family' Rhetoric in Iran." In *Islam and Assisted Reproductive Technologies: Sunni and Shia Perspectives*, ed. Marcia C. Inhorn and Soraya Tremayne, 130–156. New York and Oxford: Berghahn Books.

Tremayne, Soraya, ed. 2001. *Managing Reproductive Life: Cross-Cultural Themes in Fertility and Sexuality*. New York: Berghahn Books.

Weir, Darren. 2012. "Iran Moves to Legalize Marriage for Girls under Ten Years Old." *Digital Journal*, 25 July. Retrieved 19 September 2021 from http://iranian.com/main/news/2012/08/23/iran-moves-legalize-marriage-girls-under-10-years-old.html.

Chapter 9

Assisted Reproductive Technologies and Making and Unmaking of Kin in Iran

Transformation or Variation on a Theme?

Introduction

Major changes that have taken place in Iran during the past few decades have had a profound, lasting, and irreversible impact on some of the social institutions they have touched. But their impingement has been less transformative on others and has served the purpose of further strengthening the existing core cultural values. Global trends, among many other agents of change, have played a significant part in engendering some of these changes and, in spite of the conservative outlook of the Iranian state, both Iranians and their theocratic ruling clerics have been swift to embrace what globalization, especially the global technologies, have to offer (Lotfalian 2004). However, while some of these technologies have been adopted without the necessity for an examination of their impact on moral and ethical grounds, the application of others has required official approval and legitimization, due to their practice affecting core cultural norms and values and religious rules. Among these technologies, none has proved more challenging, complex, and controversial than the assisted reproductive technologies (ARTs) affecting procreation, which is perceived to be a divine right and beyond the powers of humans to control. Reproduction, in its foundational role for the perpetuation of family and kinship, is paramount and considered a duty rather than a choice in Iranian culture. Historically, voluntary childlessness has not been an option for individuals and failing to reproduce is deemed not only detrimental to family and kin group, but also a threat to the stability of society. It is therefore understandable that the introduction of modern technologies affecting procreation has been received with caution and has raised profound questions as to their legitimacy, engaging experts from various disciplines to explore their broader implications.

Concern about the legitimacy of ARTs is not limited to Iran and their endorsement has required the involvement of the legal, ethical and, in some cases, religious authorities of the countries where they are practiced, to explore their impact on society. However, among the social institutions, it is kinship that has been most affected by the impingement of these technologies. ARTs, through offering their users new choices, have become instrumental in broadening and/or redefining the boundaries of kinship and relatedness in many societies. In reaching specific localities, ARTs have generated a multitude of cultural, religious, and legal interpretations, by both the state and the users of these technologies. For example, ARTs are shown to be challenging the foundational assumptions about kinship in Euro-American models (Strathern 1992), mainly through the practice of third-party gamete donation, which has transformed the structure of the family from its traditional form to an unpredictable variety of configurations. As Cahn (2014: 113) argues, by choosing to use third-party donated sperm or egg, people in the West challenge the legal construction of the family and, in her words "[the traditional model of the family], historically based on the unity of biology, parenthood, and marriage, is becoming increasingly irrelevant because of the decline of marriage in the United State and Europe (Cherlin 2009; Carbone and Cahn 2014). Third-party gametes undermine the very unity of biology, parenthood, and marriage, even as they, both paradoxically and ambiguously, affirm the importance of biology (McCandless and Sheldon 2014)." While such outcomes may be true of the way the Western models of family and kinship have developed, the situation is remarkably different in other cultures, where ARTs have been allowed precisely for the purpose of preserving, perpetuating, and protecting the sanctity of the family. For example, Kahn's (2000) studies of Israel challenge these assumptions that ARTs necessarily displace a culture's foundational assumptions about kinship and shows how ARTs have been used to perpetuate the existing core values of reproduction. Inhorn's pioneering studies on infertility in non-Western societies, with particular reference to the Muslim Middle East, also offer a different perspective on what Inhorn and Van Balen (2002: 4) refer to as "non-normative reproductive scenarios and experiences." Clarke's (2009: 47) study of kinship and ARTs in the Muslim Middle East also throws light on what constitutes kinship in Islamic societies and points out the nuances involved in defining the "biological" and the "social" by arguing that "according to the vision of the Islamic establishment, relations of filiation (*nasab*) are not mutable or fluid, but are given, paradigmatically—but not exclusively—through procreation." Eich (2012), in examining the construction of kinship in the medieval Sunni Islamic texts on fatherhood and lineage, also points out that notions of kinship and lineage are flexible and there is not one particular "Islamic way" of constructing kinship. He argues that these notions have evolved over the centuries and new meanings have been found, within the various concepts, to accommodate change for example, in the case of new reproductive technologies. Finally, this chapter also shows the flexibility of kinship in accommodating change to perpetuate the kinship ties.

From what precedes, it is clear that cultural responses to ARTs are as varied as the cultures themselves and that in their encounter with the local core reproductive norms ARTs either transform them or are excluded, if they clash with and are considered a threat to the existing norms and values. However, the choice of Iran, as an example of a country which has successfully accommodated these global technologies to fit into its own conservative mold, could be used as a lens to examine the way cultures can accommodate and shape the global technologies to their advantage without losing their own core values. Such handling has placed the country in a unique position vis-à-vis most countries in the world. On the one hand, in legitimizing ARTs, Iran has followed the Islamic law (*sharia*) and restricted procreation to heterosexual married couples. In this sense, it differs from those countries where third-party donation is not limited to married couples and unmarried as well as single parents and homosexuals can procreate with help from ARTs. On the other hand, Iran differs even more from all the other Muslim countries, where the majority of Muslims are Sunni, and except for the Shia in Lebanon, none of them allows third-party donation in any form (Inhorn 2006a). The question arises as to how these apparent contradictions of preserving the strict cultural and religious principles of procreation, and, at the same time, breaking the very rules which uphold them, have affected family, lineage, and kinship in Iran.

Methodology

Data presented in this chapter are part of a larger study carried out in Yazd (central Iran) and Tehran, and among Iranian refugees in the United Kingdom, between 2004 and 2012. The sites of study were infertility clinics; I lived with host families and carried out interviews with medical practitioners, psychologists, religious leaders, and ethicists. A surprising number of cases studied were those of Iranian asylum seekers in the United Kingdom for whom I acted as expert witness in British courts. These were mainly women, whose cases related to infertility of either their husbands or themselves and who had fled the country to avoid violence or execution. The main methodology used was that of participant observation and in-depth interviews. In total, 150 cases of infertile men and women were studied over the duration of the study.

The Ebbs and Flows of the Population Policies and Voluntary Childlessness

The history of the introduction of ARTs to Iran, their legitimization, their impact on family and kinship, and their current status can be better understood in light of the drastic demographic changes which have taken place over the past three decades in the country. These changes started in the mid-1980s, with the campaign referred to as the regulation of the family, which aimed at reducing the population growth. The program proved so successful that within ten years of its implementation the rate of population growth reduced from 3.9 percent per annum in 1986, to below 2 percent by 1996, and to 1.3 by 2012 (World Bank data), a figure that is below the replacement level. According to the findings of a study on the causes of the decline carried out by the Iranian Center for Research on Asian and Oceanic Population:

> Those couples who have just married and those who have been married for up to three years show no inclination to have any children at all, or perhaps just one. This tendency over the past decade illustrates that for women of urban and rural backgrounds, from different social classes, the poor and the rich, illiterate and literate, all have a similar attitude to giving birth these days, leading to the rapid downward trend in the Iranian TFR [total fertility rate]. (Tabnak 2013)

Concerns for the population decline were first expressed during the second term (2009–13) of Mahmoud Ahmadinejad's presidency and resulted in a return to a pronatalist policy of the early 1980s. The regime resorted to both "incentives" and "disincentives" to "persuade" people to have larger families, including, inter alia, dismantling the family planning program and re-routing the funds previously allocated to the campaign to encourage people to have larger families. But these efforts received a cool response and did not yield any results. Supreme Religious Leader Ayatollah Ali Khamenei publicly announced that it was "wrong" to continue with the family planning program and the two-decade-old policy of controlled growth must end. He admitted, "One of the mistakes we made in the nineties was population control. Government officials were wrong on this matter, and I, too, had a part. May God and history forgive us" (Karami 2012).

However, the efforts to encourage married couples to have larger families fell on deaf ears, and even the authorities realized that the incentives were not working. Although the same authorities continue to blame the economic hardship as responsible for the reluctance of the unmarried people of reproductive age to marry and have children, it is by no means certain that with an improvement in economic conditions, the generation of reproductive age will actually revert to having larger families similar to their parents' generation. The policymakers' reductionist interpretation of reproduction as a monolithic variable is misleading and as Robertson (1991: 159) puts it, "any attempt to reduce it [reproduction] into a static classification which would make the task of defining it easy and convenient, would tell us as much about reproduction as a sketch of a wing tells us about how a bird flies." Young Iranians' decisions to opt for one child, or no child at all, or even to remain unmarried, have not occurred in a vacuum and stem from a complex combination of factors and may prove difficult to reverse fully. The findings of this study and research by social scientists show that an increasing number of young people now live with their partners with no immediate intention of getting married, let alone having children.[1] Whether by refusing to reproduce this generation is also rejecting all the values associated with family and kinship is a topic for further research. But changes in reproductive behavior indicate that while reproduction, in its traditional context, has been an all-encompassing concept, embodying a person's identity, it no longer acts as the only marker of personhood. The generation between twenty-five and thirty-five years old, especially women, are able to express their identity by means other than by proving themselves capable of conceiving and perpetuating their lineage and social group. Although this voluntary childlessness merits a fuller discussion, the focus of this chapter is on a different aspect of reproduction, namely that of involuntary childlessness.

Infertility Unveiled

The focus on reducing the population growth in the 1980s was so intense in Iran that the state paid little attention to the question of infertility even though the population program of 1986 had made a mention of it as an area in need of action (Hoodfar 1995, cited in Tremayne 2004). It was with the decline in population growth, along with the research revealing the extent of infertility being made public, that the state was spurred into action and saw an opportunity in promoting the ARTs for infertility treatment as part of its pronatalist policies. Among the measures taken by the state were a considerable increase in the number of public infertility clinics and providing insurance coverage, making treatment available at low cost or free for the majority of infertile couples, who could not afford the high cost of ARTs (Tremayne and Akhondi 2016). While infertility has been a major stigma in Iran, its extent had remained unknown and it was the introduction of in vitro fertilization (IVF) and ARTs, and the high demand for them, that revealed its magnitude. For example, a nationwide survey of 17,000 married couples, carried out by Avicenna Research Center in 2011, showed the rate of infertility among married couples to be as high as 20 percent in the urban areas and up to 22 percent in rural ones, a figure which is far above that of the World Health Organization's global estimate of 10–15 percent. The country, therefore, faced not only a decline in population growth, but also a significant and larger than average number of infertile people. Realizing the vital importance of reproduction in Iranian culture, soon after the introduction of IVF in the West, Iranian medical practitioners started offering IVF treatment, but in doing so, they sought the opinion of the Islamic jurists, the majority of whom approved of IVF only for married heterosexual couples. Islam forbids conception outside marriage, which it views as equivalent to adultery, and it views the resulting child as illegitimate (*valad-e zena*). Homosexuality is forbidden and punishable by law (*sharia*). At this juncture, the practice of IVF did not provoke controversial arguments among the jurists but, as ARTs developed further in the West and conception through the third-party gamete donation of sperm, egg, embryo, and surrogacy became possible on their introduction to Iran, their legitimization was deemed necessary. The use of third-party gametes being considered equivalent to the intrusion of a third party into marriage, forbidden by Islamic law, the medical practitioners sought the opinion of the Shia jurists. Although Sunni religious leaders in most Muslim countries of the Middle East had allowed the practice of IVF between married couples, they had forbidden the donation of third-party gametes (Inhorn 2006b). But the Shia jurists in Iran found solutions within Shia practices to legitimize third-party donation, without breaking any religious rules (Tremayne 2009; Inhorn and Tremayne 2012). Currently, ARTs are practiced in Iran in all their forms, from IVF between married couples; to third-party sperm, egg, and embryo donation; to surrogacy; and pre-implantation genetic diagnosis. The legitimization of ARTs is the result of close collaboration between the Shia jurists and the medical practitioners, who went to great lengths and worked closely to find a solution for the practice of third-party donation. To this end, the medical practitioners took the initiative of publicly engaging some of the leading religious authorities in the discourse. For example, a groundbreaking conference was organized by one of the pioneers in ARTs in Iran in 1996, which included experts from various disciplines to explore the legitimacy and feasibility of gamete donation and its broader implications for family and lineage.[2] However, even after extensive deliberations, the senior Shia jurists, who are the sources of emulation (*mojtahids*)[3] for their adherents, failed to reach unanimity and to date their opinions remain divided on the legitimacy of third-party donation. Since the approval or disapproval of different *mojtahids* bears equal weight among the Shia, the medical practitioners were swift to take their cue from the favorable religious edicts (*fatwa*) and started the practice of third-party donation. Temporary marriage (*sigheh*), which is unique to the Shia, was used to legitimize donation between the spouse of the infertile party and the donor. The marriage was for the duration of the successful fertilization of the egg and no sexual contact took place between the two parties (Tremayne 2009). However, temporary marriage was mainly used in cases of egg donation and far fewer cases resorted to it for sperm donation.[4] But a few years into the practice of third-party donation, in the late 1990s, Supreme Religious Leader Ayatollah Ali Khamenei (1999) endorsed the donation of both sperm and egg, without any reference to temporary marriage, and emphasized that "as long as no touch or gaze takes place, donation is allowed."

While the endorsement of egg donation did not meet with any objection, the approval of sperm donation caused uproar in a predominantly patriarchal culture (Tremayne 2009). To date, its practice is more limited and is carried out discreetly by some private clinics.[5] While some of the religious infertile couples abided by their source of emulation, who disagreed with third-party donation, and gave up the idea of treatment, some others changed their *mojtahids* and sought the advice of other *mojtahids*, whom they knew would be more favorable, the change of source of emulation being allowed in Shia practices (Inhorn and Tremayne 2012; Tappan 2012). However, not all infertile couples sought religious permission, and many were not even aware of the necessity of such legitimization. They assumed that if the clinic is performing these treatments, it must be allowed. These considerations notwithstanding, in cases of third-party donation, both the rulings of the legislators and the choices made by infertile couples on who the donor of the gamete should be, have shown that conception must ensure the continuity of biological relatedness. The examples below are the tip of the iceberg, showing the importance of the biological relatedness among users of ARTs. In one study, several infertile women interviewed in clinics were adamant that, for them, the only option is to have their own biological child (Abbasi-Shavazi et al. 2008). One woman mentioned, "I do not want anybody to know that I have resorted to a donor's egg, because people will think that my child is not my biological child and therefore he is illegitimate." Another woman said, "Using another women's egg is forbidden (*haram*), and I feel guilty for resorting to it. But, by breastfeeding the child, I become the milk mother and therefore our relationship will become legitimate." Finally, a woman who needed to resort to using a surrogate mother mentioned that if she decided to use a surrogate mother, she would not let anybody know and would pretend to be pregnant herself for the duration "because when I tried to use the ZIFT (Zygote Intrafallopian Transfer) method, all my relatives said that this was a stranger's seed and not my own, and this time I am not going to let anybody find out that I have used a surrogate mother." As one woman interviewed put it, "if people find out that this is a donor child, they will consider him as a bastard" (Abbasi-Shavazi et al. 2008). Several other women in the same study were also emphatic that "it is a sin to conceive from an outsider's gamete outside marriage and the child will not be our biological child."

Conversely, in cases of surrogacy whereby relatives had acted as surrogate mothers, no such comments were raised as the resulting child shared the same blood with the kin group (Garmaroudi Naef 2012). It is clear that, regardless of how these infertile women conceive, their shared understanding remains that the child must be biologically related to them, a major consideration by the Shia in Iran, which is also shown by Inhorn (2006a) to be the case among Sunni Muslims. For Iranian users of gametes, even if the child is not biologically related to them, he/she must appear to be so.

Likewise, the religious rulings were clear that the donor child (child born from a third-party gamete) belongs to his/her biological parent (the donor of the gamete), and that the infertile party remains the social parent. The child is also supposed to inherit from his/her biological parent and not the social parent, but takes his/her name from the social parent, the father in this case, regardless of whether he or his wife are the infertile party. In Islam, the child belongs to his/her father. The importance of biological relatedness is particularly articulated in the preference the infertile parties show in receiving gametes from their close relatives to maintain the biological continuity and the bloodline. Another clear indication of the paramount importance of reproducing for the social group is the excessive interest and involvement of the infertile couple's relatives throughout the process of fertility treatment. Close members of the kin group see it as their duty to step in and help their infertile relatives conceive in every possible way they can. This help ranges from donating gametes (sperm or egg, embryo, or surrogacy), to financial help including selling their house, car, or other belongings, or even borrowing money to pay for the treatment. This support is not entirely altruistic, as the fertility/infertility of the couple is understood to be a matter of concern for the entire kin group. As mentioned earlier, essentially, kinship in Iranian culture means biological relatedness, and although cases in this study come from a variety of cultural, socio-economic, and educational backgrounds, they all share the belief that reproduction is about having one's own biological child (see also Inhorn 2006b). According to the findings of this study, when one of the spouses is infertile and the couple needs to receive either sperm or egg from a donor, or to use a surrogate mother, the first port of call is to ask a sibling for help (Garmaroudi Naef 2012). Failing this, other close members of the kin group may be called upon too, but the choice remains a calculated one based on the degree of closeness of relatives and how the donation can be justified in biological terms (Tremayne 2015).

Consanguinity and Sibling Gamete Donation

Third-party gamete donation, especially from siblings, has led to the emergence of a complex web of relations within the kin group. For example, in case of a woman donating an egg to her infertile sister, which is fertilized with the infertile sister's husband's sperm, the resulting child will have two mothers and his cousins are his half-siblings too. Furthermore, according to the Islamic structure of kinship, the fertilization of the sister's egg with that of her brother-in-law would, in principle, be considered adultery, even though this is at a symbolic level. A brief explanation of the kinship structure in Muslim societies is as follows. Under the *sharia*, the nature and extent of the interaction between various members of the kin group are determined by a division of men and women into two social categories i.e., *mahram* and *na-mahram*. *Mahram* are those members of the family who are related by blood or marriage or through breastfeeding, and who are not considered potential marriage partners and are, therefore, free in their social, but not sexual, interactions with each other. The *mahram* group for women consists of their father, grandfather, brother, uncle, husband, son, father-in-law, grandsons, and nephews and their children. For men, *mahram* are the mother, grandmother, sister, aunt, wife, daughter, mother-in-law, granddaughters, and nieces and their children. Everybody else outside these groups of relatives is a potential marriage partner and considered a *na-mahram* and forbidden to enter into any physical contact of any kind with the opposite sex. Sexual contact between *mahram*, for example an aunt and her nephew, is incest and between *na-mahram* adultery. It follows that a child born out of wedlock or from incest or adultery is considered a bastard (*valad-e zena* or *haram zadeh*) and has no status in society. However, within these prohibitions, mechanisms exist through which *na-mahram* can become *mahram*. One such mechanism is milk kinship (*rezayi*), allowing the milk mother (*madare rezayi*) to become equal to the biological mother of the child she has breastfed. The same rules of *mahram* and *na-mahram* then extend to include not only the milk mother and the child, but also the relatives of both parties. Khatib-Chahidi's (1992) comprehensive study of milk kinship among Shia Iranians elaborates on the fact that the milk mother's milk belongs to her husband and highlights the social significance of the prohibition of marriage between the milk mother and the family of the child she breastfeeds. In his study of Islam and new kinship, Clarke (2007: 287) has explored the potential of milk kinship for third-party gamete donation as follows: "for Muslim religious specialists, milk kinship provides a way of thinking through and resolving the ethical dilemmas of the use of donor eggs and surrogacy arrangements. Rather than disappearing under modernity, then, milk kinship endures as a resource for the mediation of social relations and intellectual challenges."

Indeed, milk kinship is a convenient vehicle for the justification of the legitimacy of third-party donation, especially in cases of egg donation, whereby the infertile mother becomes the gestational one and also breastfeeds the donor child and establishes the necessary biological connectedness with the child. As discussed earlier, many infertile cases in this and other studies had already reached such a conclusion themselves and justified their use of a stranger's gamete through the biological relatedness created through milk kinship.

In the early days of the practice of gamete donation, in parallel with the ongoing debates among various experts, infertile men and women swiftly found their own solutions in finding suitable donors and resorted to their siblings or the next closest blood relatives to provide them with gametes. Although these preferences have shifted during the past two decades and many private clinics no longer allow the users to choose or select the gamete donor themselves, the actual driving force behind the choice of relatives, namely the importance of biological relatedness, has remained consistent without exception. In reality, the solutions such as temporary marriage were devised to allow gamete donation by strangers and were practiced in parallel with sibling donation, which at no stage had required legitimization and remained unopposed by all concerned. In fact, in cases of sibling donation, temporary marriage would not have been possible, as getting married, even temporarily, to one's sister's husband or to one's brother's wife, to donate a gamete, would have been considered incest or adultery. The endorsement of many leading clerics of gamete donation, who allowed it on the condition that no "touch" and "gaze" would take place, not only effectively removed any prohibition in third-party gamete donation between any two parties; it also proved instrumental in defining the parameters of donation, by giving the individuals the freedom of choosing the donor of their future child. However, since ARTs first started, donation by the kin group has diminished at the private clinics but continues in public hospitals.

Likewise, a few years into the gamete donation, the opposite sex sibling donation came to the fore and an increasing number of embryos were formed through the fertilization of a brother and sister's gametes. The information on these practices is either communicated by the medical practitioners during personal interviews, in talking with the infertile couples themselves, or appears sporadically and casually in daily papers and does not generate any interest among their readers. It is therefore not possible to know the extent of the practice in all seventy clinics in Iran. What is clear is that, faced with such requests from opposite siblings to make embryos with their gametes, the physicians often try and reason with them on the negative outcomes, but when the users insist and as there are no rules prohibiting the request, the doctors oblige. Furthermore, the medical practitioners confide that, as there are no detailed ethical codes of practice in this area, they are not sure what is ethically right or wrong and often have to use their own judgment. However, opposite sex donation has met with disapproval by most people, even by the medical practitioners, who found it repulsive. Such practices are considered to be incest, symbolically, even though no physical sexual contact takes place between the siblings. These kinds of lateral gamete donations are becoming normal practice among donors and recipient siblings, which, in the absence of explicit laws or *fatwas* forbidding them, go unopposed. There are also more recent cases of intergenerational donation, whereby fathers have volunteered to give sperm to their sons. The fact that their daughter-in-law conceives with their sperm is in no way linked to sexual transgression deviating from the norms or breaking any sexual taboos.

Finally, a brief picture of the extent of "consanguineous connectivity," a term coined by Inhorn (2012), among Middle Eastern families can help a better understanding of the motivation behind gamete donation between siblings and other biological members of the kin group. As Inhorn (2012: 135) explains, "an additional reason for this high level of family involvement is consanguineous connectivity, or tendency to marry 'blood' relatives as a signifier of family closeness." Inhorn's (2012: 235) study of 220 Muslim Middle Eastern men shows that "consanguineous unions occur in 16 to 78 percent of all Middle Eastern marriages" and "between 8 and 30 percent of these marriages are first-cousin marriages." Studies of cousin marriages in Iran also confirm similar patterns. According to a study carried out among twelve different ethnic groups across Iran, 38 percent of marriages were consanguineous, with 28 percent with parallel patrilateral cousins as the most common form (Saadat, Ansari-Lari, and Farhud 2004).

A further study also has shown that, overall, the level of marriage to biological relatives ranged from 23 percent in Gilan [northern Iran] to 78 percent in Sistan and Baluchestan [southwestern Iran]. The findings of the study show that the practice of marriage to biological relatives has remained surprisingly resilient in the face of modernizing influences and that ethnicity, province, and area of residence remain important determinants (Abbasi-Shavazi, McDonald, and Hosseini-Chavoshi 2008).

ARTs and "Kinning" and "De-kinning"

Viewed from an anthropological perspective, the infertility clinics have become a platform where the making and unmaking, or to use terms coined by Howell cited by Edwards (2014), the "kinning" and "de-kinning" of relatives unfolds and the members of the kin group assess, strengthen, articulate, contest, deny, renegotiate, and do and undo their kinship ties.

In cases of children being conceived through gamete donation by relatives, the "kinning" is nurtured through a strong relationship and connectedness with the kin group. In this "interfamilial" model of conception the possibility of the child being rejected is almost impossible, as the child will always be included and taken care of by one or the other member of the kin group. Interviews with medical practitioners confirm that as and when disputes arise between relatives, where one party is the donor of the gamete and the other the recipient, these are often about the ownership of the child and who can claim the child as his/her own. This is in contrast with the cases whereby a stranger's gamete has been used and the dispute between the donor and the recipient of the gamete is about the financial compensation.[6]

In cases of more modern nuclear families, who are increasingly able to seek treatment without their relatives' knowledge, the couple chooses the stranger's gamete so as to be able to keep their infertility a secret. In such cases, gender plays a significant role in the making of kin with the child. In general, in the case of women in this study, who had conceived through a stranger's egg, the child was treated with affection and the "making" of kin with him/her worked well. In such cases, the father being the biological father, no disharmony took place. Of the infertile men among the cases studied, many, but not all, who had used donor sperm showed different reactions, which ranged from passive protest, by withdrawing and ignoring the child, to his/her rejection, and to violence against his wife and the child (Inhorn and Tremayne 2012).

However, in cases of a stranger's gamete, the total rejection of the resulting child can and does happen too. In one case, a woman brought back the child she had conceived through egg donation, and told the staff at the clinic, "I am no longer married to this child's father and do not want him anymore. You can have him back." It is clear that the child had been conceived to guarantee the stability of the marriage and had lost its function once the marriage had fallen apart. Once more, the extent of such rejections is not known but it is likely that these examples are only the tip of the iceberg.

Finally, as time goes by, the horizon for the reasons for resorting to treatment also broadens. The changes observed in the practice of ARTs over time not only mirror the dynamics involved in reproductive practices, but also reflect the wider social and cultural changes Iranian society is undergoing. For example, among the cases studied, some young women between twenty and thirty-five years old seeking infertility treatment confided in me that they had gone through a phase of having several sexual partners, had become pregnant and had resorted to illegal abortions. Once this phase of sexual freedom had ceased to be exciting and, after getting older, they had moved on to get married and settle down. To do so, they had resorted to hymenoplasty to restore their virginity for the wedding night. Once married, they had found themselves unable to conceive, and had ended up at the infertility clinic appealing to the medical practitioners by saying, "I must have one child so that my marriage does not break up, and so that I can also tick the box and prove that I am fertile. Please help me."[7] It seems that, for these cases, after a period of rebellion, the process had come full circle and they had voluntarily returned to wishing to find their rightful place in society.

Conclusion

This chapter has focused on showing that, in spite of the major demographic transformations of the past three decades in Iran, the core values attached to reproduction and kinship have remained of essence even if they have changed their form. To do so, I have used the lens of infertility to demonstrate that although the ground supporting the values attached to family, marriage, and reproduction may be shifting, these values continue to persist among a significantly large number of people, if not among all. Seeking treatment for infertility, which remains one of the most intimate and stigmatized aspects of one's identity, has resulted in a careful (re)assessment of what relatedness means to infertile individuals and their network of kin.

The findings of this study show that, without exception, the only acceptable form of relatedness in Iranian culture is a biological one. While state-of-the-art ARTs have led to the emergence of new forms of relatedness in many cultures and have altered the traditional structure of the family, tested in the Iranian context, they have highlighted the persistence rather than the disappearance of the traditional kinship values. Regardless of the methods chosen to conceive through ARTs, their users have found ways of justifying it to themselves and proving to others that the donor child is biologically related to them. However, in the process, the infertile individuals have also implicitly revealed that it is proving the ability to reproduce that is paramount, even at the cost of compromising the actual blood ties. In this vein, the infertility clinics become the stage for the display of their commitment to retain blood ties by barren individuals. Interestingly, the clinic seems to have become the focal point for an emergent form of "de-kinning," performed publicly in the aftermath of third-party gamete donation, in cases of the separation of the parents of the child conceived through IVF.

The analysis of the data also clearly reveals that through the preference for gamete donation by family members a new form of "consanguinity" is emerging, which, potentially, could profoundly affect the relationship between the members of the kin group. In such cases, the donor child becomes a circuit for recycling the "old blood" and for maintaining the lineage, but it also remains at the intersection of a newly created web of consanguineous connections, for which no cultural, legal, or religious provisions exist. The fact of having multiple parents, half-siblings who are also cousins, and double-relatedness to other members of the kin group, which all affect the legitimacy of the interaction between the *mahram* and *na-mahram* categories, raises a host of increasingly complicated legal and social issues, which may necessitate the interference of those legislators who in the first place allowed the practice of gamete donation in the way they did. Furthermore, the decline in population growth has promoted the state's new interest in promoting ARTs to help the considerable number of infertile couples (around 20 percent of married couples) conceive; even if a portion of these couples continue to receive gametes from their close kin, further research will be needed to establish whether and to what extent family and the structure of kinship will be transformed through such practices, the biomedical implications notwithstanding.

As for the generation of reproductive age, who have opted for voluntary childlessness, and whose number is on the increase, the questions remain: to what extent values attached to reproduction, kinship, and relatedness have vanished for this group; whether these values persist but are dormant and blurred by other competing values; and finally, whether such behavior is an informed decision and there to stay or a transient phase and a variation on a theme, which will pass once the young have passed their rebellious stage.

Acknowledgments

This chapter was published originally as "Assisted Reproductive Technologies and Making and Unmaking of Kin in Iran: Transformation or Variation on a Theme?" In *International Handbook on Gender and Demographic Processes. International Handbooks of Population* Vol. 8, ed. Nancy E. Riley and Jan Brunson, 83–93. Dordrecht: Springer (2018).

Notes

1. An interview with Masserat Amir Ebrahimi, a social scientist, in Tehran in 2011 confirms the growing number of young people, especially young women, who live together or with their opposite sex partners and refuse to marry.
2. The proceedings of this conference were published in Akhondi (2001).
3. The sources of emulation (*mojtahids*) are senior Islamic scholars, learned in religion and *sharia*, who are in a position to use independent reasoning and interpret the Qur'an and issue *fatwas*.
4. For an explanation of the reasons for the rarity of the use of temporary marriage for the purpose of receiving sperm, see Tremayne (2009).
5. While in Shia Islam a child can take his lineage (*nasab*) from both his parents, he belongs to the father and his lineage, which explains the gravity of using another man's sperm instead of his own. See also Ebadi (2003) and Mir-Hosseini (2000).
6. These observations were made in the earlier days of gamete donation, and as third-party gamete donation has been in a state of flux, the relationship between family members may have also evolved accordingly.

7. Personal communications and interviews with infertile women and female students, Tehran 2012 and Oxford 2013.

References

Abbasi-Shavazi, Mohammad Jalal, Marcia C. Inhorn, Hajiieh Bibi Razeghi Nasrabad, and Ghasem Sam Toloo. 2008. "The 'Iranian ART Revolution': Infertility, Assisted Reproductive Technology, and Third-Party Donation in the Islamic Republic of Iran." *Journal of Middle East Women's Studies* 4(2): 1–28.

Abbasi-Shavazi, Mohammad Jalal, Peter McDonald, and Meimanat Hosseini-Chavoshi. 2008. "Modernization or Cultural Maintenance: The Practice of Consanguineous Marriage in Iran." *Journal of Biosocial Science* 40(6): 911–933.

Akhondi, Mohammad Mehdi, ed. 2001. *Modern Human Reproductive Techniques from the View of Jurisprudence and Law*. In Persian. Book based on papers presented in a symposium of the same title. Tehran: Avicenna Research Institute, Academic Publishing House for the Social Science.

Cahn, Naomi. 2014. "Legal Kinship and Connection in US Donor Families." In *Relatedness in Assisted Reproduction: Families, Origins and Identities*, ed. Tabitha Freeman, Susanna Graham, Fatemeh Ebtehaj, and Martin Richards, 113–129. Cambridge: Cambridge University Press.

Carbone, June, and Naomi Cahn. 2014. *Marriage Markets: How Inequality is Remaking the American Family*. Oxford University Press.

Cherlin, Andrew J. 2009. "The Origins of the Ambivalent Acceptance of Divorce." *Journal of Marriage and Family* 71(2): 226–229.

Clarke, Morgan. 2007. "The Modernity of Milk Kinship." *Social Anthropology* 15(3): 287–304.

———. 2009. *Islam and New Kinship: Reproductive Technologies and the Shariah in Lebanon*. New York: Berghahn Books

Ebadi, Shirin. 2003. *Women's Rights in the Laws of the Islamic Republic of Iran*. In Persian. Tehran: Ganje Danesh Publishers.

Edwards, Jeanette. 2014. "Undoing Kinship." In *Relatedness in Assisted Reproduction: Families, Origins and Identities*, ed. Tabitha Freeman, Susanna Graham, Fatemeh Ebtehaj, and Martin Richards, 44–60. Cambridge: Cambridge University Press.

Eich, Thomas. 2012. "Constructing Kinship in Sunni Islamic Legal Texts." In *Islam and Assisted Reproductive Technologies: Sunni and Shia Perspectives*, ed. Marcia C. Inhorn and Soraya Tremayne. New York and Oxford: Berghahn Books.

Garmaroudi Naef, Shirin. 2012. "Gestational Surrogacy in Iran: Uterine Kinship in Shia Thought and Practice." In *Islam and Assisted Reproductive Technologies: Sunni and Shia Perspectives*, ed. Marcia C. Inhorn and Soraya Tremayne, 157–194. New York and Oxford: Berghahn Books.

Hoodfar, Homa. 1995. "Population Policy and Gender Equity in Post-Revolutionary Iran.' In *Family, Gender, and Population in the Middle East: Policies in Context*, ed. Carla Makhlouf. Cairo: American University of Cairo Press.

Inhorn, Marcia C. 2006a. "Making Muslim Babies: IVF and Gamete Donation in Sunni Versus Shia Islam." *Culture, Medicine and Psychiatry* 30(4): 427–450.

———. 2006b. "He Won't Be My Son." *Medical Anthropology Quarterly* 20(1): 94–120.

———. 2012. *The New Arab Man: Emergent Masculinities, Technologies, and Islam in the Middle East*. Princeton: Princeton University Press.

Inhorn, Marcia C., and Frank Van Balen, eds. 2002. *Infertility around the Globe: New Thinking on Childlessness, Gender, and Reproductive Technologies*. Berkeley: University of California Press.

Inhorn, Marcia C., and Soraya Tremayne. 2012. "Introduction: Islam and Assisted Reproductive Technologies." In *Islam and Assisted Reproductive Technologies: Sunni and Shia Perspectives*, ed. Marcia C. Inhorn and Soraya Tremayne, 1–21. New York and Oxford: Berghahn Books.

Kahn, Susan Martha. 2000. *Reproducing Jews: A Cultural Account of Assisted Conception in Israel*. Durham: Duke University Press.

Karami, Arash. 2012. "Khamenei on Population Control: 'May God and History Forgive Us.'" *Al-Monitor*, 17 October. Retrieved 19 September 2021 from https://www.al-monitor.com/pulse/fr/contents/articles/originals/2012/al-monitor/iran-population-control.html.

Khamenei, Ali. 1999. *Ojoubeh Al-Esteftaat*. Questions 1271 to 1277. Tehran: Amir Kabir.

Khatib-Chahidi, J. 1992. "Milk Kinship in Shi'ite Islamic Iran." In *Anthropology of Breast-Feeding: Natural Law or Social Construct*, ed. Vanessa Maher, 109–132. Oxford: Berg.

Lotfalian, Mazyar. 2004. *Islam, Technoscientific Identities, and the Culture of Curiosity*. Washington, DC: University Press of America.

McCandless, Julie, and Sally Sheldon. 2014. "Genetically Challenged: The Determination of Legal Parenthood in Assisted Reproduction." In *Relatedness in Assisted Reproduction: Families, Origins and Identities*, ed. Tabitha Freeman, Susanna Graham, Fatemeh Ebtehaj, and Martin Richards, 61–78. Cambridge: Cambridge University Press.

Mir-Hosseini, Ziba. 2000. *Marriage on Trial: A Study of Islamic Family Law*. Revised ed. London: I.B. Tauris.

Robertson, A.F. 1991. *Beyond the Family: The Social Organization of Human Reproduction*. Cambridge: Polity Press.

Saadat, Mostafa, Maryam Ansari-Lari, and Dariush Farhud. 2004. "Consanguineous Marriage in Iran." *Annals of Human Biology* 31(2): 263–269.

Strathern, Marilyn. 1992. *After the Nature: English Kinship in the Late Twentieth Century*. Cambridge: Cambridge University Press.

Tabnak. 2013. "Iran's Population Crisis Awaits the Iranian People." In Persian.

24 September. Retrieved 19 September 2021 from www.tabnak.ir/fa/news/346841.

Tappan, Robert. 2012. "Ethical Decision-Making in Iranian Fertility Clinics." In *Islam and Assisted Reproductive Technologies: Sunni and Shia Perspectives*, ed. Marcia C. Inhorn and Soraya Tremayne, 103–129. New York: Berghahn Books.

Tremayne, Soraya. 2004. "'And Never the Twain Shall Meet': Reproductive Health Policies in the Islamic Republic of Iran." In *Reproductive Agency, Medicine and the State: Cultural Transformations in Childbearing*, ed. Maya Unnithan-Kumar, 181–202. New York: Berghahn Books.

———. 2009. "Law, Ethics, and Donor Technologies in Shia Iran." In *Assisting Reproduction, Testing Genes: Global Encounters with New Biotechnologies*, ed. Daphna Birenbaum-Carmeli and Marcia C. Inhorn, 144–164. New York and Oxford: Berghahn Books.

———. 2015. "Whither Kinship? Assisted Reproductive Technologies and Relatedness in the Islamic Republic of Iran." In *Assisted Reproductive Technologies in the Third Phase*, ed. Kate Hampshire and Bob Simpson. New York: Berghahn Books.

Tremayne, Soraya, and Mohammad Mehdi Akhondi. 2016. "Conceiving IVF in Iran." *Reproductive Biomedicine & Society Online* 2: 62–70.

Part IV

Fertility, Religion, Technology

Chapter 10

Law, Ethics, and Donor Technologies in Shia Iran

The population policies of the Islamic Republic of Iran won international acclaim for their success in reducing population growth in the ten-year period from 1986 to 1996. Indeed, in 1998, Iran received the United Nations Population Award for its achievements. Within a span of ten years, population growth dropped from 3.8 percent in 1986, to 2.5 percent in 1991, to 1.5 percent in 1996, where it stands to the present day (Statistical Center of Iran 1998; Tremayne 2004: 181–185).[1] The secret to this success was a well-coordinated campaign on the part of health policymakers who showed an acute awareness of the cultural sensitivities in trying to persuade people to have fewer children. The campaign also received the full endorsement and involvement of clerics at the highest level. Islam and Iranian culture are assumed to value fertility, so in order to preempt public objections to the campaign, policymakers avoided the use of words such as "reduction" or "control" and instead used "regulation of the family" (*tanzim-e-khanevadeh*). At the same time, the campaign emphasized it was not only about reducing family size, but was also about the treatment of infertility, and therefore, special attention would be given to infertile couples (Hoodfar 1995: 114).[2] This gained great favor with those objecting to the campaign's anti-natal stance. Following such approval, which coincided with the spread of new assisted reproductive technologies (ARTs) worldwide, the past two decades have witnessed a rapid flourishing of infertility treatment in Iran, and centers making use of ARTs are opening at an increasing rate in the major cities. Currently, around fifty centers exist and range from private to semi-sponsored to almost-free treatment clinics.

ARTs have spread around the world, beyond technologically advanced countries, but "perhaps nowhere is this globalization process more evident than in the twenty-two nations of the Muslim Middle East" (Inhorn 2005). According to Marcia C. Inhorn (2005), "Iran is definitely in the lead among the Muslim countries in the Middle East in the application of these technologies." For those less familiar with Shia Islam, the speed and relative ease with which Iran has adopted ARTs come as a complete surprise. For a conservative theocracy not only to allow interference in matters of divine creation, but also to race ahead remains a puzzle. This is even more so given that the secular Western countries from which these technologies have come are still struggling to resolve some of the emerging ethical problems.

The use of ARTs in Muslim countries has been made possible by the approval of religious leaders because, as "in all of the Middle Eastern Muslim countries, Islamic *fatwas* have profoundly affected the practice of IVF (in vitro fertilization) in ways that are not commonly seen in the West" (Inhorn 2006). Although the application of ARTs in the West is under the scrutiny of various medical, legal, and ethical committees, in the Muslim countries of the Middle East the responsibility for such endorsement has remained largely with religious leaders regardless of whether the state is secular or theocratic. "Infertile couples in these countries are usually extremely concerned about making their test-tube babies in the Islamically correct way. To that end, they seek 'official' Islamic opinion on the practice of IVF in the form of a *fatwa*" (Inhorn 2006). The religious leaders in these countries have therefore taken the center stage and play an active role in examining and legitimizing the use of ARTs. In doing so, Sunni and Shia leaders have reached different conclusions. In this chapter, I explain some of the built-in mechanisms available to the Shia sect that pave the way for the legitimization of ARTs without breaking any divine rules. In addition, with Iran being a theocracy, decisions made by religious authorities are all-encompassing; once they have issued a *fatwa*, no further approval is required by secular or even other religious authorities. However, *fatwas* themselves are based not just on lengthy debates between religious authorities, but also on a thorough engagement with secular experts. Although ruling clerics have officially approved the use of ARTs, differences of view remain among jurists as well as senior clerics as to the limits of their application and interpretation of their use (for Ayatollah Madani's views, see Mir-Hosseini 2000).

This chapter focuses on Iran's process of legitimizing the donation of sperm, eggs, and embryos, and explores the interaction between the three main players involved in the practice of ARTs: religious leaders; biomedical practitioners, who are the ultimate source of knowledge for the application of ARTs; and infertile couples, whose choices of donors are based on their understandings of what constitutes lineage and kinship. I argue that the flexibility of the Shia religion allows sufficient scope for manipulation by all three parties, which, if continued, can lead to a change in the landscape of kinship. The speed with which ARTs continue to invade the market, infertile couples' high demand for them, religious leaders' lack of consistency regarding their use, and the failure of the ruling religio-legal *fatwas* to keep pace with new situations arising from these practices have all created rifts regarding the ethical aspects of the practices and cultural norms. The research conducted so far suggests that the practice of ARTs remains in a state of flux. Only when the "new babies" come of age will the nature and extent of problems, ranging from ethical issues to kinship and gender relations, emerge.

The data presented in this chapter are part of a larger study spanning two years (2003–05) in Iran. The main sites of study were Tehran and Yazd, in central Iran, with some data from Gorgan, in the northeast, and Ardebil, in the northwest. Several clinics in Tehran and Yazd were selected on the basis of being private, semi-governmental, or public, in order to gain access to infertile couples of different social and economic backgrounds. The majority of clinics in both cities, especially the public clinics, focus on female infertility. Preliminary interviews were also carried out at a clinic catering to men whose infertility had resulted from spinal injuries occurring during the Iran–Iraq War. A total of sixty couples were interviewed. Forty-five were recruited from clinics, and others were through personal contacts. The main method used was participant observation. In-depth interviews were carried out with medical staff, psychologists, and ethical experts at the fertility clinics, as well as with senior clerics.

Assisted Reproductive Technologies

ARTs are expanding so quickly in Iran and demand is so high that keeping pace with them has become a major task for all involved. Islamic jurists are often faced with new ARTs being practiced without their approval and have to catch up with this fait accompli rather than determine their legal use in advance. In the early days, the practice of IVF took place between a wife and a husband and was considered merely another medical technology helping infertile couples reproduce. No third party was involved, and questions related to lineage, kinship, and the changing relationship between wife/husband and parents/children did not arise. However, with rapid advances in ARTs and the emergence of multiple choices, such as third-party donation, legitimization has proved a major challenge to Islamic jurists, who are faced with the dilemma of whether and how to allow ARTs without breaking incest taboos and parentage rules.

Islamic law (*sharia*) is clear about lineage (*nasab*), and *sharia* meticulously defines the relationship of the kin group. In this system, a child belongs to his or her father and is his property. The mother is only a caretaker and has no rights over her children (Mir-Hosseini 1998; Ebadi 2003). The law of inheritance follows such a stance. Marriage, incest, and adultery are also clearly explained, and social and sexual interaction between men and women is defined by dividing them into two categories, *mahram* and *na-mahram*. Briefly, *mahrams* are parents and siblings, among others (see Khatib-Chahidi 1981). As they are not potential marriage partners, close social contact is allowed. *Na-mahrams* are potential marriage partners, and therefore close social and sexual interaction between them is forbidden (*haram*). *Na-mahrams* are not allowed to come into close contact with or touch each other, and *na-mahram* men are not allowed to see a woman's body except for her face, nor can they touch her. Breaking any of these rules involves severe sanctions. In such circumstances, it is not difficult to imagine the extent to which the application of some ARTs would violate these rules, especially that of lineage, and lead to complicated situations for which *sharia* has no simple answers or solutions. According to Sunni religious leaders in Egypt and Lebanon, ARTs are limited to IVF between a married couple, and no third-party donation of gamete or embryo is allowed (Inhorn 2003, 2005). Shia clerics in Iran also ruled that ARTs should only be available to those within the marital union but resorted to interpreting the Qur'an (*ijtihad*), a practice unique to the Shia sect, which in turn led to *fatwas* allowing third-party donation.[3]

Shia Islam and Sperm and Egg Donation

In vitro fertilization has been practiced for nearly twenty years in Iran, but it was not until the late 1990s that supreme religious leader Ayatollah Khamenei (1999: 281–283) endorsed its use between a married couple, as well as third-party donation, by answering the following questions: "Is the application of IVF between a wife and husband allowed?" and "In case of the infertility of the wife or husband, leading to difficulties in marriage and mental problems, is the use of another man or woman's sperm or egg, which is fertilized outside the womb, allowed?" His replies were, "IVF is not in and of itself legally forbidden as long as no haram acts such as gaze or touch take place." He extended his approval for both egg and sperm donation on the same basis, emphasizing there is no legal prohibition from receiving an unknown man's sperm as long as no touch or gaze take place. In answer to the question, "If a wife is unable to produce eggs (because of menopause or other reasons) can the husband's second wife, whether permanent or temporary, donate her egg to be fertilized and planted inside the infertile wife?" he replied, "In principle such action is not forbidden and there is no difference between the nature of marriage whether it is permanent or temporary" (Khamenei 1999: 281–283). Although Ayatollah Khamenei did not explicitly mention temporary marriage as a solution to legitimize gamete donation, his answers were taken as a cue, and the definition of wife and husband was expanded to accommodate temporary marriage to carry out ARTs.

Temporary marriage (*mut'a* in Arabic and *sigheh* in Persian), a practice particular to the Shia sect, occurs when a man and woman agree to enter into marriage within a time limit, which can be from one hour to ninety-nine years (see Haeri 1989). To legitimately receive gametes from a third party, the husband of an infertile woman will nominally—meaning that no touch or gaze will take place—marry the donor for one day. Donors should be widows or divorcees and ideally already have children of their own. Such conditions, in theory, prevent virgins and married women from donating eggs. Once the egg has been donated, it is fertilized with the husband's sperm, outside the womb, and the embryo is planted inside the infertile wife's uterus. Khamenei's (1999: 282) *fatwa* on egg donation states that "both the egg donor and the infertile mother must abide by the religious codes regarding parenting. Thus, the child of the egg donor has the right to inherit from her, since the infertile woman who received the eggs is considered to be like an adoptive mother." In the case of sperm donation, the child takes the name of the sperm "owner" (the infertile father) rather than the sperm donor. However, as with egg donation, the child inherits from his biological father, the sperm donor, as the infertile father is considered to be like an adoptive father. These rulings, however, are not always followed in practice. In addition to the Supreme Leader's written questions and answers (*esteftaat*) and *fatwas*, special permission on specific issues can be obtained by telephone consultation, but these are not made public.[4] However, such endorsements, especially sperm donation from unknown men, have been met with the strong disapproval of some senior clerics, and in the case of the husband's infertility, the couple usually resorts to two options. In the first, the couple receives an embryo from another married couple, and this embryo will be planted inside the wife's uterus. The second option is for the wife to divorce her husband and wait for three-and-a-half months (*edeh*), to ensure she is not pregnant. She then nominally marries the sperm donor for a day, receives his sperm, which is fertilized with her egg, outside the womb, and planted in her uterus. She then remarries her own husband. Temporary marriage for women is rare despite some known examples. The director of one of the fertility clinics in Yazd, who is a pioneer in this field, mentioned that temporary marriage for infertile women has never happened in the city, which is labeled as the most conservative in Iran.

Initially, the ethical, moral, and legal problems that emerged from the practice of temporary marriage as a means of legitimizing third-party donation were not anticipated. All three of the parties engaged in gamete donation—the practitioners, the donors, and the recipients—are frequently faced with new situations, and in the absence of clear religious instructions resolve them as best they can. The examples observed so far indicate that the balance of relationship in the majority of cases leaves women worse off regardless of whether they are the donors or recipients. For example, a considerable number of women donors who had sold their eggs through temporary marriage found it impossible to detach from the child and doggedly pursued the recipient families. In one case, the donor so persistently harassed the couple that they allowed her to live with them. They used her for a second egg donation and when faced with the doctor's puzzled expression said, "She is not leaving us alone, [so] we may as well use her to have a second child." In a reverse case, an infertile woman arranged for her husband and the donor to temporarily marry from a remote village. The donor became so attached to the child that in order to stay close to him, she became totally subservient to the couple, who ruthlessly exploited her. In some cases, men who had temporarily married the egg donor decided to extend the duration of the marriage and keep the donor as a second wife. Occasionally, the infertile husbands of wives receiving sperm from temporary husbands experienced serious psychological problems after the children were a few years old, developing hatred for and rejecting these children.[5]

Practitioners, Ethics, and *Sharia*

In theory, the issue of third-party donation of sperm and egg seems to have been resolved officially through the supreme leader's *fatwas* and questions and answers despite strong objections by some senior leading clerics. However, research reveals a more complex and complicated picture that shows discrepancies between the religious rulings and actual practice, as well as the ease with which *fatwas* become instrumental in the hands of medical practitioners and donors and recipients to suit their purposes. Although Ayatollah Khamenei has given clear instructions on parenting, lineage, and inheritance (namely, that a child belongs to his biological parents and should inherit from them), whether the identity of donors and recipients is kept confidential depends entirely on the clinic and its practices, and the lines between "confidentiality" and "anonymity" depend on each clinic's interpretation. Some clinics require donors and recipients to sign forms agreeing not to ask for each other's identity or pursue one another in the future. Other clinics allow donors and recipients to decide whether they wish to remain anonymous, and in such cases the clinics and recipients encounter myriad ethical and legal problems. For example, some infertile couples use their close relatives as donors, a practice often leading to unforeseen situations and conflicts, which the clinics must resolve. As the head of a specialized embryology team at a fertility clinic mentioned, "In the past most of our donors were relatives of the recipients, and this created conflicts and tensions, but now the donors are anonymous, and we have no further problems." In some clinics, the matching of donors and recipients is carried out entirely by a medical expert, and the recipients have no say in the choice of donor. In such cases, records of the donors are buried so well that it is almost impossible for the recipients or the future children to find them.

The question of anonymous donation remains problematic globally. In the United Kingdom, gamete donation had been anonymous since its initiation, but the law was reversed (in 2005), making it compulsory for donors to give their names. This has led to a decline in the number of sperm donors. In Iran, the leading clinics' increasing tendency to move toward anonymous donation goes against the very rules that are the basis for gamete donation, namely, that donation is only allowed within the marital union. Temporary marriage, which was initially used as the key to third-party donation, becomes a façade. Temporary marriage's unique feature is that it is based on a direct agreement between a man and a woman, and the application of total anonymity is in defiance of this basic rule. Furthermore, legislators and medical practitioners, in the absence of clear, detailed instructions, are faced with the dilemma of how to protect the child's identity and rights to his biological lineage and inheritance while keeping the donor's anonymity in order to prevent serious future ethical and legal problems.

Motivations behind Gamete Donation

In Iran, the application of ARTs has predominantly been determined by deeply rooted cultural values and notions of maintaining one's lineage. Whenever possible, the recipients select close members of their families as donors. In doing so, they do not commit incest or adultery. Modern technologies for the treatment of infertility seem to remove some of the barriers of *mahram* and *na-mahram* and *halal* (what is permitted) and *haram*, which normally apply to fertile couples. The strong desire to reproduce and ensure the continuity of the lineage becomes the driving force behind the decisions of infertile couples.

The solutions carry an inherent contradiction with Islamic rules of incest but ironically conform with Ayatollah Khamenei's rulings that as long as touch and gaze are not involved, donation by a third party is allowed. Often, donors are brothers or sisters of the infertile wife or husband. Although having intercourse with or marrying one's brother-in-law or sister-in-law is forbidden and considered incest (*zena*) in Islam, these rules do not apply to infertility treatment. When a woman donates an egg to her sister, there is no hint of sexual union between the donor and her sister's husband. Likewise, men call on their brothers for sperm donation. In one clinic, I came across a man who made a deal with his doctor to use his own brother's sperm without his wife's knowledge. In this way, he killed two birds with one stone, namely, no one would discover he was the infertile party, and the continuity of his lineage was ensured. Although a man can receive his wife's sister's egg and a woman can receive her husband's brother's sperm, only siblings of the same sex donate gametes to spouses. No known donation has taken place between a brother and his sister's husband, or parents and children.

Likewise, rules requiring that egg donors should be widows or divorcees who have been proven fertile by having children of their own have been bent to suit the recipients. Most patients may disregard these rules by resorting to family members they know and trust regardless of their marital status but who also have children of their own. As long as these relatives meet age and health requirements, all concerned parties accept them as donors. In one case, an infertile woman brought her husband's brother's wife for donation, insisting on her eggs "because she has three lovely children, and I want her to donate her egg. Besides, her husband is my husband's brother, and it will all be within the family." The doctors tried to draw her attention to the possibility that their children may fall in love with one other and wish to marry. Although marriage between cousins is desirable, in this case a half-brother and half-sister would be marrying. However, the doctors' concerns fell on deaf ears, as the possibility was in the remote future whereas the need to have a child was immediate. In the case of donations between the kin group, especially between two brothers or two sisters, temporary marriage is not performed, and donation does not involve any ceremonies to legitimize it. As confusing as it may sound, marrying one's wife's sister or husband's brother would be considered incest. As Simpson (2004: 44) puts it, "beyond the paradigm of Euro-American kinship, however, 'contestations' over what can be brought together in the name of procreation invoke different ideas of kinship; different ways that is, of understanding how persons see themselves as connected by substances to one another, to their past and to their future." Donation of gametes between relatives, especially siblings, merits a separate study.

Following the importance of kinship, the fertility of the couple is still seen as a matter for the larger kin group and even the community. In this sense, close relatives remain actively involved in the treatment of their kin group and in the fertility decisions they make. For example, much to the dismay of a psychologist from one of the clinics, some clinics do not allow the wife and husband to attend the initial consultation session together. In several such cases, the husband's mother or another senior woman from his family insists on being present. The husband's family is often suspicious of how his wife will be impregnated and fears undesirable practices by the clinic. They also want to find out whether the daughter-in-law is the infertile party, as male infertility is still a stigma. In other cases, older brothers interfere in the reproductive decisions of their brothers and their wives, arguing with the doctors to persuade them to yield to the wishes of the couple, even if these are against clinic rules. Fertility, in general, remains a matter for the extended family and entitles the other members, especially those from the husband's side, to be drawn in for consultation and action. However, the fact that the larger kin group feels it their duty to get involved in the reproductive lives of their relatives does not mean that infertile couples necessarily make their problems known to their kin groups. The stigma of infertility remains so strong that some infertile couples seek treatment secretly and therefore must resort to unknown donors. Some of the people I interviewed in Tehran were from the provinces and had not told their relatives they were receiving treatment in Tehran. When their babies were born, they said they had been given some blessed meat from the Holy City of Mecca. Others said they had sought the help of holy men and healers.

Those who resort to using their own relatives for donation obviously come from a similar social and cultural background. The relationship between the two parties is initially friendly, with the financial, legal, and kinship disagreements usually emerging later. The ensuing difficulties between relatives have led to such complicated and confusing situations that most clinics have dissociated themselves from the religious and legal aspects by asking the patients to clarify these aspects with their own *mojtahid* (a senior cleric) before coming for treatment. *Mojtahids* themselves are not unanimous, as each follows one of the senior ayatollahs, who are sources of emulation (*maraje-e taqlid*) and may differ in their views. If one *mojtahid* does not approve of the treatment, patients may sometimes go to one who is more flexible.

Those infertile couples without a donor of their own may resign themselves to the rules of the clinic and allow the practitioners to choose a donor for them without inquiring too deeply about the technical details of the treatment. For example, genetic tests are not always carried out in some clinics, but the recipients are not aware of such basic steps and do not raise any questions.[6] The majority of donors not related to the infertile couple come from more modest social layers of society and often have low levels of education. Their main incentive remains financial, and they have little interest in questioning the technical aspects of infertility treatment. The combination of the recipients' strong desire to have children and donors' equally strong financial needs allow considerable scope for medical practitioners to take charge, shifting the power of decision making and control from the patients to the clinics.

However, recipients' and donors' lack of knowledge does not imply a lack of agency on their parts. Whenever possible, they try to shape procedures. During an interview with a clinic director, his mobile rang. A woman whose egg was going to be fertilized with her husband's sperm told him that her husband's sperm was going to be washed, and she asked if he could put in a good word so that the technicians would wash it properly.[7] Even though he replied that the washing process was the same for everyone and there was no need for a special recommendation, she insisted, "All the same, please make sure of it." It was clear she had not realized the meaning of washing in this context but wanted to use her friendship with him for a "special favor."

To improve the knowledge of both donors and recipients, a few private clinics have taken the initiative to educate donors and recipients. Medical practitioners refer to such education as "creating a culture" (*farhang sazi*) of infertility treatment. These clinics' waiting rooms have giant television screens transmitting the fertilization of the egg.[8] With her permission, the woman's name is shown on the screen while the doctor's voice explains the procedure. All present in the waiting room usually watch with no surprise or adverse reaction to the public display of the woman's reproductive organs. In the minds of the audience, the entire operation belongs to the realm of scientific knowledge and medical technology and is not a display of the intimate parts of a woman's body. The screening, therefore, does not invoke any thoughts of the violation of the sexual taboos of *mahram/na-mahram* nor the prohibition of gaze by men. When I asked what the patients think about these direct transmissions, a midwife replied, "We think it is good for them to be informed," and one of the clinic directors joked, "In Islam, it is the outside of the body of a woman which should be covered. Nowhere has it been said that the inside could not be shown." Faced with my astonishment, he continued, "To tell you the truth, we have not even thought about this aspect. Our intention has been to educate people." The lack of patient reaction and the attitude of the medical staff made it clear that for all parties involved there was no connection between religious and sexual taboos and the scientific and technological world of biomedicine.

In general, practitioners are often patronizing to donors and recipients and humiliate them for their "ignorance." One of the senior psychologists in a private clinic said, "We think because we make people fertile, we have a right to treat them like animals." However, in their desperation to have a child, patients remain oblivious to the treatment and humiliations they receive. Patients who believe God has punished them with infertility even see this maltreatment as a chastisement. Medical staff extended a similar reaction to me when I inquired about some of their ethical and cultural practices that breached the boundaries of *mahram*/*na-mahram* and incest by donors and recipients. The doctors took a sarcastic view of these and said, "Surely, as an educated person, you do not believe in all this, which from a scientific point of view is all nonsense."

To return to the motivations behind gamete donation, beyond the cultural bonds, another determining factor is that of emotions, either among relatives or between strangers. Two women are prepared to give and receive eggs without any compensation, either from an emotional bond but also perhaps because they do not necessarily place a high value on their eggs. In a study of egg donations in London clinics, Konrad (1998: 651) mentions that women were prepared to donate their eggs as a gift because they did not view their donation as "providing unique autonomous and individualized genetic material. These women perceived themselves as donating body parts that were without inherent biogenetic properties." In Konrad's (1998) study, one woman told the doctor she did not think the egg was hers and that she did not think of her eggs as eggs. Another woman said, "My eggs were like fingernails or something; they are just a normal part like any other part." My study in clinics in Tehran confirms these findings, as women sometimes told the doctors to "please give some of my eggs to this poor woman, I have too many, and she has none." The doctors would say, "But this is your body, how can you just give your eggs away so easily?" The women simply could not understand what was so precious about their eggs. In Konrad's (1998: 652) words, "the gifts of eggs that women donate are given to help other women conceive, in generalized terms, rather than being thought of as already formed halves of new genetic identities. Donors see themselves as simply furnishing a means for 'starting off' a process that the recipients will 'finish.'" Among the cases I studied in Iran, saving their "poor new friend" the high expense of an egg was also a consideration, and the donors offered their eggs for free.

A third reason to donate a gamete is purely financial. Although gamete donation should be free and given as a gift, considerable financial transactions take place between the donors and recipients. Infertile couples who do not have relatives as donors or do not wish their relatives to find out they are infertile and/or receiving treatment for infertility, which is still a major stigma, have no choice but to purchase gametes. In such cases, a donor can be found among the couples attending the clinics, and negotiations are carried out between the two parties, or the clinics act as the go-between and suggest fees, which are often large sums, calculated as "costs" to be paid to the donors. The sum is effectively the amount of the ongoing price of the gamete, which is exclusive of the clinic's charges. The average sum paid for an egg is around five million rials (approximately US$550). This is equivalent to four months' salary for a schoolteacher.

Embryo Donation

As explained earlier, the legitimization of gamete donation has proved far from perfect in dealing with the inevitable and unforeseeable problems that arise. In the case of embryo donation, when it became clear that *ijtihad* and *fatwas* alone could not justify its practice, a law was passed in August 2003. The law's background is interesting in itself. In 1998, one of the leading infertility clinics organized a symposium titled "Modern Human Reproductive Techniques from the View of Jurisprudence and Law."[9] The religious deliberations made by senior Islamic clerics at this symposium and similar conferences organized by the leading clinics played an important role in presenting a bill to parliament. The ayatollahs' favorable verdicts influenced parliament's decision in approving the bill for embryo donation. As with all laws in Iran, this was sent to the Guardian Council (*Shorayeh Negahban*) for careful scrutiny, and with final approval it became law. The composition of the members of the Guardian Council is noteworthy. Of its twelve members, six are clerics selected by the Supreme Leader, Iran's head of state; the other six are lawyers proposed by the head of the judicial branch (selected in turn by the Supreme Leader) and voted in by the

Iranian legislature. This effectively means that embryo donation was met with the approval of clerics at the highest level, with both legislative and enforcement powers. The law's opening paragraph is paraphrased as:

> The consolidation of the institution of the family, which is the main factor underpinning the social structure, has been one of the most important aims of human beings historically, and any action taken to support the institution of family will lead to its unity and consequently to its equilibrium. One of the most beautiful manifestations of the application of science to reach its spiritual aim is in the field of infertility treatment, including the techniques concerning the donation of embryos to infertile couples.

The law specifies that with the court's permission, clinics are allowed to treat infertile couples by transferring the embryo, which has been fertilized outside the womb, to the infertile couple. To obtain this permission, infertile couples have to prove they are in good health but infertile. They must be of sound mind, be healthy, not have any incurable diseases or addictions, and be nationals of Iran. The law, however, remains unclear in several areas, and due to this lack of clarity, some clinics are reluctant to treat infertile couples in need of embryo donation. For example, although the law specifies that only people of the same religion can donate to each other (Muslims can donate to Muslims and Zoroastrians to Zoroastrians, but donation cannot take place between Zoroastrians and Muslims), it is not clear whether Sunnis can donate to Shia. In addition, in spite of the law clearly stating that embryos should be gifts, some clinics build up the "costs" of the transaction to considerable sums that should be paid by the recipients and given to the donors.

Demand for embryos is so high that it has already created undesirable and illegal practices. One clinic director was alarmed when contacted by a woman who had set up an agency for embryo donation, charging recipients large sums of money. The director found evidence that the embryos sold by the agency did not belong to married couples, as the law specifies they must be; instead, the eggs had come from prostitutes and fertilized by strangers' sperm. An embryo that is the result of the union between a prostitute and a stranger's sperm is effectively an illegitimate child. So far, no law enforcement agency has looked too closely at the implementation of embryo donation. As with sperm and egg donation, the interface between the law/*fatwa*, the medical practice, and infertile couples' choice of donors has not been scrutinized too closely. Another unclear aspect of the law regarding embryo donation is that the donation is a gift, and no money should change hands. Cases abound whereby embryos are traded for money. In one case, a clinic that had developed five embryos from the same donor couple asked the couple for permission to donate the other four embryos to infertile couples. The donor couple became suspicious of the clinic and accused it of trying to make money from their embryos and asked for payment for all five embryos. As it happened, only one of the five embryos survived.

As discussed previously, the existing gaps between the laws and *fatwas* with regard to sperm and egg donation created a confusing situation and blurred the lines between "confidentiality" and "anonymity." This also applies to embryo donation. For example, obtaining a birth certificate is proving to be a major problem, as it is not clear under whose name the birth certificate should be obtained. The real parents are supposed to be the biological parents, but the laws of confidentiality prevent their names from being revealed, and the social or carrier parents are not supposed to apply for birth certificates. Although embryo donation is supposed to be confidential, one clinic director said, "In the present cultural atmosphere it is impossible to protect confidentiality." The only solution, according to that director, is for a code to be devised so the child will be able to locate the biological parents at a later date. A clinic director highlighted another unclear area of the law when she mentioned that she is faced with a serious dilemma when two different infertile couples have received embryos from the same donor, and she does not know whether to let the recipients know their children have siblings. Uncertainties of this kind abound, and, in the absence of clear and detailed guidelines, practitioners are forced to use their own judgment as best they can. These few examples are the tip of the iceberg and are far from being solved, hence some practitioners' reluctance to carry on embryo donation, at least until the law becomes more comprehensive and covers most of the foreseeable eventualities.

Surrogacy

Surrogacy is the most recent ART in Iran, and no specific law endorsing or forbidding it has been decreed as yet. Evidence has emerged that the first cases of surrogacy were carried out after receiving permission from family-court judges, who endorsed surrogacy in the name of the happiness of the family and gave couples permission to proceed by making use of the same law as that for embryo donation. By February 2005, twelve couples had applied for the use of surrogate mothers. Although surrogacy, or a rented mother/womb, could be a financially profitable undertaking, few volunteers have been forthcoming. For infertile couples, the main disincentives have been the absence of a law protecting them from a breach of contract, such as a surrogate not returning the baby, and the high costs involved (around US$3,000). As for potential surrogates, the real problem is a cultural one. At the moment, few women are prepared to act as surrogates. Virgins, unmarried women, and widows would find it very difficult to explain their pregnancies, which would stigmatize them. Surrogacy methods are still relatively unknown in Iran, and no one would believe these women were just surrogates. According to infertility clinic staff, most of the women who become surrogate mothers are relatives or acquaintances of infertile couples. I have not been able to interview those involved in surrogacy.

Although from a legal point of view surrogacy may appear to be a more complex procedure than embryo donation, clinics find it easier. The child's biological parents are known and can apply for a birth certificate in their own names despite the fact that the birth mother usually must apply for the birth certificate. The matter can be solved through court permission. However, surrogacy is still new, and information on its application is sparse.

Moral and Legal Dilemmas

From the brief previous accounts, it is clear that in Iran two powerful sources of authoritative knowledge, religion and biomedicine, determine the practice of ARTs. These two cooperate at times and compete at others. The discrepancies between them provide room for donors and recipients to use their own agency and make their own reproductive decisions. These decisions are often a reflection of cultural priorities, and the way these are negotiated and resolved ultimately shapes the outcome of ARTs. So far, donors and recipients have been able to resort to one or the other sphere of knowledge as necessary and by moving between the two worlds with relative ease to ensure the continuity of their lineage wherever possible. However, this active role is gradually diminishing as the clinics move toward a policy of preventing donors and recipients from meeting and by treating information regarding both parties as confidential. Some of the major leading clinics are now beginning to move toward complete anonymity of the donors.

Although ethical and legal experts at major clinics are still wrestling with the issues, most clinics' main preoccupation remains the biological well-being of their patients and their success rates rather than concerns over the ensuing moral and ethical eventualities. That ARTs create happy families is beyond question, but in a large number of cases this has been accomplished by negotiations between the patients and the practitioners and at times by breaching some of the ethical and legal rules. The doctors at the clinics are open about these shortcomings. According to them, in some of the semi-sponsored clinics, control over the ethical and legal aspects of treatment is left to the clinics, and no law-enforcing body inspects the procedures. For example, in some of the clinics used by less wealthy patients, genetic tests are not routinely carried out before the eggs are transferred. According to a doctor in one of the major public hospitals in Tehran, a veterinary surgeon was allowed to carry out infertility treatments because "he had pulled strings." A counselor at a major clinic cited the example of a couple who, after achieving pregnancy from a different clinic, came to the clinic where she works. After the examination, it became clear there was no way this couple could have had a baby, and "God alone knows how this woman [had] conceived!" It was obvious the couple had no idea which methods the previous clinic had used to produce positive results.

Conclusion

The flexibility of Shia practices has allowed the adoption and accommodation of ARTs through religious rulings that were the result of senior clerics' lengthy engagement with other religious and secular experts, and through the proper Islamic procedures of independent reasoning. Once the *fatwas* are issued, they become the ultimate source of authoritative knowledge and above questioning from secular legal frameworks. However, these religious edicts remain inadequate in their details, as they cannot predict every eventuality arising with the practice of ARTs but are powerful enough and so all-encompassing that they have succeeded in legitimizing the practice of ARTs in a relatively short time.

In reality, the lack of clarity in religious rulings has left a wide gap in the ethical, moral, and legal aspects of ARTs. The overall protection such approvals provide has inadvertently created a confusing situation for medical practitioners, who face complex situations not covered by religious rules. They therefore make their own rules to suit their priorities, without any apparent breach of religious edicts. Between the spiritual guidance of religion and the scientific knowhow of biomedicine, those utilizing ARTs will try to find solutions that will ensure the continuity of their lineage, which remains their ultimate priority. By trying to accommodate and justify the use of ARTs, the *fatwas* have unintentionally undermined kinship rules as well as social and cultural norms and taboos. The relaxation of third-party donation has led donors and recipients to examine their own understandings of kinship and relatedness. In the process, they often break the very rules underpinning kinship that they are anxious to protect. The duality between the text and practice and the liberty taken by users have led to complex and undesirable situations, which ruling clerics attempt to remedy with additional *fatwas*.

So far, the hiatus created by the shortcomings of the religious rulings has allowed ART users to make their own reproductive choices. However, when these gaps emerge and medical practitioners cooperating closely with the "liberal" religious rulers try to close them, the balance of power shifts in favor of biomedical knowledge as the determining and authoritative source of wisdom as far as ARTs are concerned. In the meantime, after nearly two decades of infertility treatment, it is only now that some of the more acute problems are beginning to surface and the need for a completely new set of ethical and legal rules becomes apparent.

Acknowledgments

This chapter was published originally as "Law, Ethics, and Donor Technologies in Shia Iran." In *Assisting Reproduction, Testing Genes: Global Encounters with New Biotechnologies*, ed. Daphna Birenbaum-Carmeli and Marcia C. Inhorn, 144–163. New York: Berghahn Books (2009).

Notes

1. Although the Iranian government took credit for the decline in population growth, many other factors were also responsible (see Tremayne 2004).
2. The World Health Organization estimates that the rate of infertility worldwide is between 12 and 15 percent. There are no accurate figures for Iran, but according to the Ministry of Health, around 15 percent of Iranian couples are infertile. Obviously, not all of these couples seek treatment from clinics, but an increasing number do so.
3. Through Islamic reasoning and interpretation of the Qur'an, senior clerics can reach new decisions, which are given as *fatwas*. Such edicts have been given since the Islamic Revolution in 1979, on a broad range of issues, including ARTs. The history of *ijtihad* is an interesting one; for more information see, for example, Keddie and Richard (2003), Mottahedeh (1985), and Mir-Hosseini (2000).
4. Personal communication, April 2004.
5. Personal communication from Dr. Fahimeh Ramezani Tehrani at the Reproductive Disruptions Conference, Ann Arbor, Michigan, May 2005.
6. A doctor in one of the clinics in Tehran confidentially told me that no genetic tests are carried out in his clinic and in some other hospitals.
7. Washing sperm is a procedure to separate sperm from semen and select active sperm.
8. I asked one of the clinic technicians for a copy of a transmitted operation, which they did willingly. On scrutinizing it, it occurred to me that this was general Western software that does not show the actual operation being performed on the infertile woman whose name is written on the screen, but a general one used to explain the procedure. However, the patients in the waiting room do not know this.
9. An edited volume of the same name was published as the result of the symposium by the Avicenna Research Institute in 2001.

References

Ebadi, Shirin. 2003. Interview with *Yas-e-No*. 10 October.

Haeri, Shahla. 1989. *Law of Desire: Temporary Marriage in Shi'i Iran*. London: I.B. Tauris.

Hoodfar, Homa. 1995. "Population Policy and Gender Equity in Post-Revolutionary Iran." In *Family, Gender and Population in the Middle East: Policies in Context*, ed. Carla Makhlouf. Cairo: American University Press.

Inhorn, Marcia C. 2003. *Local Babies, Global Science: Gender, Religion, and In Vitro Fertilization in Egypt*. New York: Routledge.

———. 2005. Opening speech. Reproductive Disruptions Conference. Ann Arbor, Michigan. 18 May.

———. 2006. "Local Babies, Global Science: Gender, Religion, and Gamete Donation in Egypt and Lebanon." Gamete and Embryo Donation in Infertility Treatment Conference, Tehran, 2 March. Tehran: Avicenna Research Institute.

Keddie, Nikki, and Yann Richard. 2003. *Modern Iran: Roots and Results of Revolution*. New Haven: Yale University Press.

Khamenei, Ali. 1999. *Ojoubeh Al-Esteftaat*. Questions 1271 to 1277. Tehran: Amir Kabir.

Khatib-Chahidi, Jane. 1981. "Sexual Prohibitions, Shared Space and 'Fictive' Marriages in Shiite Iran." In *Women and Space: Ground Rules and Social Maps*, ed. Shirley Ardener. London: Croom Helm.

Konrad, Monica. 1998. "Ova Donation and Symbols of Substance: Some Variations on the Theme of Sex, Gender and Partible Body." *Journal of the Royal Anthropological Institute* 4(4): 643–664.

Mir-Hosseini, Ziba. 1998. *Marriage on Trial: A Study of Islamic Family Law*. London: I.B. Tauris.

———. 2000. *Islam and Gender: The Religious Debates in Contemporary Iran*. London: I.B. Tauris.

Mottahedeh, Roy. 1985. *The Mantle of the Prophet: Religion and Politics in Iran*. New York: Simon and Schuster.

Simpson, R. 2004. "Localizing a Brave New World: New Reproductive Technologies and the Politics of Fertility in Contemporary Sri Lanka." In *Reproductive Agency, Medicine and the State: Cultural Transformations in Childbearing*, ed. Maya Unnithan-Kumar. New York: Berghahn Books.

Statistical Center of Iran. 1998. *Statistical Yearbook of Iran*. Tehran: SCI Publications.

Tremayne, Soraya. 2004. "'And Never the Twain Shall Meet': Reproductive Health Policies in the Islamic Republic of Iran." In *Reproductive Agency, Medicine and the State: Cultural Transformations in Childbearing*, ed. Maya Unnithan-Kumar, 181–202. New York: Berghahn Books.

Chapter 11

Conceiving IVF in Iran

Introduction

The history of in vitro fertilization (IVF) in Iran has been shaped by the interaction between the pioneers of IVF and an interdisciplinary group of experts, together with the endorsement and strong support of the Shia jurists (*foqaha*), referred to as "jurists" throughout this chapter. As a result, the practice of IVF has been legitimized in all its forms in the country and the alliance between biomedical science and religious ideology has placed Iran at the forefront of Muslim countries in the field of assisted reproductive technologies. As Inhorn (2005) points out, "Iran is definitely in the lead among the Muslim countries in the Middle East in the application of these technologies." Inhorn (2007: 193) later reiterates, "Iran is currently the country to watch, as it has been on the 'cutting edge' of new reproductive technologies."

However, the evolution of IVF in Iran is inextricably linked with the broader and continued interest and involvement of the state in the reproductive life of its citizens. The direct or indirect attempt by the state to control the population, to either increase or decrease its growth, dates back to the nineteenth century under the late Qajar Dynasty (1785–1925), which aimed to encourage the population to grow (Kashani-Sabet 2011). The state's concern continued under the Pahlavi Dynasty (1925–79), which attempted to reduce population growth (Abbasi-Shavazi 2001); and under the Islamic Republic of Iran (1979–present), which has reversed its population policies three times since coming to power (Abbasi-Shavazi 2001; Hoodfar 1995; McDonald et al. 2015; Tremayne 2004). However, the most significant transformations, which have deeply affected the reproductive behavior of Iranians, have taken place under the current Islamic regime, which has put in place one of the most remarkable family planning programs ever recorded, and has induced a sea change among the generation born after the implementation of the population policies, which started in 1986. It is noteworthy that at no point have the state policies resorted to coercive measures and that the success or failure of the policies have depended on the responses of individuals guided by their own cultural values and religious beliefs. Such a strong dependence on cultural norms and religious beliefs, in turn, has justified the direct or indirect involvement of the jurists in the reproductive life of their adherents, regardless of the nature of the regime or the policies.

This chapter argues that, controversial policies notwithstanding, the core values attached to fertility and childbearing have remained paramount in Iranian culture and that the involvement of the jurists has proved crucial in the success or failure of reproductive policies. To this end, the chapter will explore the process by which the pioneers of IVF, and the jurists who sanctioned them, succeeded in making these technologies compliant with the Islamic imperatives of procreation. Data presented in this chapter are based on primary sources and on research carried out by both authors during the past two decades. Contributions from some of Iran's pioneering physicians of IVF are also included.

The Ebbs and Flows of Population Policies

The history of the involvement of the Iranian state with the reproductive life of its citizens dates back to the nineteenth century, when the state linked women's health to the building of a healthy and strong nation. According to US-based Iranian historian Kashani-Sabet (2011), under the Qajar Dynasty, when concerns surrounding the depletion of the population were most strident, the state's pronatalist policies did not resort to formal laws regarding childbirth and its arguments were not solely based on Western concepts. The state's discourse on the importance of mothers' health appealed to Iranians because such themes could be adapted to the more familiar Islamic injunctions regarding parenting and maternity. As the author observes, "the awareness of women's health and infant mortality, which can be situated in the nineteenth century, brings maternalism to the heart of modern Iranian thought, concepts of nationhood, and tasks of a modern government" (Kashani-Sabet

2011: 5). Following the Qajar Dynasty, under the later part of the Pahlavi regime, Iran also underwent a process of reform aimed at the modernization of Iranian society, which included the inception of a government-sponsored family planning program in 1967 to reduce the population growth of 3.1 per annum. Iran's participation in the Third International Population Conference in Bucharest in 1974 strengthened the country's commitment to reducing population growth by linking the issue of population to economic development (Tremayne 2001). Interestingly, amid efforts to bring population growth down, being mindful of the importance of fertility in Iranian culture, a clause was added to the enactment of family protection law (Article 8) in 1974, which gave men and women an additional right to divorce their spouse if he or she proved to be infertile. However, the family planning program under the Pahlavi rule (1967–79) was primarily intended for the urban middle classes and was not as successful as it might have been due to its top-down policies and to a distinct lack of sensitivity toward the persisting positive core values attached to high fertility (Hoodfar 1995; Tremayne 2004).

After the Islamic Revolution in 1979, the regime initially took a pronatalist stance by promoting larger families, closing family planning centers and lowering the age of marriage to nine for girls and to fifteen for boys, in keeping with the Islamic law (*sharia*). The regime also offered maternity benefits, provided incentives for families to have more children and outlawed sterilization and abortion, which is not allowed unconditionally under Iranian law. As a result, in 1986 the country's census showed that the population had grown from 33.7 million to 49.4 million between 1976 and 1986, at an annual growth rate of 3.9 percent (Statistical Center of Iran 1986). These figures caused alarm among the policymakers, who feared that such rapid increase could undermine the development efforts, especially after the eight-year war with Iraq (1980–88), which had thrown the country into social and economic crisis. The government embarked upon a massive reconstruction program, which had the implementation of an effective family planning program as its top priority. Mindful of the importance of reproduction and aware that such a campaign may not be received favorably by the majority of Iranians, a population conference held in 1988 resulted in the adoption of an "Islamic" population program, which, within less than a decade of its implementation, succeeded in bringing down population growth from 3.9 percent per annum in 1986 to around 2.1 by the mid-1990s. By 2012, population growth was

TABLE 11.1. Population Census Results.

Census Year	Population	Average Annual Growth Rate (percent)	Populations Density/km²	Proportion Urban (percent)	Household Size
1956	18,954,704	—	12	31.4	
1966	25,785,210	3.1	16	~37.5	
1976	33,708,744	2.7	20	47	5.02
1986	49,445,010	3.9	30	~54.0	5.11
1996	60,055,488	2	36	~61.0	4.84
2006	70,495,782	1.6	43	68.5	4.03
2011	75,149,669	1.3	46	71.4	3.55

Source: United Nations (2016)

reported at 1.3 percent,[1] a decline to below the replacement level. Fluctuations in population growth in Iran between 1956 and 2011 are presented in Table 11.1.

A notable feature of the family planning campaign was the cooperation between the health policy planners and the jurists without whose endorsement and active support the policies would not have succeeded. In aiming to reduce population growth, the campaign avoided any form of coercion and, to demonstrate that it was not anti-natalist, the campaign included the provision of treatment for infertility as part of its program. The campaign also asked for the cooperation of the people of Iran, which, inter alia, stressed the importance of the reciprocity between the state and the citizen and their mutual responsibilities and obligations. Some of the jurists, in their deliberations on the permissibility of family planning and in resorting to the work of the Islamic scholars, concluded that Islam does not necessarily advocate large families, but encourages better quality of life and health for mothers and babies, which can be achieved by having fewer children (Elgood 1978: 273–274; Hoodfar 1995; Makhlouf-Obermeyer 1991). The policies further argued that it was the duty of the citizens to help the state build a strong, independent (of foreign interference and colonialism), healthy, and well-educated Muslim nation by reducing the size of families, thus linking reproduction to national identity (Hoodfar 1995; Tremayne 2004: 185).

A noticeable outcome of the campaign has been the emergence of uniformity in the childbearing values and behavior among all layers of society, as shown by the findings of a study carried out by the Iranian Center for Research on Asian and Oceanic Population:

> Those couples who have just married and those who have been married for up to three years show no inclination to have any children at all, or perhaps just one. This tendency over the past decade illustrates that for women of urban and rural backgrounds, from different social classes, the poor and the rich, illiterate, and literate, all have a similar attitude to giving birth these days, leading to the rapid downward trend in the Iranian TFR [total fertility rate]. (Tabnak 2013)

Following the drop in population growth to below the replacement level, the authorities have re-introduced some of the pronatalist policies of the early 1980s, as reported by Population Policy: "Iran is dramatically changing its population policy. Iranian President Ahmadinejad announced a new policy to encourage population growth saying that previous family planning was ungodly and a Western import. The new policy will pay families for newly born children and deposit money into their bank accounts through to their eighteenth birthday."[2]

Further measures taken by the state included the dismantling of the family planning program and the re-routing of funds to promote pronatalist policies. Thus far, the generation of reproductive age has ignored the state's plea to have more children and although the authorities blame economic hardship as the cause of the decline in childbearing, other factors, such as the effective family planning of the 1980s and 1990s and a successful literacy campaign, have played a major role in a profound transformation of the country's reproductive practices, which previously valued high fertility (Tremayne 2004). And, when Supreme Religious Leader Ayatollah Khamenei announced publicly that it was "wrong" to continue with the family planning program and that the two-decade-old policy of controlled population growth must end, he was challenging these, by now, deep-seated values in the generation of reproductive age, who had grown up to believe in the advantages of having fewer children. The Supreme Leader admitted that "one of the mistakes we made in the nineties was population control" and stressed the necessity of building a strong nation and that Iran's goals were to reach a population increase from the current 80 million to 150 million by 2050 (Tabnak 2013). Interestingly, the justification for having larger families to form a strong nation is identical to the argument used in the 1980s family planning campaign, advocating smaller families for the purpose of building a stronger nation.

While the family planning program of the 1980s delivered most of its promises, it failed to address infertility, which remained unfulfilled. The sporadic efforts of the Ministry of Health to address infertility proved negligible and more of a symbolic gesture than a genuine commitment. For example, the allocation of a small budget of $10,000 per infertile couple to be sent abroad for treatment, among other similar efforts, proved a drop in the ocean in the face of the magnitude of demand. Other attempts were made by both the public and private sector: for example, in 1985, in the Shariati Hospital (affiliated with the Tehran University of Medical Sciences), which had just been equipped with ultrasound, experts took the first measures to treat infertility. However, no evidence about the practice and its success is available. In 1988, a similar practice was performed in the IVF section of Aban Hospital in Tehran. However, the relevant documents about the results are not available. Therefore, in the absence of local modern medical facilities and faced with persistent pressure from family, kin, and society to reproduce, infertile couples continued to resort to traditional options such as treatment from local healers, polygyny, or informally adopting children from among family members. Although adoption has been allowed and practiced in Iran since the 1960s, it has not been considered as a genuine substitute for having one's own biological children. While the stigma of infertility may be widespread throughout the world (Inhorn and Van Balen 2002), it varies in degree and having children remains an imperative in the Middle Eastern cultures, where biological relatedness remains the only acceptable form of procreation. Procreation, for the purpose of perpetuation of family and kinship, which are fundamental, sacrosanct institutions, acting as the guiding principle of social organization, has been paramount in Iranian culture. Traditionally, voluntary childlessness has not been an option and failing to reproduce has been a stigma and considered not only detrimental to family and kin group, but also a threat to the stability of society. Even though in the past few decades, modern medical technologies have created a new understanding of the causes of infertility and have raised the hopes of infertile couples that conception is possible, and in spite of family size having shrunk considerably, the deeply rooted values attached to viewing infertility as shameful and as a "failure" have not been dislodged accordingly. While choosing not to reproduce is frowned upon, the inability to reproduce is regarded as a damnation for which the infertile individual pays a heavy price (Inhorn and Tremayne 2012: 1–21).

The History of IVF

IVF was introduced to Iran against the backdrop of the family planning program of the 1980s. At its inception, the physicians, who were mindful of the Islamic beliefs, which consider procreation to be within divine power only, sought the opinion of the jurists, the majority of whom approved of the practice of IVF on the condition that it remained limited to married heterosexual couples, as conception outside marriage in Islamic law (*sharia*) is equivalent to adultery and the resulting child is considered illegitimate or a bastard (*valad-e zena*). At this juncture, debates on IVF for married couples did not lead to strong controversial arguments among the jurists, but it was the introduction of third-party gamete donation which led to a more profound exploration of the permissibility of these state-of-the-art technologies and their implications for the entrenched beliefs surrounding reproduction. The use of a third party to procreate seemed discordant with the prohibition by Islamic law of conception outside marriage, as mentioned earlier, and with the position that the only acceptable form of reproduction is through heterosexual marital union, resulting in one's own biological children (Inhorn 2006b; Inhorn and Tremayne 2012). Conception through third-party donation therefore proved problematic as it obstructed the possibility of using reproductive technologies to help infertile couples conceive with a stranger's gamete. The jurists, therefore, needed to find valid arguments to justify the legitimacy of third-party donation, which could be a potential threat for the purity of lineage and yet allowed the continuity of the family line. However, although some solutions were eventually found, the deliberations did not lead to a unanimous verdict and, to date, the opinions of jurists remain divided on this issue, as discussed below (see section on legitimization of IVF, below).

The Application of IVF

The first definite step taken toward the application of IVF begins with a congress held on obstetrics in 1987, which was hosted by Iran's University of Medical Sciences (IUMS) in cooperation with the Iranian Center for Education, Culture, and Research (ACECR). At the congress' invitation, Professor Safaa Al-Hassani, one of the leading IVF experts in Germany, introduced IVF technology to the congress. Professor Al-Hassani's crucial role in introducing and training local physicians in IVF, and in setting up infertility clinics, won him the title of "the leader of IVF" in Iran. Simultaneously, attempts were made by ACECR to establish infertility clinics in Tehran. Subsequently, Dr. Aflatounian, director of the hospital housed in Shahid Sadughi University of Yazd (central Iran), invited Professor Al-Hasani to help establish the first IVF clinic in the city. The location of Yazd itself is indicative as the city epitomizes the interface between tradition and modernity. In the 1980s Yazd was officially classified as the most conservative city in the country on the basis of its lowest rate of divorce. A comparative study of four Iranian provinces, Gilan, Sistan and Baluchestan, Western Azerbaijan, and Yazd, showed that Yazd had retained most of its traditional and religious characteristics, in spite of its highest levels of socioeconomic development in the country, and a relatively high level of female literacy at around 80 percent (where literacy rate refers to the percentage of people with the ability to read and write; Abbasi-Shavazi, McDonald, and Hosseini-Chavoshi 2003). The study showed that women in Yazd placed more emphasis on education as a means of enhancing marriage and that the rate of early marriages was higher in Yazd than in any of the other four provinces (Abbasi-Shavazi, McDonald, and Hosseini-Chavoshi 2003; Tremayne 2006). The findings implicitly confirmed the persisting importance of reproduction above all other institutions, regardless of the degree of social and economic development.

The development of IVF technologies in Yazd led to the training of the first group of Iranian physicians, who were sent to Germany to train under Professor Al-Hasani, and the opening of the first IVF clinic in the city's Afshar Hospital, where the first IVF baby was born in 1990. However, prior to the above, the first successful pregnancy through IVF took place in Tehran, in Aban Hospital in 1989, which resulted in a miscarriage in the second month of pregnancy. In late 1989 the second attempt of IVF by Aban Hospital resulted in pregnancy, but the six-months-pregnant woman died in a car crash. The first IVF babies, a set of twins, were born in Tehran, on 27 December 1991, in Aban Hospital. All the IVF treatment of the patients and the Caesarean section, carried out at Aban Hospital, were performed by Dr. Mohajeri, Dr. Aboutaleb Saremi, and Dr. Jalil Pakravesh.[3] The second IVF baby to be born in Tehran was born on 23 July 1993 at the Royan Institute.

To return to the consequence of the Afshar Hospital's success, mentioned earlier, the spread of the news and the subsequent overwhelming response by infertile couples, who swarmed to Yazd from all over the country, revealed the tip of the iceberg as far as demand for infertility treatment was concerned and led to the training of further groups of physicians in Germany and Denmark. The first clinic to open in Tehran, in 1991, was the Royan Institute, where the first IVF baby was born in 1993. The first infertility treatment section established in Tehran was at Aban Hospital in 1987, followed by the Research and Clinical Center for Infertility at the Shahid Sadughi University of Medical Sciences, established in 1989 in Yazd. Currently sixty-one infertility clinics (twenty-four public and thirty-seven private) operate in the capital, Tehran, as well as in some major cities such as Isfahan, Shiraz, Tabriz, and Mashhad. The majority of the public clinics are housed within the public hospitals and work under the supervision of university medical departments. Two of these establishments merit a brief mention as pioneers of assisted reproductive technologies in Iran and because of their continuing role in introducing the most recent developments and familiarizing the public with them. The Royan Institute and the Avicenna Research Institute, which are both affiliated to ACECR, have remained the leaders and most influential institutes in the field of reproductive technologies in Iran. As mentioned above, the Royan Institute was the first infertility clinic established in Tehran (1991) where the first IVF baby was born (1993) in the city. Today, this institute is not only one of the most popular infertility clinics in Tehran, it is also well known internationally by specialists and academics in the field of bioreproductive technologies for its Annual International Congress on Reproductive Biomedicine, which it has held successfully for almost sixteen years. The Avicenna Research Institute was established by one of the founding members of the Royan Institute, Dr. Mohammad Mehdi Akhondi, who, mindful of the distinct absence of coordination and development of existing expertise and facilities, founded the Avicenna Research Institute in 1998. The objectives of the Institute, the first of its kind, are education, research, and treatment, all of which are channeled through its research groups on reproductive genetics, reproductive immunology, reproductive infection, embryology, and bioethics and law. However, currently most of these services are offered by the private clinics only and at relatively high cost. Even the public clinics, operating as small units within public hospitals, are not free and the patients have to meet treatment costs. Amid the expansion of infertility clinics, the state's occasional interest in infertility has stemmed from its focus on nation-building rather than the actual treatment of infertility. For example, to reward war heroes who had suffered spinal injuries, and become infertile as a result, during the Iran–Iraq War, the government allocated a special infertility unit to treat them. Interestingly, even this clinic was not completely free and the war veterans themselves had to meet a portion of the cost based on the extent of the injuries they had suffered. Nevertheless, the state's lack of interest in infertility treatment did not discourage Iranian physicians from introducing the latest IVF technologies, as they developed elsewhere, as is shown in the following chronology:

1992 – Birth of the first baby following retrograde ejaculation using intrauterine insemination (IUI) first started in 1989 in Aban Hospital by Dr. Jalil Pakravesh.[4]
1994 – Birth of the first baby resulting from intracytoplasmic sperm injection (ICSI) and the birth of the first baby through egg donation carried out in Yazd by Dr. Mohmmad-Hossein Amir Arjomand.[5]
1996/97 – Use of ICSI+ percutaneous epididymal sperm aspiration (PESA) resulting in the birth of a baby at Shariati Hospital, Tehran, carried out by Dr. Hojat-Allah Saeedi.[6]
1998 – First case of transferring an embryo produced from testicular spermatozoon by microinjection carried out by Dr. Akhondi.[7]
2004 – Birth of the first baby born following pre-implantation genetic diagnosis (PGD) at Royan Institute, Tehran, carried out by Dr. Leila Karimian.[8]

Indeed, the use of IVF in a range of contexts, such as PGD (as a preventive measure for diseases with a genetic basis or for sex selection); sperm, egg, and embryo donation; surrogacy; fertility preservation; and animal conservation (freezing of egg, sperm, and embryo), is commonplace in Iran.

In the section "The Ebbs and Flows of Population Policies" above, it is stated that the expansion of IVF clinics took place during the family planning campaign of 1986–96. In line with the policies of the campaign, the Ministry of Health focused on population reduction and infertility remained low on its list of priorities and was classified as cosmetic surgery. As a result, infertility did not qualify for coverage by any of the approved health insurance schemes. Furthermore, the extent of infertility itself remained unknown until a survey carried out by Avicenna Research Institute, which studied 17,000 households, showed that the prevalence of infertility among married couples in the general population was 20.2 percent (19.9 percent in urban areas and 22 percent in rural areas) (Akhondi et al. 2013). These facts gradually began to focus the attention of the health planners and through active campaigning by the physicians and the recent pronatalist policies, the Ministry of

Health has shown a more serious commitment to infertility treatment. For example, it has encouraged insurance companies to cover the expenses of medical and diagnostic tests and to meet the cost of the medication for the treatment. The Ministry also plans to increase the number of infertility clinics in the public sector. Finally, the lack of the state's interest in infertility treatment has led to an improvement and expansion of IVF centers in the private sector, and through increased competition, to an equilibrium in the charges made by the clinics.

Legitimization of IVF, Lineage Recast

Unlike most secular countries, where the responsibility for the legitimization of biotechnologies, including assisted reproductive technologies, is the responsibility of a secular committee of experts and the parliament, in Iran their legitimization has fallen on the Islamic jurists (*foqaha*, sing. *faqih*), as was mentioned earlier. In doing so, the jurists engaged with the medical practitioners to better understand the broader ethical implications of assisted reproductive technologies for lineage, family, and kinship, which Ebrahim Moosa (2003), cited in Inhorn and Tremayne (2012: 3), explains as follows:

> In terms of ethics, Muslim authorities consider the transmission of reproductive material between persons who are not legally married to be a major violation of Islamic law. This sensitivity stems from the fact that Islamic law has a strict taboo on sexual relations outside wedlock (*zena*). The taboo is designed to protect paternity (i.e. family), which is designated as one of the five goals of Islamic law, the others being the protection of religion, life, property and reason.

In elaborating further on the bioethics concerning assisted reproductive technologies, Richard Tappan (2012: 103), a scholar on Islamic ethics, theology, and law, demonstrates that, in seeking justification and legitimization for the use of bioethics, "clinicians and bioethics consultation groups consider a range of justificatory sources, including civil laws, *fatwas* (edicts), reason, and bioethical cases from the West" to come to a decision. Morgan Clarke (2009, 2012), a social anthropologist specializing in Islamic bioethics and contemporary Islamic legal discourse and authority, also argues that to understand bioethics in the Muslim Middle Eastern context more fully, a broader approach is required beyond the sole focus on religion.

It was, therefore, being mindful of the need to address the full implications of reproductive technologies, that on the introduction of IVF, the jurists, the medical practitioners, and the ethicists and others from related disciplines engaged in an extensive examination of the congruence of these technologies with the rules attached to Islamic ideas of procreation. To this end, the jurists, who are the sources of emulation (*maraje-e taqlid*) of the Shia followers, resorted to the interpretation of the Islamic sources (*ijtihad*) and issued their religious edicts on the permissibility of IVF technologies and, more specifically, on third-party donation. However, these rulings differed from each other, and at times were contradictory, but all remained equally valid and left to the followers to choose those edicts, which suited them best. As Tappan (2012: 105) explains, "there is a religious duty incumbent upon each Shia believer to follow the rulings of one high-ranking [source of emulation]. This leads to a plurality of equally authoritative religious rulings, which might differ greatly from one another, and may vary from the state law as well." The diversity of opinions, especially on the question of third-party donation, persists to date and has opened up a gap, which allows room for maneuvering by both the medical practitioners and by the infertile to make choices on the most suitable use of assisted reproductive technologies as befits them (Tremayne 2009).

In general, the edicts of these sources of emulation fall into three groups: (i) those which forbid the use of IVF in any form, especially third-party donation, which is viewed as the intrusion of a third person into the marriage, and as such is forbidden (*haram*) and which also leads to confusion in the purity of the lineage (for example the late Ayatollah al-Ozma Madani Tabrizi 2009); (ii) those opinions which are favorable toward the use of some assisted reproductive technologies based on "conditional permission" and depending on the circumstances (Khomeini 2001); and (iii) the edicts that permit the application of assisted reproductive technologies in all their forms (Yazdi 1996). In the latter set of opinions, assisted reproductive technologies are interpreted as a means of mediating between God and his subjects to allow procreation and not as interfering in God's design. These proponents argue that conception in a petri dish bypasses any suggestion of an intrusion by a stranger and that this form of conception plays an instrumental role in resolving some of the theological concerns that would otherwise arise from third-party donation. These concerns include the possibility of the parties involved in IVF—the practitioners, the donors, and the recipient of gametes, most of whom are strangers to each other—coming into bodily contact with each other; and the ensuing implications, for adultery and incest, according to the Islamic law. The proponents favoring IVF also ruled that one of the distinguishing features of the Shia branch of Islam is its openness toward science and technology, and a lack of automatic objection to innovation. Effectively, the engagement between the medical experts and the jurists resulted in a better understanding, by the latter, of the ethical dimensions of IVF practice and led to them concluding that IVF belonged to the domain of science and was not a matter for ethical-theological considerations (see also Tappan 2012). Thus, concerns about the "manipulation of nature" or trying to "play God," through procreation by IVF, were alleviated by the argument in favor of IVF practices in Shia Iran, unlike among the Sunni Muslims or in Catholicism (Eslami 2007; Inhorn, Patrizio, and Serour 2012).

In order to legitimize third-party gamete donation, some of the jurists put various solutions forward. One such suggestion was that of temporary marriage (Haeri 1989), a uniquely Shia practice, which is similar to permanent marriage but has a time limit agreed between the two parties and can be between one hour and ninety-nine years (Tremayne 2009). This would allow the infertile party to receive gametes from the donor, who would be the temporary spouse and therefore a legitimate donor. The gametes would then be fertilized on a petri dish, but without any bodily contact taking place between the two parties. Other Islamist jurists allowed donation on the condition that no form of bodily contact, such as "touch" or "gaze," should take place between the recipient of the gamete and the practitioner of the opposite sex, as these could potentially be the instigators of forbidden (*haram*) relations between the two parties, who are not married to each other and therefore prohibited from coming into close contact (Khamenei 1999; Sistani 1999).

The fundamental premise upon which all the jurists, regardless of their stance, based their edicts has been the implications of third-party donation for lineage and inheritance, the latter being automatically linked to lineage in the Islamic law (*sharia*). Although a fuller explanation of lineage and inheritance are beyond the remit of this chapter, a brief clarification may help illustrate the connection between the two and the complexities involved in determining the hitherto unresolved issues of inheritance in cases of third-party donation. Lineage (*nasab*) as defined by Coulson (1971: 22), cited in Mir-Hosseini (2000: 134), is described as follows:

> Sharia legal notions of kinship and filiation are encapsulated in the concept of *nasab* (lineage), which translates not only as parentage and kinship, but also as filiation and descent status. While the child takes its *nasab* from both sides, it is the paternal side which has ascendancy over the maternal. In all schools of Islamic law the primary significance of *nasab* is that of paternity, closely tied to legitimacy, through which a child acquires its legal identity and its religion.

Under such notions, the child belongs to his father's lineage, which extends beyond the father and includes the paternal grandfather, who also has equal rights over the child. In the absence of the father or grandfather, the rights go to the paternal uncles (Ebadi 2003; Mir-Hosseini 2000). Such rights are reciprocal, and the child can also claim his rights from his biological father and grandfather. Lineage, therefore, consists of a complex web of relatedness, involving duties and obligations, which cannot be described or understood in simple terms. In addition, under the Islamic law, inheritance rights are exclusively linked to biological relatedness and to marriage as between the wife and the husband, except for the one-third of the heritage on which there is a right (for the deceased) to bequeath (to make a will). It is therefore understandable that, on the introduction of third-party gamete donation, the Islamist jurists' main concern was the implications of such technologies for lineage and inheritance. An example of the deliberations on these issues can be found in a publication by the Avicenna Research Institute (2001), which was the outcome of a conference bringing a number of leading religious and legal experts together to examine the consequences of these technologies, above all, on lineage and inheritance. The clear proof of the persistence of the exclusivity of the right of blood relatives to inheritance is seen in the case of adopted children. Although adoption has been allowed in Iran for several decades now, the adopted child does not have an automatic right to inherit from his adoptive parents.

Following on from the paramount importance of biological relatedness, those jurists opposed to IVF ruled out recognition of a child conceived through third-party donation as legitimate. In their opinion, biological relatedness is the only acceptable form of procreation. The jurists in favor of IVF, on the other hand, took a different route by redefining relatedness. According to this definition, the parent, in agreeing to donate his/her gamete, transfers the parental rights to the adoptive parent and forgoes any claim on the resulting child (Sanei 1998). In the process, a new representation of relatedness has emerged, replacing the biological link as the basis of relatedness with that of permission/consent on the part of the parent. For the opponents of third-party donation such justification of parentage is equal to a challenge to the foundation of lineage, family, and kinship, as explained earlier.

The question of mutual rights between biological parents and children and inheritance remains unresolved to date based on the absence of any laws and due to a number of controversial rulings. For example, several of the favorable edicts, in defining the status of the child, have ruled that the child belongs to its biological parent and inherits from him/her, but takes its name from the "adoptive" parent (Sanei 1998). This would have been in line with the rules defining lineage and right to inheritance. But, at the same time, the required rules of confidentiality often lead to the anonymity of the parent and thereby make it impossible for the child to know the identity of the parents, and therefore have the possibility of inheriting from them (Gooshki and Allahbedashti 2015). In addition, amid these controversies, medical practitioners face a number of other emerging ethical and legal questions, which they either resolve by further consultation with the jurists, or as best they can, using their own judgment and in consultation with their colleagues. These issues include the permissibility of financial transactions between the recipients and donors of gametes (considering that donation is supposed to be a gift), the use of supernumerary embryos, sex selection, and fertility preservation.

The Medicalization of Infertility

As discussed above, with the arrival of each new reproductive technology, medical practitioners engaged in a dialogue with the jurists to inform them on the scientific aspects of IVF practices. Some of the medical pioneers, for example the Avicenna Research Institute, also took the initiative to educate the public by organizing conferences, carrying out research, making films, and appearing in the media and by extensive publication of informative booklets for their patients to explain the medical causes of infertility. The publicizing of infertility proved so effective that, as I observed, infertile women were seen on the television speaking openly about their infertility and its treatment through IVF. Men, however, remained more reluctant to do so, as male infertility remains a more serious stigma to date, as does the open admittance of sperm donation, which by and large is frowned upon by the conservative layers in society (Abbasi-Shavazi et al. 2008; Tremayne 2012). Consequently, the fervent debates and the diversity of opinions engaging the jurists with experts in medical, legal, ethical, and psychological disciplines resulted in the question of infertility, which is one of the most intimate and stigmatized aspects of life, coming to the public forum and being discussed openly, a process which resulted in the medicalization of infertility, but in the public arena only. In private, the anonymity of treatment through assisted reproductive technologies paved the way for infertile couples to conceal their infertility fully even from the nearest members of their kin group, leading to stigmatizing infertility further, but at the same time reducing the pressure to conceive by the kin group.

The medical practitioners, in their enthusiasm to promote the use of the emerging reproductive technologies, continued to play an active role by opening up debates on the use of those technologies, which could not be justified solely by religious edicts, and thus smooth the path for their legitimization. For example, on the introduction of embryo donation in Iran, as no amount of religious interpretation could justify its practice, the Avicenna Research Institute took the lead by organizing a conference which proved instrumental in the presentation of a bill to parliament and the passing of a law in 2004 related to embryo donation to infertile couples. Likewise, it was through the initiative of the same research institute that the agenda for the recognition of infertility as a disability came to the public arena and led to the provision of insurance for infertility treatment. With the introduction of surrogacy, questions similar to those surrounding third-party gamete donation were raised, and surrogacy was allowed on the basis of the same edicts issued for third-party donation. Stem cell research received a favorable *fatwa* (Hosseini 2015; Makarem Shirazi 2015), as did sex selection, but only on the condition that its use is restricted to the avoidance of sex-linked medical conditions rather than for choosing the sex of the child or discriminating against a particular sex (Akhondi and Rasekh 2011a, 2011b). Currently, research is taking place on mitochondrial gene therapy and its application. Effectively, to date, all the reproductive technologies have been legitimized but these approvals apply to married heterosexual couples only and no single or homosexual individual qualifies for treatment (Law on Embryo Donation to Infertile Couples, Act 1). In addition, the concerns of some individuals, that by resorting to IVF they may be breaching the cultural and religious taboos and committing a sin, have been alleviated through the favorable religious edicts.

Discussion and Conclusion

From what precedes, it is clear that since the nineteenth century the Iranian state's interest in the reproductive life of its citizens has been shaped by its broader ambition of nation-building, rather than out of a concern for the well-being of the population. Central to the success or failure of state policies has been the direct or indirect involvement of the jurists in matters concerning the reproductive life of the citizens. Under the Qajar Dynasty, pronatalist debates, advocating the necessity of building a healthy nation, were received favorably as they coincided with the prevailing religious and cultural values attached to reproduction. Under the Pahlavi regime, the policies to reduce population growth failed to gain popularity at the grassroots level as they were aimed predominantly at the urban middle classes and also conflicted with the norms and values favoring high fertility and had no support from the religious leaders. However, the same anti-natalist policies proved effective under the Islamic Republic's regime, which supported them and had as one of its core arguments the benefits of a smaller nation as key to the state's security and prosperity. Likewise, the active engagement of the jurists with IVF technologies has been crucial in their legitimization. One of the unintended outcomes of the complex process through which assisted reproductive technologies has been legitimized and practiced has been the fact that Iran has gained a distinctive position in assisted reproductive technologies among many countries in the world. On the one hand, Iran, which is an Islamic state following the Islamic law (*sharia*), limits procreation to heterosexual married couples. In this sense, it differs from those countries where third-party donation is available to married and unmarried couples, single parents, and non-heterosexuals. On the other hand, Iran differs even further from other Muslim countries, where the majority of Muslims are Sunni and do not allow third-party donation in any form (Inhorn 2006a).

However, the determination by the jurists to legitimize the practice of assisted reproductive technologies has resulted in a broadening and redefinition of lineage, from that of an inexorable blood link between the parent and the child, to include relatedness via the transfer of parental rights from the biological parent to the social/adoptive parent. Such re-casting remains controversial to date, not only among the jurists, but for some of the infertile users of assisted reproductive technologies too.

A further outcome of assisted reproductive technologies has been a shift in the public perception of infertility, from the realm of a predetermined affliction to the domain of the medical sciences as a treatable condition. Such a move has proved to be a double-edged sword as, on the one hand, the medicalization of infertility has helped normalize it and diminish its stigma in the public arena, while on the other hand, the privacy offered by IVF clinics has made it possible to keep infertility a secret and has reinforced the shame associated with barrenness. Both responses merely confirm the importance of reproduction, which is shown to remain paramount in essence if not in form.

Finally, faced with a population decline, the role of assisted reproductive technologies has become increasingly important for the state, which views the rise in voluntary childlessness as a national challenge and is resorting to every legitimate means, including facilitating infertility treatment through IVF, to persuade those of reproductive age to contribute their share of children to the nation.

Acknowledgments

This chapter was published originally, with Mohammad Mehdi Akhondi, as "Conceiving IVF in Iran," *Reproductive Biomedicine and Society Online* 2: 62–70, Elsevier (2016). It is the result of the joint co-operation between Dr. Soraya Tremayne, who provided the historical and anthropological content and analysis, and Professor Mohammad Mehdi Akhondi, who provided the history of the introduction of IVF, its legitimization, and its current practice in Iran. Both authors have carried out extensive research in their separate fields of expertise, and the data in this chapter are based on larger studies, extending over three decades. Both authors have read and approved this chapter.

The authors would like to thank the following for their help in identifying the relevant sources of information, translating parts of the chapter from Persian to English, and for commenting on the draft: Dr. Alireza Milanifar, Dr. Mohammad Rasekh, Ms. Zohre Behjati Ardakani, Ms. Golanna Ashtari, Ms. Homa Mahmoodzadeh, Ms. Faezeh Ameri, and Mr. Amir Hossein Khodaparast.

Notes

1. For more information, refer to World Bank population data: http://data.worldbank.org/indicator/SP.POP.GROW?locations=IR.
2. https://www.populationinstitute.org/resources/populationonline/issue/8/53/.
3. Personal interview with Dr. Jalil Pakravesh, Tehran, 2015.
4. Personal communication.
5. Personal communication.
6. Personal communication.
7. The co-author.
8. Personal communication.

References

Abbasi-Shavazi, Mohammad Jalal. 2001. "La Fécondité en Iran: L'autre Revolution" [Fertility in Iran: The other revolution]. *Population et Societé* 373.

Abbasi-Shavazi, Mohammad Jalal, Marcia C. Inhorn, Hajiieh Bibi Razeghi-Nasrabad, and Ghasem Toloo. 2008. "The 'Iranian ART Revolution': Infertility, Assisted Reproductive Technology, and Third-Party Donation in the Islamic Republic of Iran." *Journal of Middle East Women's Studies* 4(2): 1–28.

Abbasi-Shavazi, Mohammad Jalal, Peter McDonald, and Meimanat Hosseini-Chavoshi. 2003. "Changes in Family, Fertility Behaviour and Attitudes in Iran." Working Paper in Demography 88. Demography and Sociology Program, Australian National University.

Akhondi, Mohammad Mehdi, Koorosh Kamali, Fahimeh Ranjbar, Mahdi Shirzad, Shiva Shafeghati, Zohreh Behjati Ardakani, Abolfazl Goodjani, Mahboubeh Parsaeian, and Kazem Mohammad. 2013. "Prevalence of Primary Infertility in Iran in 2010." *Journal of Public Health* 42(12): 1398–1404.

Akhondi, Mohammad Mehdi, and Mohammad Rasekh. 2011a. *The Reports on Friendly Meetings of Infertility Specialists in Iran: Symposium on Sex Selection.* Tehran: Avicenna Research Institute.

———. 2011b. *The Reports on Friendly Meetings of Infertility Specialists in Iran.* 2nd ed. Tehran: Avicenna Research Institute.

Avicenna Research Institute. 2001. *Modern Human Reproductive Technologies from the View of Jurisprudence and Law.*

Clarke, Morgan. 2009. *Islam and New Kinship: Reproductive Technologies and the Sharia in Lebanon.* New York and Oxford: Berghahn Books.

———. 2012. "Islamic Bioethics and Religious Politics in Lebanon." In *Islam and Assisted Reproductive Technologies: Sunni and Shia Perspectives,* ed.

Marcia C. Inhorn and Soraya Tremayne, 261–284. New York and Oxford: Berghahn Books.

Coulson, Noel J. 1971. *Succession in the Muslim Family*. Cambridge: Cambridge University Press.

Ebadi, Shirin. 2003. *Women's Rights in the Laws of the Islamic Republic of Iran*. In Persian. Iran: Ganje Danesh Press.

Elgood, Cyril. 1978. "Safavid Medical Practice, Or the Practice of Medicine, Surgery and Gynecology in Persia between 1500 A.D. and 1750 A.D." Translated by Mohsen Javidan. Tehran: Tehran University Press.

Eslami, H. 2007. *Human Cloning from the Perspective of Catholicism and Islam*. 1st ed. Qom, Iran: The Center for Religions Studies.

Gooshki, Ehsan Shamsi, and Neda Allahbedashti. 2015. "The Process of Justifying Assisted Reproductive Technologies in Iran." *Indian Journal of Medical Ethics* 12(2): 57–96.

Haeri, Shahla, 1989. *Law of Desire: Temporary Marriage in Shi'i Iran*. Syracuse, NY: Syracuse University Press.

Hoodfar, Homa. 1995. "Population Policy and Gender Equity in Post-Revolutionary Iran." In *Family, Gender and Population in the Middle East: Policies in Context*, ed. Carla Makhlouf, 80–105. Cairo: American University of Cairo Press.

Hosseini, Tehrani. 2015. Fatwa on Piety. Retrieved 25 September 2021 from http://motaghin.com/fa_question_1113.aspx.

Inhorn, Marcia C. 2005. Opening Speech. Reproductive Disruptions Conference. Ann Arbor, Michigan. 18 May.

———. 2006a. "Making Muslim Babies: IVF and Gamete Donation in Sunni versus Shia Islam." *Culture, Medicine and Psychiatry* 30(4): 427–450.

———. 2006b. "He Won't Be My Son." *Medical Anthropology Quarterly* 20(1): 94–120.

———. 2007. "Reproductive Disruptions and Assisted Reproductive Technologies in the Muslim World." In *Reproductive Disruptions: Gender, Technology, and Biopolitics in the New Millennium*, ed. Marcia C. Inhorn, 181–199. New York and Oxford: Berghahn Books.

Inhorn, Marcia C., Pasquale Patrizio, and Gamal I. Serour. 2012. "Third-Party Reproductive Assistance around the Mediterranean: Comparing Sunni Egypt, Catholic Italy, and Multisectarian Lebanon." In *Islam and Assisted Reproductive Technologies: Sunni and Shia Perspectives*, ed. Marcia C. Inhorn and Soraya Tremayne, 223–261. New York and Oxford: Berghahn Books.

Inhorn, Marcia C., and Soraya Tremayne, eds. 2012. *Assisted Reproductive Technologies: Sunni and Shia Perspectives*. New York and Oxford: Berghahn Books.

Inhorn, Marcia C., and Frank Van Balen, eds. 2002. *Infertility around the Globe: New Thinking on Childlessness, Gender, and Reproductive Technologies*. Berkeley: University of California Press.

Kashani-Sabet, Firoozeh. 2011. *Conceiving Citizens: Women and the Politics of Motherhood in Iran*. Oxford University Press.

Khamenei, Ali. 1999. *Ojoubeh Al-Esteftaat*. Questions 1271 to 1277. Tehran: Amir Kabir.

Khomeini, Ruhollah. 2001. *Tahrir-Al-Vasilah*. Qom: Islamic Publishing.

Madani Tabrizi, Yousef. 2009. *Al-Massael-al-Mostahadasseh* 3. Tehran: Ayatollah Madani Tabrizi's Office, 212–228.

Makhlouf-Obermeyer, Carla. 1991. "Women, Islam and Population: Is the Triangle Fateful?" Working Series Paper No. 6. Harvard: Harvard School of Public Health, Harvard University.

McDonald, Peter, Meimanat Hosseini-Chavoshi, Mohammad Jalal Abbasi-Shavazi, and Arash Rashidian. 2015. "An Assessment of Recent Iranian Fertility Trends using Parity Progression Ratios." *Demographic Research* 32: 1581–1602.

Mir-Hosseini, Ziba. 2000. *Marriage on Trial: A Study of Islamic Family Law*. Revised ed. I.B. Tauris.

Moosa, Ebrahim. 2003. "Human Cloning in Muslim Ethics." *Voices across Boundaries* (Fall): 23–26.

Sanei, Ayatollah. 1998. Fatwa on Marriage. Retrieved 23 September 2021 from http://www.saanei.org/?view=01,00,00,00,0#01,05,13,76,0.

Sistani, Ayatollah. 1999. Fatwa on Artificial Insemination. Retrieved 7 May 2022 from http://www.sistani.org/persian/book/53/238/ and http://www.sistani.org/persian/book/50/3731/.

Statistical Center of Iran. 1986. *Statistical Yearbook of Iran*. Tehran: SCI Publications.

Tabnak. 2013. "Iran's Population Crisis Awaits the Iranian People." In Persian. 24 September. Retrieved 23 September 2021 from www.tabnak.ir/fa/news/346841.

Tappan, Robert. 2012. "Ethical Decision-Making in Iranian Fertility Clinics." In *Islam and Assisted Reproductive Technologies: Sunni and Shia Perspectives*, ed. Marcia C. Inhorn and Soraya Tremayne, 103–129. New York: Berghahn Books.

Tremayne, Soraya. 2001. "Introduction." In *Managing Reproductive Life: Cross-Cultural Themes in Fertility and Sexuality*, ed. Soraya Tremayne. New York and Oxford: Berghahn Books.

———. 2004. "'And Never the Twain Shall Meet': Reproductive Health Policies in the Islamic Republic of Iran." In *Reproductive Agency, Medicine and the State: Cultural Transformations in Childbearing*, ed. Maya Unnithan-Kumar, 181–202. New York: Berghahn Books.

———. 2006. "Modernity and Early Marriage in Iran: A View from Within." *Journal of Middle East Women's Studies* 2(1): 65–94.

———. 2009. "Law, Ethics, and Donor Technologies in Shia Iran." In *Assisting Reproduction, Testing Genes: Global Encounters with New Biotechnologies*, ed. Daphna Birenbaum-Carmeli and Marcia C. Inhorn, 144–163. New York: Berghahn Books.

———. 2012. "The 'Down Side' of Gamete Donation: Challenging the 'Happy Family' Rhetoric in Iran." In *Islam and Assisted Reproductive Technologies: Sunni and Shia Perspectives*, ed. Marcia C. Inhorn and Soraya Tremayne, 130–157. New York and Oxford: Berghahn Books.

United Nations. 2016. *Demographic Yearbook*: "Demographics of Iran." Retrieved 19 September 2021 from http://www.worldometers.info/world-population/iran-population/.

Yazdi, Mohammad. 1996. "Infertility Treatment and its Jurisprudential Approach." *Figh-e-Ahl-e-Beit* 5: 5–6.

Chapter 12

Third-Party Gamete Donation, Anonymity, and the Conundrum of Lineage

Introduction

The history of the introduction, legitimization, and application of assisted reproductive technologies (ARTs) in Iran has been documented and analyzed extensively (Tremayne 2009, 2015; Clarke 2009; Inhorn and Tremayne 2012; Tremayne and Akhondi 2016). The treatment of infertility using ARTs was legitimized in Iran with the assistance and approval of leading Shia Islamic jurists. In allowing third-party gamete donation, these jurists, who were mindful of the paramount importance of biological relatedness and lineage purity, emphasized that a child conceived through gamete donation inherits from his/her biological parent but takes his/her name from the social parent (Tremayne and Akhondi 2016). They also underscored the importance of confidentiality in protecting the identity of the gamete donor and the dignity of the child. However, the ruling on confidentiality remained open to the interpretation of the infertility clinics, many of which chose to keep the donor's identity anonymous rather than confidential. The anonymity of the donor parent, therefore, prevented the child from being able to identify his/her biological parents and affected his/her inheritance rights. These contradictory rulings, while fomenting confusion for all parties involved, also enabled infertile couples to manipulate the situation to suit their own agendas. For example, in the early days of the practice of gamete donation, couples turned to relatives or other known donors for gamete donation, an act that made it impossible to maintain anonymity or confidentiality. Two decades later, gamete recipients had moved to favor anonymous donation, aiming to keep their infertility struggles confidential. The ambiguity of these religious verdicts combined with the recent proclivity of couples toward anonymous gamete donation impacted the traditional Iranian value of biological lineage purity. This chapter examines the aftermath of the practice of donor technologies in Iran, which "has led to a brave new world of reproductive possibility never imagined when these technologies were first introduced to the Middle East exactly thirty years ago" (Inhorn and Tremayne 2016: 429).

The Legitimization of ARTs

The introduction of in vitro fertilization (IVF) to Iran in the 1980s by pioneering medical practitioners was met with the approval of most Islamic jurists, who limited its practice to married heterosexual couples[1] (Tremayne and Akhondi 2016). But the introduction of third-party donor technologies proved more controversial. In the absence of the state's interest in alleviating infertility, these techniques were legitimized through interactions between medical professionals and Shia jurists (*foqaha*), who endorsed and supported them by issuing legal opinions (*fatwas*) on infertility treatment. These religious edicts function in accordance with the Iranian legal system and, in the absence of related stipulations within the existing legal code, are legitimate. These edicts also reassured ARTs users, many of whom were devout Muslims, that they were not breaching any religious laws in seeking assisted conception (Tremayne and Akhondi 2016). In their deliberations on the legitimacy of third-party gamete donation, the Islamic jurists were mainly concerned about the impact of these technologies on the continuity and purity of lineage, which would be disrupted by the intrusion of a third party. However, the jurists were not unanimous in their verdicts, differing from and even sometimes contradicting one another. The rulings in favor of ARTs focused on finding solutions to allow the use of a stranger's gamete without breaching the sanctity of marriage and interrupting lineage continuity, which is forbidden in Islam (Inhorn 2006a, 2006b; Inhorn and Tremayne 2012; Tremayne 2012; Shabana 2015). However, while some solutions were found (Tremayne 2009), these rulings did not foresee, or they remained silent on, the implicit and at times negative aftermath of third-party gamete donation on lineage, the very institution they were anxious to protect.

Conception through third-party gamete donation and its implications for the deeply rooted norms and values surrounding reproduction led to the emergence of a range of opinions among leading Islamic jurists. The involvement of a third party in procreation seemed discordant with Islam's prohibition on conception outside marriage and with its position that the only acceptable form of reproduction is through heterosexual marital union, resulting in one's own biological children. The objection to third-party donation by some leading Shia jurists is based on the same reasoning as that of Sunni jurists, who rejected third-party donation in all its forms and have allowed IVF only for married couples (Inhorn 2006a; Inhorn and Tremayne 2012; Shabana 2015). As the physicians who brought ARTs to Iran realized that their implementation transcended the realms of biomedicine and religion, they reached out to ethicists, legal experts, social scientists, and psychologists to explore the congruence of ARTs with the norms and values attached to reproduction and their consequences for family, kinship, and society in general. Experts and Islamic jurists needed to find valid arguments to justify the legitimacy of third-party donation, which, while a potential threat to the purity of lineage, would facilitate the continuity of the family line. While jurists have proposed some solutions, overall, to date, their opinions remain divided on this form of procreation. For example, initially the legitimization of third-party gamete donation required a temporary marriage (*sigheh*) between gamete donors and recipients, without any actual physical contact taking place between the two parties.[2] In issuing their opinions on whether to accept or reject ARTs, the jurists, who are the sources of emulation (*maraje-e taqlid)* for the Shia followers, based their verdicts on interpretations of the Islamic sources (*ijtihad*), each arriving at their own independent reasoning (*fatwa*).

Faced with these contradictory edicts, followers were left to choose the opinions that appealed to or concurred with their own sensibilities. As Robert Tappan (2012: 105), a scholar in Islamic ethics, theology, and law, explains, "There is a religious duty incumbent upon each Shia believer to follow the rulings of one high-ranking [source of emulation]. This leads to a plurality of equally authoritative religious rulings, which might differ greatly from one another, and may vary from the state law as well." The diversity of opinions, especially on the question of third-party donation, persists to date and has opened a gap, allowing the parties involved to make decisions that befit them (Tremayne 2009).

In general, the edicts of the *maraje-e taqlid* fell into three groups: (i) those that deem forbidden (*haram*) the use of IVF in any form, especially third-party donation, which is viewed as intruding on the sanctity of marriage (see also Inhorn 2006a) and as confusing the purity of lineage (for example, the late Ayatollah al-Ozma Madani Tabrizi (2009)); (ii) those that permit the use of some ARTs in certain circumstances (Khamenei 1999); and (iii) those that permit the application of ARTs in all forms (Yazdi 1996). The lenient sources interpret ARTs as a means of mediating between God and God's subjects to allow procreation and not as a means of interfering in God's design (Tremayne and Akhondi 2016: 67).

As already discussed, regardless of the verdicts on the permissibility or otherwise of ARTs, the premise upon which all the jurists based their edicts has been the implication of third-party gamete donation on lineage and inheritance, values automatically linked in Islamic law (*sharia*). It is noteworthy that even among those jurists who viewed third-party donation favorably, egg donation was largely accepted, but sperm donation was not. The permission of sperm donation provoked a strong reaction from many conservative quarters, among the majority of *ulama* (Muslim legal scholars) in the parliament, and among the general public; to date, its practice is carried out discreetly by some private clinics. As explained elsewhere, "sperm donation is seen defying deeply rooted patriarchal values in Iran, including patrilineal kinship reckoning, in which the father assumes priority and rights of ownership over the child" (Inhorn and Tremayne 2015).

Further clarifying this adversity to sperm donation, Coulson defines lineage (*nasab*) as follows (Coulson 1971: 22, cited in Mir-Hosseini 2000: 134):

> Sharia legal notions of kinship and filiation are encapsulated in the concept of *nasab* (lineage), which translates not only as parentage and kinship, but also as filiation and descent status. While the child takes its *nasab* from both sides, it is the paternal side which has ascendancy over the maternal. In all schools of Islamic law the primary significance of *nasab* is that of paternity, closely tied to legitimacy, through which a child acquires its legal identity and its religion.

According to Islamic law, a child belongs to his father's lineage, which extends beyond the father to include the paternal grandfather, who shares equal rights over the child. In the absence of a father or grandfather, these rights go to the paternal uncles (Ebadi 2003; Mir-Hosseini 2000). Such rights are reciprocal, and the child can also claim rights from his/her biological father and grandfather. Lineage, therefore, consists of a complex web of relatedness, involving duties and obligations, predominantly involving the paternal side.

Furthermore, inheritance in Islam is exclusively linked to biological relatedness, and only blood relatives can inherit from each other. It is therefore understandable that the Islamic jurists were concerned not only for the continuity of the lineage, but also for the child's right to inherit from its biological parents—the gamete donors (Tremayne and Akhondi 2016). For a child to inherit from a biological parent, he/she must know the identity of this parent; yet an increasing number of infertility clinics, resorting to those *fatwas* advocating confidentiality, have moved to keep the identity of the donor anonymous if the latter is not a relative or a known person to the infertile couple. In addition, the infertile couples have also moved to seek treatment as anonymously as possible, aiming to keep their infertility a secret. Proof of the exclusivity of the right of blood relatives to inheritance can be seen in the persisting debates on adoption. Although the adoption of strangers, which is generally forbidden in Islam, has been allowed in Iran for several decades, dating back to the Pahlavi era, the adopted child does not have any legal claim to inherit from his adoptive parents. According to the same principle, until 2009, the wife of a deceased man, not being a blood relative, could inherit only one-eighth of his movable belongings. But this has now been revised, and a law was passed in 2009 (Article 946, Section 5 of the Civil Code of the Islamic Republic of Iran) that allows a woman to inherit property from her husband and removes the limits on the proportion of movable property a women can inherit.[3]

Social and cultural norms and values mirror these religious and legal factors and agree that the only acceptable form of relatedness is through the blood line. As a result, in the absence of rules explicitly forbidding gamete donation between blood relatives, in the early days of the practice of gamete donation, it was assumed that donation between siblings or other relatives was allowed. As far as the users of ARTs were concerned, receiving gametes from their blood relatives, mainly their siblings, was the ideal way to conceive. As I have discussed elsewhere (Tremayne 2015: 75), couples often chose relatives as donors in attempts to keep the donation "in the family" and to avoid mixing one's blood with that of a stranger.

Evidence from various research on infertility treatment confirms these findings: having one's own biological child is so important that, unless the donor of the gamete is a relative, the recipients of strangers' gametes do not reveal their decision and instead pretend that the child is theirs biologically (Inhorn 2006b; Abbasi-Shavazi et al. 2008).

While gamete donation by siblings initially seemed like a win-win solution, over time, problems emerged. Conflicts arose between the related gamete donors and recipients, between unrelated donors, whose identities were known to the recipients, and between gamete recipients and donors and clinics. These arguments ranged from disputes over ownership of the child to financial claims by gamete donors. As a result, clinics became tribunals for establishing kinship rights and ownership of the resulting child, providing counseling to the "losing" party, and determining the financial losses and gains of gamete donors and recipients. These conflicts forced each clinic to adjudicate its own solutions. In the absence of laws, these disputes, especially those concerning the ownership of children, can end up in court, where judges usually base their verdicts on *fatwas* issued by their own *maraje-e taqlid*. One such example, among many others, recounted in a personal interview, is the case of two sisters, one of whom had donated an egg to her infertile sister. The infertile sister conceived and had a son. When the boy was seven years old, the son of his aunt—who was also his biological mother—died in a car accident. The aunt then claimed "her" son from her sister and the case ended up in court, which gave the son to his biological mother, based on a *fatwa* ruling that the child belongs to his biological parent. It is noteworthy that conflicts on the ownership of the child arise only when the identities of gamete donors and recipients are known, hence the tendency to avoid them through anonymous donation.

In other cases, concerning the ownership of children, whereby the *fatwas* are unclear, judges refer to Islamic rulings, which consider biological relatedness as the guiding principle for establishing the right to parenthood. The only case of conflict over third-party donation whereby Iranian law supersedes religious edict is that of embryo donation. No amount of *ijtihad* could justify embryo donation, which parliament legalized in 2003.

In the early days of ARTs in Iran, couples tended to rely on relatives over strangers to donate gametes because, while many couples simply preferred to use relatives' gametes, few strangers were volunteering to donate. Although infertility was a huge stigma kept secret whenever possible, infertile couples often had no choice but to involve their kin group by seeking help. This help could extend from gamete donation to financial contributions toward high treatment costs. Examples abound of relatives selling their cars or even houses to help pay for the infertility treatment of their infertile kinfolk. This high degree of involvement, inevitably, justified the interference of relatives in all stages of treatment, and the infertility of one couple became that of the whole kin group, which caused additional problems for clinics. In addition, in the absence of law enforcement, each clinic was able to establish its own rules on gamete donation, based on the preferences of clinic directors and which jurists' *fatwas* he/she followed. Interestingly, gamete donation by same-sex siblings or relatives had also expanded over time to include donations from opposite-sex siblings or even donations from different generations in the same family, whereby brothers gave sperm to their sisters' infertile husbands, or fathers to their sons. Effectively, fertilizing a woman's egg with her brother's or her father-in-law's sperm crosses red lines of sexual prohibition and is tantamount to incest and adultery. The Islamic concept of *mahramiat* (closeness/privacy)[4] regulates practices of social and sexual interaction between men and women (Tremayne 2015; Inhorn and Tremayne 2015). In sum, this combination of donor selection and clinician perspective has determined the practice of ARTs in Iran for three decades. Another factor, allowing room for maneuver, is the flexibility of the relationship between the *marja* and his followers. While each believer can follow the advice of one *marja*, if the views of that *marja* go against the adherent's own agenda, the latter can change his *marja* and follow another one, whose views are more compatible with his or her own. For example, one infertile couple mentioned that their *marja*, who was against third-party gamete donation, told them, "I am against it, but go to such and such *marja*, who agrees with it, and you can then seek treatment." That said, many couples seeking treatment are not necessarily religious and do not seek permission from a *marja*. In addition, many infertile couples, religious or otherwise, are unaware of the involvement of the religious leaders and their approval or disapproval as they consider infertility treatment a medical intervention.

Adulterating Lineage?

In light of these complications, some leading infertility clinics in Iran decided to stop the widespread practice of gamete donation between known donors. Many clinics moved to take control of the situation by matching gamete donors and recipients, ensuring the anonymity of the donors, while keeping track of it in their own records. The larger and better-equipped clinics took great care to match donors with recipients. Donors who were strangers were financially motivated even though altruism is a fundamental condition for gamete donation in Iran. In practice, most "volunteer" donors received money, justified as compensation for travel and accommodation "expenses," an amount calculated by the clinics. In most cases these donors were not told who the recipient of their gamete may be nor did they express an interest in finding out. As an example, a practitioner in one of Tehran's infertility clinics told me that one egg donor to their clinic went from one clinic to the next, donating her eggs. When she was told of the risks and negative outcome of her actions, she just shrugged her shoulders, unwilling to relinquish what had become a profitable endeavor. I came across some practices whereby infertile couples had brought their own relatives as donors, but the clinics decided to freeze the gametes for use on another infertile couple and had chosen an anonymous gamete for the infertile party without informing the parties involved. In another case, an infertile man persuaded the doctor to use his brother's sperm to impregnate his wife without the wife's knowledge, and the doctor obliged (Tremayne 2015).[5] In an interview with one of the practitioners responsible for matching the donors and recipients, she mentioned an exceptional (in her experience) case whereby the donor had asked about the identity of the gamete's recipient. The donor then insisted that the clinic withhold his gametes from anyone who lived within a few specific provinces, naming these locations. When the physician asked the reason, the donor replied, "I have many relatives in these provinces and many of them are infertile. I do not want them to receive my gamete accidentally. If the treatment works and a child is born and looks like me, everybody will know that the child is mine." Although there is no further information on this case, several assumptions could be made, namely the embarrassment of others knowing that she was earning money by selling her eggs, the possibility of parenting a child with one of her relatives without their prior knowledge and consent, as well as myriad other complications.

As a result of these practices, health care practitioners sought further clarification from religious authorities on questions of confidentiality and anonymity. For example, they wanted to know how the *fatwa* on "the child belongs to its biological parent and inherits from him/her but takes his name from the 'social' parents" (Sanei 1998)[6] could be reconciled with the idea of keeping the identity of the gamete donors a secret. As Gooshki and Allahbedashti (2015) point out, the contradictory rulings espousing that the child's biological origins must be known and at the same time advocating confidentiality led to blurred lines between confidentiality and anonymity and prevented children from tracing the identity of their biological parents to inherit from them.

However, these jurists revisited the problem and issued further *fatwas* acknowledging the changing circumstances, as follows:

> The jurists in favor of IVF, on the other hand, took a different route by redefining relatedness. According to this definition, the parent, in agreeing to donate his/her gamete, transfers the parental rights to the adoptive parent and forgoes any claim on the resulting child (Sanei 1998). In the process, a new representation of relatedness has emerged, replacing the biological link with that of permission/consent on the part of the parent. (Tremayne and Akhondi 2016: 68)

Opponents of third-party donation objected to the above rulings, which they saw as challenges to the foundations of lineage, family, and kinship (Tremayne and Akhondi 2016). Questions of mutual rights between biological parents and children and anonymity or the lack of it, as well as the inheritance rights, remain unclear and unresolved due to the absence of related legislation and the existence of many controversial religious rulings.

Although debate surrounds the ethical aspects of practicing ARTs, with some of the larger clinics having their own in-house ethicists, in the absence of clear official guidelines, individual practitioners are left to establish their own ethical parameters. What emerges from the flexible climate in which ARTs are practiced is the persistence of the wide gap between the perceptions of the medical practitioners, who view ARTs as medical interventions, and those of users of these technologies, who act according to their own understandings of what constitutes relatedness. However, this situation has changed over time, revealing an even more profound motivation behind the decisions made by infertile individuals. The motivation to procreate supersedes belief in the importance of maintaining "the continuity and purity of lineage."

Three decades after IVF was first introduced into Iran, with infertility treatment becoming more known to the general public, a shift has taken place. Urban, educated, and less conservative infertile couples in larger cities are increasingly seeking gamete donation from strangers who remain anonymous. This has been facilitated by a considerable increase in the number of gamete donors, which enables recipients to seek treatment without the knowledge or involvement of their closest relatives, including their parents. Increasingly, couples do not even admit to seeking treatment, and, if successful, the conception appears natural. As Iran does not yet have a national DNA database, it is impossible for a child conceived in this manner to trace his/her biological lineage in the unlikely event that he/she finds out that his/her parents are not his/her biological ones. That said, many infertile couples, rural or less well-off urban inhabitants, and those from conservative and religious backgrounds are unable or unwilling to seek treatment secretly or resort to third-party gamete donation. For these groups, receiving an anonymous gamete secretly and pretending to have conceived their own biological child is still a distant possibility. Furthermore, many among these groups cannot afford the costs of the treatment and continue to depend on their kin group for financial support. Although as part of its pronatalist policies the state is now covering the costs of three free cycles of IVF, the additional expenses are beyond the financial ability of this group. Furthermore, there are others who may prefer to continue using their consanguineous relatives, and, so far, no rule prevents them from doing so. Many also choose to forgo third-party donation altogether, viewing it as a sin to bring a stranger's lineage into the family. Nevertheless, infertile couples in Iran now have a few options: refuse third-party gametes and live with the stigma of infertility; disclose their infertility, admit to receiving gametes from a third-party and thus to compromising biological purity, and live with the embarrassment of having bred a stranger's child; or secretly resort to anonymous donors and pretend to be the biological parents with the advantage of being able to register their children in their own names. As ongoing research indicates, the number of infertile couples opting for anonymous gamete donation is increasing.

In tandem with these shifts in attitude, the state's pronatalist policies are contributing to the success of infertility treatment in the country. Practitioner interviews confirm that these policies are actively encouraging the use of third-party gamete donation. The state's contributions range from revising its approach to infertility and moving to consider it a disability, to increasing the number of new public infertility clinics, which currently number around 100, to covering the costs of three free IVF cycles for those who cannot afford them.

Because the practice of ARTs was in flux, prior to the 2021 presidential elections, leading medical practitioners had seized the opportunity to actively cooperate with legislators to redefine its parameters. For example, it is with their encouragement that a white paper was drafted and submitted to the parliament to legitimize anonymous gamete donation. However, since the submission of the white paper, Iran has undergone several crises, inter alia, the financial hardship resulting from the sanctions imposed on the country by the West, the COVID-19 pandemic, and the rise to power of an ultra-conservative government, so for now debating the bill on anonymity has given way to more urgent matters. Although the legalization of anonymous gamete donation is not guaranteed, it would not occur without consequences. By accepting this proposal, lawmakers would in effect be rejecting the rulings of the senior sources of emulation who permit third-party donation. Moreover, by endorsing gamete donation generally, these lawmakers would also be rejecting the rulings of the jurists who oppose third-party donation altogether. Ironically, this acceptance will also counter the work of leading practitioners, perpetuating the stigma of infertility by allowing couples to mask their infertility.

However, the current Iranian parliament, which consists of a majority ultra-conservative members, could reject third-party gamete donation altogether, anonymously or otherwise, as has been the case in Turkey and Italy, which have reversed their policies on third-party donation (Inhorn, Patrizio, and Serour 2012; Gürtin-Broadbent 2012). Such a possibility raises questions about what might happen to the state's pronatalist policies, which rely on the success of ARTs, including third-party gamete donation.

The legal aspects of ARTs and the state's pronatalist policies notwithstanding, the prevalence of third-party gamete donation introduces a conundrum: on one hand, it aims to alleviate—and eventually eliminate—the stigma of infertility. On the other hand, it enables couples to conceal the shame of their infertility, thereby perpetuating and reinforcing its stigma. As a result, outwardly the burden of barrenness is removed while inwardly the sanctity of the purity of lineage gradually vanishes into a convenient myth. Over time, anonymous gamete donation could prove instrumental in diminishing the true significance of the "purity of lineage," which would exist only symbolically among its users.

Conclusion

This chapter examines the implications of third-party gamete donation on the integrity of lineage, a paramount value in Islam and in Iranian culture. The chapter further explores the gradual shift of attitudes among ARTs users: while third-party gamete donation began as an open exercise between recipients and donors, with close members of the kin group being the preferred donors, it has evolved to recipients now resorting secretly to anonymous gamete donation whenever possible. Although the use of anonymous gametes is meant to dispel the stigma of infertility and hide the shame of compromising lineage purity, the outcome has been twofold: first, users are unintentionally challenging the rulings of leading jurists by effectively disrupting their own blood lines; second, in using anonymous gametes, recipients are able to uphold the myth of the authenticity of their lineage. Reproducing anonymously seems to have reinforced rather than weakened the cultural norms and values attached to reproduction. Put differently, it is not the existence of ARTs, but the ways in which they have been used, that have shaped attitudes toward infertility in Iran. Ironically, should anonymous gamete donation be legalized, this would dissipate the authority of both the jurists who endorsed third-party donation on the condition that the purity of lineage be preserved, and the jurists who opposed any form of third-party donation. Finally, the legalization of anonymous gamete donation could have the unintended effect of polarizing biological reproduction and lineage continuity, which together form the cornerstone of Iranian society. However, the possibility of finding a solution to these seemingly unresolvable questions, through further *fatwas* and in the name of the good of the nation, cannot be ruled out.

Acknowledgments

An earlier version of this chapter was written as a paper presented at the "Family Structure in the Wake of Genetic and Reproductive Technologies" International Symposium at Georgetown University in Qatar on 7–8 October 2018.

Notes

1. Interestingly, with the legitimatization of sex reassignment surgery in Iran, individuals who have undergone the procedure have been allowed to resort to surrogacy (Najmabadi 2013).
2. Temporary marriage, which is unique to the Twelver Shia Muslims, is a type of marriage in which the two parties agree to enter into marriage set to expire automatically at a set time, between one hour and ninety-nine years. In cases of gamete donation, the marriage agreement would last for a maximum of a few days until the gamete donation proved successful. However, this practice is increasingly rare.
3. The 2009 law's enactment was catalyzed by a *fatwa* by Grand Ayatollah Sanei and undermined the claim that the current state of legislation concerning female inheritance correctly adhered to Islamic principles.
4. *Mahramiat* determines the boundaries of interactions between men and women in Iranian society. Accordingly, men and women are divided into two groups, the *mahram* and *na-mahram*. The *mahram* are relatives, who are not potential marriage partners and with whom one may freely interact (not sexually). Any sexual relationship between the members of the *mahram* group therefore constitutes incest. The *mahram* group includes one's siblings, parents, grandparents, aunts and uncles, and children and grandchildren.
5. This information is based on personal interviews with experts at infertility clinics between 2004 and 2012.
6. Social children have no claims to inheritance; only biological relatives can inherit from each other. If the child is not known to be the result of gamete donation, the problem does not arise. However, there are a number of ways through which even an adopted child or one who is the result of gamete donation can inherit from his/her adoptive or social parents. Going into these details is beyond the remit of this chapter.

References

Abbasi-Shavazi, Mohammad Jalal, Marcia C. Inhorn, Hajiieh Bibi Razeghi-Nasrabad, and Ghasem Toloo. 2008. "The 'Iranian ART Revolution': Infertility, Assisted Reproductive Technology, and Third-Party Donation in the Islamic Republic of Iran." *Journal of Middle East Women's Studies* 4(2): 1–28.

Clarke, Morgan. 2009. *Islam and New Kinship: Reproductive Technologies and the Sharia in Lebanon*. New York and Oxford: Berghahn Books.

Coulson, Noel J. 1971. *Succession in the Muslim Family*. Cambridge: Cambridge University Press.

Ebadi, Shirin. 2003. *Women's Rights in the Laws of the Islamic Republic of Iran*. In Persian. Iran: Ganje Danesh Press.

Gooshki, Ehsan Shamsi, and Neda Allahbedashti. 2015. "The Process of Justifying Assisted Reproductive Technologies in Iran." *Indian Journal of Medical Ethics* 12(2): 57–96.

Gürtin-Broadbent, Zeynep. 2012. "Assisted Reproduction in Secular Turkey: Regulation, Rhetoric, and the Role of Religion." In *Islam and Assisted Reproductive Technologies: Sunni and Shia Perspectives*, ed. Marcia C. Inhorn and Soraya Tremayne, 285–311. New York and Oxford: Berghahn Books.

Inhorn, Marcia C. 2006a. "Making Muslim Babies: IVF and Gamete Donation in Sunni versus Shia Islam." *Culture, Medicine and Psychiatry* 30(4): 427–450.

———. 2006b. "He Won't Be My Son." *Medical Anthropology Quarterly* 20(1): 94–120.

Inhorn, Marcia C., Pasquale Patrizio, and Gamal I. Serour. 2012. "Third-Party Reproductive Assistance around the Mediterranean: Comparing Sunni Egypt, Catholic Italy, and Multisectarian Lebanon." In *Assisted Reproductive Technologies: Sunni and Shia Perspectives*, ed. Marcia C. Inhorn and Soraya Tremayne, 223–261. New York and Oxford: Berghahn Books.

Inhorn, Marcia C., and Soraya Tremayne, eds. 2012. *Assisted Reproductive Technologies: Sunni and Shia Perspectives.* New York and Oxford: Berghahn Books.

Inhorn, Marcia C., and Soraya Tremayne. 2016. "Islam, Assisted Reproduction, and the Bioethical Aftermath." *Journal of Religion and Health* 55(2): 422–430.

Khamenei, Ali. 1999. *Ojoubeh Al-Esteftaat*. Questions 1271 to 1277. Tehran: Amir Kabir.

Madani Tabrizi, Yousef. 2009. *Al-Massael-al-Mostahadasseh* 3. Tehran: Ayatollah Madani Tabrizi's Office, 212–228.

Mir-Hosseini, Ziba. 2000. *Marriage on Trial: A Study of Islamic Family Law.* Revised ed. London: I. B. Tauris.

Najmabadi, Afsaneh. 2013. *Professing Selves: Transsexuality and Same-Sex Desire in Contemporary Iran*. Durham: Duke University Press.

Sanei, Ayatollah. 1998. Fatwa on Marriage. Retrieved 23 September 2021 from http://www.saanei.org/?view=01,00,00,00,0#01,05,13,76,0.

Shabana, Ayman. 2015. "Foundations of the Consensus against Surrogacy Arrangements in Islamic Law. *Islamic Law and Society* 22: 82–113.

Tappan, Robert. 2012. "Ethical Decision-Making in Iranian Fertility Clinics." In *Islam and Assisted Reproductive Technologies: Sunni and Shia Perspectives*, ed. Marcia C. Inhorn and Soraya Tremayne, 103–129. New York: Berghahn Books.

Tremayne, Soraya. 2009. "Law, Ethics and Donor Technologies in Shia Iran." In *Assisting Reproduction, Testing Genes: Global Encounters with New Biotechnologies*, ed. Daphna Birenbaum-Carmeli and Marcia C. Inhorn, 144–163. New York: Berghahn Books.

———. 2012. "The 'Down Side' of Gamete Donation: Challenging the 'Happy Family' Rhetoric in Iran." In *Islam and Assisted Reproductive Technologies: Sunni and Shia Perspectives,* ed. Marcia C. Inhorn and Soraya Tremayne, 130–157. New York and Oxford: Berghahn Books.

———. 2015. "Whither Kinship? Assisted Reproductive Technologies and Relatedness in the Islamic Republic of Iran." In *Assisted Reproductive Technologies in the Third Phase,* ed. Kate Hampshire and Bob Simpson, 69–83. New York: Berghahn Books.

Tremayne, Soraya, and Mohammad Mehdi Akhondi. 2016. "Conceiving IVF in Iran." *Reproductive Biomedicine & Society Online* 2: 62–70.

Yazdi, Mohammad. 1996. "Infertility Treatment and Its Jurisprudential Approach." *Figh-e-Ahl-e-Beit* 5(6): 105.

Conclusion

The chapters in this volume were selected to counter the perspectives of a profusion of new studies that argue that exposure to modernity and globalization have changed Iran's fundamental cultural norms and practices. The ethnographic studies in this book, spanning over three decades of research, challenge these assertions by adopting a chronological and comparative perspective on whether, why, how, and to what extent Iran's core cultural values have changed. These chapters were also chosen for their thematic consistency around the study of reproduction in all its manifestations, encompassing family, marriage, kinship, patriarchy, fertility, population, and the state's body politic and its relationship with the nation. By exploring change over time, these studies show the variety, subtlety, and complexity of the underlying cultural responses to these innovations, revealing how Iranians have received, understood, and tailored them to local practices. While some of the chapters show that deviating from tradition by adopting a "modern" perspective has provoked resistance, others point to the fact that lasting change has succeeded only in cases where it has been implemented in harmony with local beliefs and practices. Put together, the findings of this research challenge the general perception that Iranian culture has undergone "inconceivable" and radical change.

These studies do not claim to serve as universal verdicts applicable across Iran, a multi-cultural and multi-ethnic country with ideological differences. However, they consistently indicate that social change, albeit in different forms and to varying degrees across all layers of Iranian society, has not eroded the underlying values that surround reproductive life. They are evidence of the multitude of ways that core cultural norms accommodate modernity.

Every chapter in this book highlights the need to distinguish between social transformation and fundamental cultural change in the norms and values surrounding reproduction. Several points emerging from this collection show the diverse ways that reproductive practices have responded to modernity when modernity has been perceived as a threat to core cultural values. Examples of the centrality of marriage abound and prove that, despite fluctuations, the institution of marriage is firmly grounded albeit under different guises.

Child marriage is shown to be increasing, especially among conservative families faced with economic hardship or with the threat of transgression by their young children, who may be tempted by the "misguided" freedom the modernity offers. However, while these factors may be overarching causes, many child marriages in Iran are customary and occur without coercion. While modern human rights activists see the practice of child marriage as a form of child abuse and rights violations, local communities understand childhood, age, and maturity differently. They consider children adult enough to marry but young enough to need the guardianship of fathers or other male relatives, through patrilineal connection. Furthermore, most customary marriages take place between relatives or in close-knit communities and serve to maintain and strengthen the bonds of the kinship.

Consanguineous marriages, too, which have traditionally formed a high percentage of all marriages, are shown to be increasing in number. The drastic rise in divorce rates, threatening the stability of the institution of family, has strengthened the kin network in an attempt to ensure the stability of marital relationships through the bounds of relatedness.

A new form of cohabitation called "white marriage" has also emerged among those couples who do not wish to formalize their union. Although Islamic rule sees white marriage as equivalent to adultery, punishable by law, and although conservative layers in society frown on its practice, the word "marriage" gives it an aura of legitimacy and respectability, and even the authorities seem to overlook the "transgression" by and large.

Temporary marriage, practiced uniquely by Shia Muslims, is also used in creative ways to reconcile modernity with tradition. For example, Islamic jurists suggest temporary marriage as a way to legitimize otherwise controversial forms of infertility treatments, such as third-party gamete donation, which is viewed by many as tantamount to adultery, as discussed in Chapter 10. Furthermore, unmarried couples use temporary marriage to formalize their relationships and to avoid the risk of punishment for adultery. Faced with delays in marriage, some clerics suggested this form of union as a way to allow people to "satisfy" their sexual needs. This practice extends to people visiting brothels, who resort to temporary marriage to avoid breaching Islamic prohibitions on intercourse outside the marital union (Tate 2007).

Finally, the importance of marriage is also shown in a separate study on people with thalassemia in Iran, who, in spite of being fully aware of the risks involved in having children, choose to marry, conceive, and have abortions, if needed, rather than relinquishing their marriages (Hosoya 2017: 28).

The studies on fatherhood provide correctives to those claims that, in general, patriarchal values and practices in Iran have weakened. They show that, while the meanings and functions of fatherhood may have been altered in their modern contexts, its ideals have survived, rather than eroded, and are disguised in a variety of forms. These variations range from becoming familiar with technological innovations to surveil family activity, to creating strong bonds of affection with or using financial control over their children. In some cases, fathers are even emigrating out of the country with their families in order to keep better control of their children in new environments.

Kinship's pervasive influence also emerges in several chapters, for example on infertile couples seeking third-party gamete donation. Couples usually choose to receive gametes from blood relatives to maintain the continuity of their lineage. However, over time, some gamete recipients are also turning to anonymous donors, secretly from the kin group. While this decision may be perceived as breaching the sanctity of lineage, curious as it may seem, it is fully in line with the ideals that underpin kinship and the continuity of the blood line, as the resulting child is seen as the biological child of the couple. From the examples in these studies, it is clear that, whereas children born as a result of relatives' gamete donations are fully integrated into their kin groups, those children known to be conceived with the help of strangers' gametes, not those of blood relatives, are never accepted as equal by their kin groups and are considered outcasts by conservative families. This has been witnessed time and again, including in cases of adoption whereby even the law deprives adopted children of inheriting from their adopted parents. In addition, keeping the nature of the conception a secret also protects the child in the future. It then follows that Iranian society remains conservative, by and large, about third-party gamete donation. Recent studies show that, even decades after its legitimization, the involvement of a stranger in procreation is shown to be unacceptable by the majority of Iranian society. For example, in a survey asking the general public about third-party gamete donation, the majority disapproved of the practice in general and of sperm donation more specifically (Bamdad and Ahmadi 2014). Such attitudes extend to conservative and/or religious physicians who refrain from practicing sperm or embryo donation, even though embryo donation was legalized through an act of the parliament.

The extent to which a couple's kin group influences—and even shapes—its reproductive decisions, explained in this volume, is further evidence of the endurance of the underlying structures that determine and cement social relations, and act as gate keepers to prevent any general deviation. The studies on infertility in this volume merely confirm that not only have values and practices attached to kinship not vanished or weakened under modernity, but they help ensure the cohesion of the kin group.[1]

The centrality of purity, as a core value in reproduction, is shown to transcend lineage and extend to female sexuality and control of women. The studies in this volume refer to an increasing number of unmarried, sexually active girls who restored their virginity through modern technologies, in the form of hymenoplasty, thus appearing pure and "marriageable" to their future husbands and their husbands' kin groups. Such solutions might justify the Foucauldian argument that these actions can be interpreted as forms of resistance against the power of the state, especially when even a leading Islamic jurist, defeated by the drastic increase in numbers of girls seeking hymenoplasty, issues a *fatwa* allowing it. However, this could also indicate a need to be seen as conforming rather than rebelling. As an in-depth study of female university students (Khalajabadi, Månsson, and Cleland 2018) shows, most young women interviewed mentioned that they preferred to be virgins at marriage. Although it is not clear whether these young women were upholding virginity as an ideal or genuinely believed in it, or whether they had undergone hymenoplasty, nevertheless, what emerges from the study is the continuation of the concept of purity itself. Furthermore, virginity remains so important that, until a few years ago, young men living in the diaspora used to travel to Iran in search of virgin girls to marry.[2]

A common point emerging from the chapters is the ingrained gender inequalities in a society caught at the crossroads of tradition and modernity. Modernity, including socio-economic developments, has improved the position of women considerably, and women have marked their presence in almost every public sphere, including those that were traditionally male. Furthermore, women now transcend socio-cultural barriers, and their acts of defiance also regularly appear in the media in the form of, for example, venturing into the forbidden areas of choosing men as casual sex partners, regardless of the men's ages or levels of education or income, but as experimental objects. However, examples of gender inequality are conspicuous throughout the chapters, confirming the persisting beliefs and practices of men's rights in women's procreative powers. Men's virility and reproductive abilities in the patrilineal Iranian kinship system are crucial, as a man's progeny belongs to him and to his male relatives, even though lineage comes from both parents. Therefore, male infertility is still seen as a total failure, which explains why the woman assumes blame for the couple's success or failure to conceive. Women are shown to be subject to atrocious treatment, mostly among conservative groups, not only by their husbands but also by their own fathers and brothers, in cases of conception through third-party donation. Such examples are by no means exceptional and rarely become public, outside the immediate family.

The chapters on infertility have also shed light on the body politic of the various Iranian states, who have targeted reproduction as the most effective institutional tool to serve their nation-building policies. Interestingly, although the only truly effective population policies, implemented during the 1980s and 1990s, succeeded in changing the reproductive attitudes to childbearing among the generation of reproductive age, in terms of the size of the family and revisiting the value of children, these changes have not shifted the fundamental values attached to marriage and family. A longitudinal study of couples who have opted to remain childless shows that, after a few years, these couples ultimately formed families, each with at least one child. Such inconsistencies could indicate that voluntary childlessness might be more of a passing phase than a permanent shift in reproductive value. This merits a longer-term study to examine changes in attitudes toward childbearing.

In sum, the studies in this volume yield several general observations. First, the behavior of Iranians across all generations remains consistent in its compliance with reproductive norms. The generation of reproductive age forms the largest age group in the population pyramid in Iran, with those between the ages of twenty-five and fifty-four forming the largest group at 48.94 percent of the total population, and with the age group between twenty-five and forty-five being the largest.[3] Considering that individuals within this latter age group, the main agent of reproductive change, embrace innovation with open arms and are more likely to rebel and deviate from norms, the question becomes: how and why do they ultimately comply with the core reproductive norms, often to an unexpected degree? The seemingly contradictory and puzzling behavior is interpreted as "paradoxical," "rebellious," and even "inconceivable," and young people are perceived as "disturbed" and "confused" about their identity. However, as the findings of the studies in this volume suggest, the "confusing" and "inconsistent" behavior of this group tends to be more of a coping strategy—a modus vivendi that helps these individuals reconcile modernity with tradition.

Second, a chronological perspective reveals the extent of the resilience or fragility of reproductive norms in their encounters with innovation. Case studies show that many cohabiting couples, while initially digressing from social norms, ultimately break up under the pressure of prevailing cultural imperatives. Similarly, many educated women, who have gained some independence and chosen to delay marriage, find themselves under the control of their families perpetuating the status quo. Moreover, a considerable number of divorced women who willingly enter temporary marriages with men, many of whom are already married, anticipating a sense of freedom, find their freedom severely restricted by their "temporary" husbands.

Third, this volume reveals an otherwise overlooked aspect of the "confusing" behaviors of all the actors on the reproductive scene. These findings lift the veil on the fact that transgression and conformity are not necessarily polar opposites but rather subtle ways to bridge the gap between tradition and modernity. Transgression, in the context of reproductive behavior, attitudes, and modernity, including reproductive technologies or sexuality, has been contextual and has not threatened the social order. As examples throughout the book have shown, breaking up biological lineage by endorsing third-party gamete donation or resorting to hymenoplasty to restore one's virginity are phenomena that have developed specifically to facilitate conformity with the fundamental cultural norms associated with reproduction. In effect, conformity and transgression have become interchangeable to suit the agendas of the actors. Shia jurists, by allowing third-party donation, break away from certain Islamic rules by breaching the sanctity of marriage and allowing "adultery," so that they can uphold the Islamic values of creating stable and happy families. Likewise, infertile couples breach the same rules by secretly receiving anonymous gametes from strangers, thereby committing "adultery," so that they can be seen as maintaining the purity of their blood lines and creating biologically and socially acceptable family units.

Finally, the examination of the different Iranian states' population policies depicts their failures not as deliberate rejections of the state's political and ideological agenda but as proof that, when the state's policies do not fit into the people's own vision of an ideal society, they are bound to be ignored or bypassed, as is the case with the latest pronatalist policies. In sum, reproduction and its surrounding institutions of marriage, family, and kinship have so far acted as the custodians of the core cultural norms and values, in their encounters with modernity and innovations that inadvertently threaten the cohesion and stability of Iranian society. However, whether and for how long these norms, beliefs, and practices remain valid for successive generations requires continued in-depth investigation.

Notes

1. See also Tremayne (2017).
2. See also Zavieh (2017).
3. https://www.populationpyramid.net/iran-islamic-republic-of/2020/; see also https://www.indexmundi.com/iran/age_structure.html.

References

Bamdad, Sara, and Aliyar Ahmadi. 2014. "Public Perspectives Towards Third-Party Reproduction in Iran." European Population Conference, Budapest, Hungary, 25–28 June 2014. Retrieved 4 February 2022 from https://epc2014.princeton.edu/papers/140601.

Hosoya, Sachiko. 2017. "Changes in Attitudes Towards Marriage and Reproduction among People with a Genetic Illness: A Study of Patients with Thalassemia in Iran." *Journal of the Anthropology of the Middle East* 12(2).

Inhorn, Marcia C., and Nancy J. Smith-Hefner, eds. 2021. *Waithood: Gender, Education, and Global Delays in Marriage and Childbearing*. Berghahn Books.

Khalajabadi Farahani, Farideh, Sven-Axel Månsson, and John Cleland.

2018. "Engage In or Refrain From? A Qualitative Exploration of Premarital Sexual Relations among Female College Students in Tehran." *The Journal of Sex Research* 56(8): 1009–1022.

Tate, Robert. 2007. "Iranian Minister Backs Temporary Marriage to Relieve Lust of Youth." *The Guardian*, 4 June. Retrieved 2 February 2022 from https://www.theguardian.com/world/2007/jun/04/iran.roberttait.

Tremayne, Soraya. 2017. "Introduction." Special Issue, Emerging Kinship in Changing Middle East. *Journal of the Anthropology of the Middle East* 12(2).

Zavieh, Zahra Ghassemi. 2017. "Reproducing the Virginity Imperative: Women's Collusion and Men's Complicity among Young Iranians Living in Montreal." MA thesis. Montreal, CA: Concordia University.

INDEX

www.ingramcontent.com/pod-product-compliance
Ingram Content Group UK Ltd.
Pitfield, Milton Keynes, MK11 3LW, UK
UKHW020726230926
8686IPUK00002BB/4

9 781800 736719